BDJ Clinician's Guides

This series enables clinicians at all stages of their careers to remain well informed and up to date on key topics across all fields of clinical dentistry. Each volume is superbly illustrated and provides concise, highly practical guidance and solutions. The authors are recognised experts in the subjects that they address. The *BDJ Clinician's Guides* are trusted companions, designed to meet the needs of a wide readership. Like the *British Dental Journal* itself, they offer support for undergraduates and newly qualified, while serving as refreshers for more experienced clinicians. In addition they are valued as excellent learning aids for postgraduate students.

The BDJ Clinicians' Guides are produced in collaboration with the British Dental Association, the UK's trade union and professional association for dentists.

Brett Duane

Editor

Sustainable Dentistry

Making a Difference

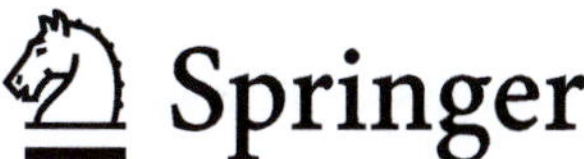 Springer

Editor
Brett Duane
School of Dentistry
Trinity College Dublin
Dublin, Ireland

ISSN 2523-3327　　　　　　　　ISSN 2523-3335　(electronic)
BDJ Clinician's Guides
ISBN 978-3-031-08001-2　　　　ISBN 978-3-031-07999-3　(eBook)
https://doi.org/10.1007/978-3-031-07999-3

This Springer imprint is published by the registered company Springer Nature Switzerland AG
The registered company address is: Gewerbestrasse 11, 6330 Cham, Switzerland

Acknowledgements

I would like to acknowledge the hard work of all the authors who wrote this textbook. This big group of inspired people have embraced sustainability within their fields.

Particular note to:

The conversations with my office member Caoimhin Mac Giolla Phadraig about sustainability over many years—finally, he was convinced to write about sustainability within managing the anxious patient.

"My" two previous Centre for Sustainable Healthcare fellows Darshini and Sara for continuing to drive the sustainability agenda as they both specialise—and for Ingeborg Steinbach and Rachel Stancliffe, my centre for sustainable health care colleagues.

Eleni Pasdeki-Clewer for her friendship, mentorship, wit, drive and passion (one day we will meet).

Gavin Ballentyne for being innovative enough to move temporarily from pollination to biodiversity in a dental setting.

To my new academic friends Amarantha (Fennell Wells), Sheryl Wilmott, to Nick Armstrong (who met me after the BDJ papers and was roped into this book) to Colombian colleagues Ricardo and Viviana (who along the way also helped me with my Spanish!—Muchas Gracias).

To Graham Ball for allowing me to choose carbon footprint dentistry as part of my training and to Derek Richards without whom I couldn't have been a specialist.

To my mentors Alison Dougal and Professor Blanaid Daly (those coffees where you supported and inspired me).

To my UCL colleagues and friends Lexy Lyne and Paul Ashley for starting a whole publishing agenda!

To my Fife colleague Liz Fissenden who spent weeks reading the book and making it readable.

And finally to my family, my father and mother who said I could do whatever I wanted (I miss you Dad)—and although not true, (ha) were a driving force in my life. And to my grown-up children for their love, and to Maree and for those save the planet conversations and for driving me to travel less!

Contents

List of Figures

List of Tables

List of Boxes

Sustainable Dentistry: An Urgent Need for Change

Brett Duane, Julian Fisher, Paul Ashley, Sophie Saget,
and Eleni Pasdeki-Clewer

1.1 An Urgent Need for Change

> **Box 1.1 Climate Change Is Widespread**
> Climate change is widespread, rapid, and intensifying across every part of the planet. So published the International Conference on Climate Change (ICCC) as we write this book [1].

> **Box 1.2 Planet Is Deteriorating**
> We all know the planet is deteriorating. We are using more resources than ever before, the world's population continues to rise, more and more coastal cities are flooding as a result of global warming, and we hear increasingly that "the world is burning".

B. Duane (✉) · S. Saget
Trinity College Dublin, Dublin, Ireland
e-mail: brettdu@tcd.ie; sagets@tcd.ie

J. Fisher
Charité Zahnklinik, Berlin, Germany
e-mail: julian-marcus.fisher@charite.de

P. Ashley
University College London, London, UK
e-mail: p.ashley@ucl.ac.uk

E. Pasdeki-Clewer
Amersham, England, UK

In parallel with the industrialisation of countries, the world population increased from 1 billion in 1804 to 7.7 billion [2]. During this time, carbon emissions increased from 283 ppm to the 2021 level of 444 ppm. To put these carbon emissions in perspective, the last time atmospheric CO_2 amounts were this high was more than 3 million years ago, when the temperature was 2°–3 °C (3.6°–5.4 °F) higher than during the pre-industrial era, and the sea level was 15–25 m (50–80 ft) higher than today [3]. At the time of writing, the planet had 6 years to halt carbon emissions before we find ourselves forced to accept a 1.5° rise in temperature [4].

All these changes aren't just affecting the planet we live on. We know that exploiting nature's resources has implications for all parts of the life we live especially, and most notably, the health of every life form that lives on this planet. Increasingly, we are aware of the growing relationship between changes to the structure and function of the Earth's natural systems and human health. "The concept of planetary health is based on the understanding that human health and human civilisation depend on flourishing natural systems and the wise stewardship of those natural systems" [5]. Health effects from environment degradation are posing a serious challenge to human health, and more worryingly for the health of future generations. If the planet health is harmed, so is human health. No longer can we continue to imagine that humanity is immune or somehow insulated to the risks of planetary health [6].

Climate change has profound implications for human health. These impacts, however, do not derive solely or simply from climatic events but also from the way in which social, economic, and political condition's structure exposure and vulnerability, the risks and effects of climate change, as well as the ability to respond to them, and these risks vary greatly from country to country. The basic health of a country or community is the single largest determinant of the likely effects of climate change and the cost of adapting to it. This reinforces the need for global action on the social determinants of health and the interconnected and interdependent nature of the problem and potential solutions [7, 8].

In 1992, the WHO Commission on Health and Environment published a landmark report— "Our planet, our health"—which drew attention to the complex ways in which the environment interacts with human health. It was one of a number of international reports that began to investigate and document the rapid deterioration of the planet's ecosystem and biodiversity due to human activity and, specifically, the configuration of political and socio-economic systems [9].

The WHO World Health Assembly resolutions and a series of reports on climate change and health call for action and stress the urgency of addressing climate change through health partnerships in all policy approaches [10, 11].

The WHO document, "One Health", suggests approaches to designing and implementing programmes, policies, legislation, and research in which multiple sectors communicate and work together to achieve better public health outcomes [12]. These documents make the case that the risks the world faces are not abstract physical risks created by external forces beyond our control, rather they are risks that we, as societies, have created for ourselves. This framing also strengthens the

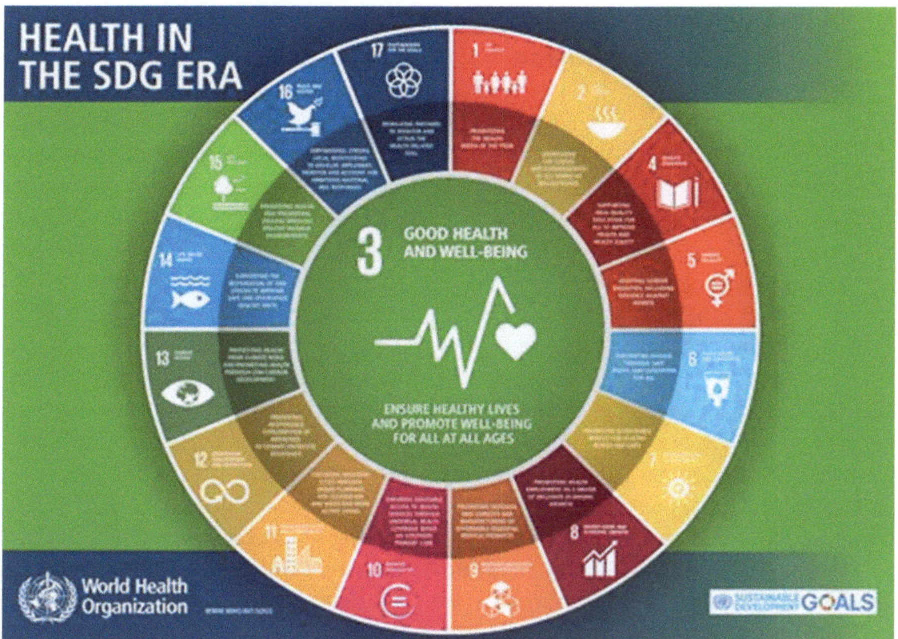

Fig. 1.1 Health in the sustainable development goal era

call for action on the eco-social determinants of health, which provides a clear pathway linking complex global problems to solutions through the UN 2030 Agenda on Sustainable Development and the 17 Sustainable Development Goals which have been adopted by all United Nations Member States [13, 14] (see Fig. 1.1).

The aims of the Sustainable Development Goals are to provide a "shared blueprint for peace and prosperity for people and the planet, now and into the future". As the evidence underpinning the relationship between human health and the health of the planet (planetary health) continues to grow, the goals are necessarily crucial to systematically reduce our impact on the environment. This relationship affects population health and well-being through its impact on infectious and non-communicable disease, nutritional outcomes, displacement, conflict, and mental health outcomes. One example of this pattern is the deterioration in air quality which is linked to a worsening global burden of disease.

The Sixth Assessment Report of the Intergovernmental Panel on Climate Change provides the most up-to-date physical understanding of the climate system and climate change. It notes that "With further global warming, every region is projected to increasingly experience concurrent and multiple changes in climatic impact-drivers". Changes in several climatic impact-drivers would be more widespread at 2 °C compared to 1.5 °C global warming and even more widespread and/or pronounced for higher warming levels [15].

1.2 Healthcare Systems Cause Planetary Health Deterioration

The relationship between our own health and healthcare systems is complicated. Our own health is a beneficiary of healthcare system influences and is an indicator of sustainable development. From an environmental perspective, however, the health system is a significant contributor to deteriorating planetary health.

This harm comes from the way in which buildings are managed (energy), how we access healthcare services (travel), and the products healthcare systems buy (procurement) [16]. Much can be done to make healthcare systems more sustainable through changes that do not compromise the quality or outcomes of patient care (e.g. wise use of resources and reducing inappropriate care). However, sometimes changes are made which exacerbate planetary and therefore population harm. A significant contributor to environmental and planetary harm is the growing infection prevention and control (IPAC) sector, introduced to reduce healthcare-associated infections and keep people safe. An integral part of IPAC is the instruments we use. Single-use instruments (SIs) are rapidly replacing traditional multi-use medical instruments. The IPAC industry suggest SIs be used to reduce infection rates, but there is no substantial evidence for this; we do, however know that the manufacture, travel (distribution), and disposal of SIs cause planetary and population harm.

> **Box 1.3 Health Care Is Harming the Planet**
> Established to facilitate the improvement of population health, health care is harming the planet contributing on average 5% of annual national carbon dioxide emissions [16–18].

> **Box 1.4 Defining Dentistry**
> In this chapter, we use the word dentist in line with the American Dental Association's definition of the (abridged)…" evaluation, diagnosis, prevention and/or treatment of diseases, disorders and/or conditions of the oral cavity, maxillofacial area and/or the adjacent and associated structures. We use the word dentistry to mean the practice of dentistry. The term oral health however we keep in line with that used by the FDI, i.e. oral health means the health of the mouth.
>
> The oral health system contributes around 1% of the total healthcare system expenditure [19].

In 2010, the editor of this book undertook what was believed to be the first carbon footprint of the dental service in a small health board in Scotland (Fife) [20]. It was calculated that, for dentistry, travel was the greatest source of carbon (45.1%), followed by procurement (35.9%), and building energy (18.3%). Regarding travel, 21.7% of our footprint came from patient travel with a similar amount surprisingly

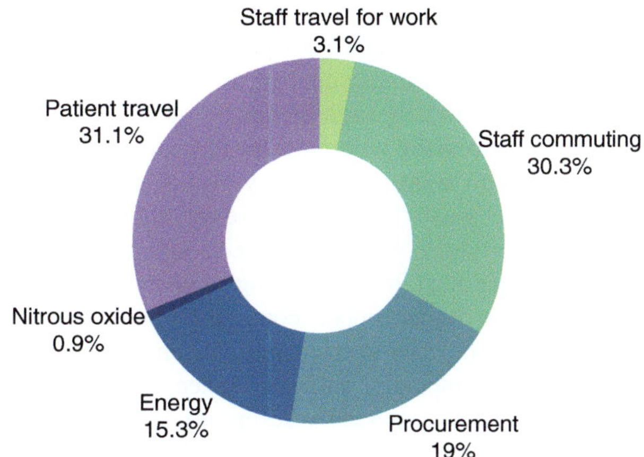

Fig. 1.2 Carbon footprint of the English NHS Dental service 2014–2015

from staff travel. Energy included electricity which accounted for 9.4% of our carbon footprint, followed by gas at 8.8%.

In the 11 years since this data was collected, the amount of research has increased considerably from a low baseline. A carbon footprint of dentistry in England was carried out producing similar results to the Scottish study (see Fig. 1.2).

In 2019, the authors of this book had a series of articles published in the BDJ (British Dental Journal) which looked at the various ways dentistry could adapt to become more sustainable. In many ways, this book highlights the rapid changes that have taken place in the last 3 years since these articles were published. Clinicians, academics, industry leads, educationalists, and policy makers are turning to current research to support the sustainability of dentistry. Recently, the FDI (*World Dental Federation*) started a project in sustainability dentistry and with my colleague, James Field, and a large group of international collaborators, we worked with ADEE (Association for Dental Education in Europe) to develop a consensus in sustainable dentistry [21, 22].

Climate change and oral health may seem far removed from routine general dental practice but, as recent extreme weather events are illustrating, dentistry is not immune to drought and water scarcity, nor fires, and power outages. These are complex global problems with solutions that lie outside the health sector and will require coordinated multi-sectoral action at global, national, regional, and community levels.

Healthcare systems need to fundamentally change to enable systems to deliver appropriate, affordable, and sustainable health care. In our Journal of Dental Research paper, we advocate the need in dentistry for more research, for more sustainability-based dental education, and for policy changes [23]. These suggestions closely align with WHO calls for a new research agenda that is oriented towards public health programmes, population-based interventions, learning health systems, workforce models, digital technologies, and the public health aspects of oral diseases and conditions. Healthcare systems need to become focussed on prevention, undergo broad system analysis and change. These changes will need to be attentive to how dental care is integrated within systems of universal, needs-based access to care [24]. Dentistry needs to change on a practice-wide level and within the system of health care.

As clinicians, we need to advocate and influence sustainability across all oral health systems. Chapter 12 describes in greater detail what systemic changes might look like. Such changes could be as simple as influencing our own dental practice or working nationally to influence the dental education system, the governance of dentistry, or working with industry to facilitate change.

We need to adapt to planetary events, for example, rising temperatures, more frequent heat waves, potential flooding, and supply changes (e.g. where we source our dental products from). Chapter 12 will cover these adaptations in more detail.

One of the most important things a dental practice can do is focus on prevention, including how it can support community-based prevention programmes. We discuss this in this chapter. We also recognise that how we manage patients from a behavioural perspective is important with the choice of adjunct (e.g. nitrous oxide, behavioural management, GA—general anaesthesia) and the way that adjunct is applied is crucial to both the patient's quality of care and the subsequent impact on planetary health.

In a number of chapters, we consider the term ASARA (as sustainable as reasonably achievable see Sect. 1.1), a phrase coined by a colleague Caoimhin Mac Giolla Phadraig when incorporating sustainability into clinical practice which implies finding a balance between what is effective, acceptable, and also environmentally sustainable.

In Chap. 3, we highlight how a practice can influence the high travel-related footprint, particularly concentrating on the role of technology and telecommunications in delivering dentistry. In Chap. 9, we look at how practices can influence our procurement footprint in line with how they can reduce their waste footprint. In Chap. 11, we highlight how manufacturers can consider innovation. This innovation Chap. 11 supports the idea of the development of innovations in practice—how the dental team can experiment with new ways of doing things, evaluate their impacts, and pursue niche change.

From an energy perspective we realise that there are two different practice scenarios: (1) the need for most practices to retrofit their practices to save on energy, or to be more energy efficient, or to generate their own energy (see Chap. 4) or (2), bearing in mind the environmental consequences of a total rebuild, to build a sustainable dental practice (see Chap. 2). In this book, we have combined the latter with how to also build biodiversity into a dental practice.

It is important that the decontamination of dental premises is carried out to the standard advised by national authorities. Our decontamination Chap. 7 makes several recommendations for the clinical team to consider regarding reducing their decontamination environmental footprint; to find better alternatives to the disinfectant wipe; and with the help of our manufacturing colleagues reduce, reuse, and recycle the plastic within our products. Within the same area of patient and clinician safety, in our personal protective equipment (PPE) Chap. 6, we outline how we can reduce our PPE usage (including rationalising glove and apron use, and sessional use of PPE where appropriate), how we can consider reusable alternatives, including how to optimise manufacture and distribution processes.

In our final chapter (Chap. 12), we discuss building a sustainable healthcare system for the future, including the role of professional associations, regulatory bodies, and educational authorities in creating and embedding change. For a graphical representation of the book (see Fig. 1.3).

Chapter	Chapter title		Chapter	Chapter title	
1	**An urgent need for change**	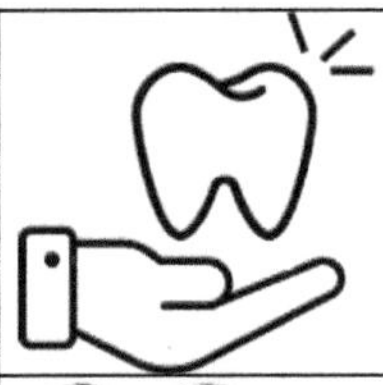	7	Responsible decontamination	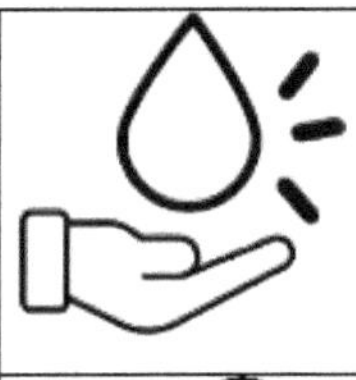
2	**Building a sustainable dental practice (Considering the need to rebuild, material, location)**	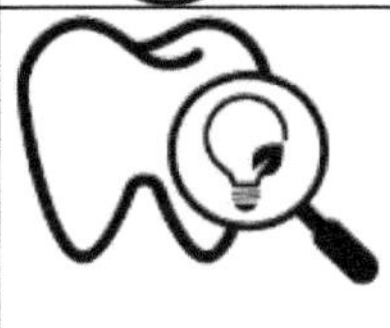	8	Supporting people and their behaviour in the dental setting as sustainably as reasonably achievable	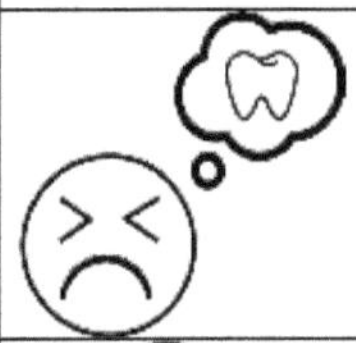
3	Planning the location, skills mix and method of delivery of care and reducing your travel emissions for sustainable dentistry	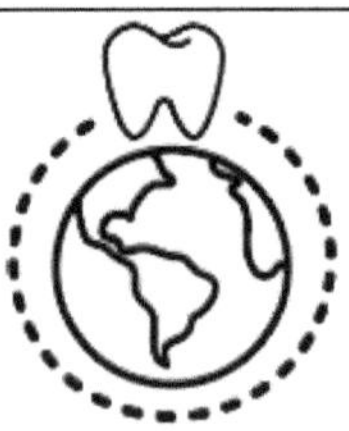	9	Buying sustainably and ethically for the dental practice (procurement)	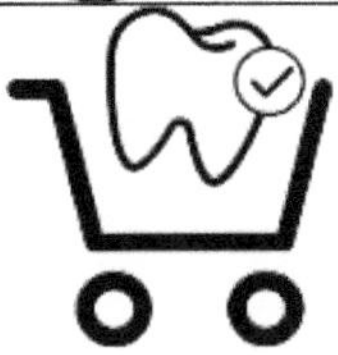
4	Reducing the energy needs of your dental practice	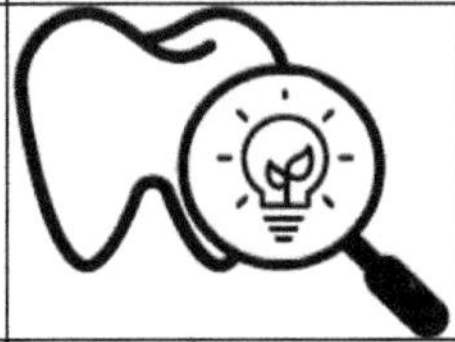	10	Responsible waste management; Using resources efficiently/responsibly.	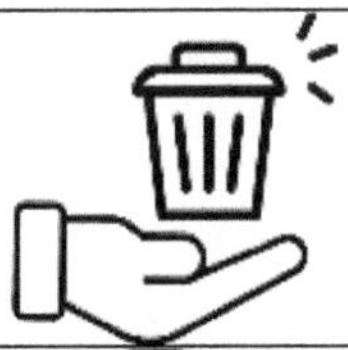
5	Prevention; the sustainable practice initiative	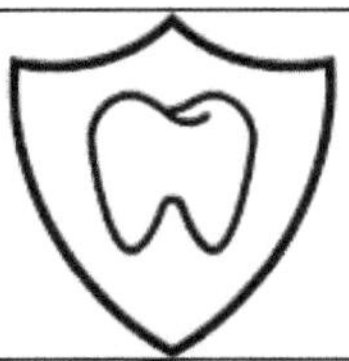	11	The future of dentistry products; How can we redesign the products we create	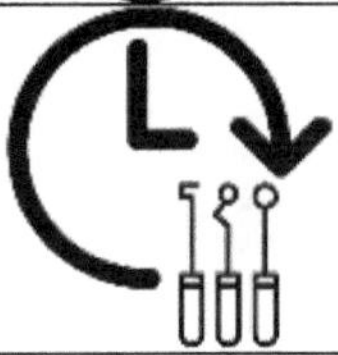
6	A guide to how to reduce the impact of PPE in your dental practice	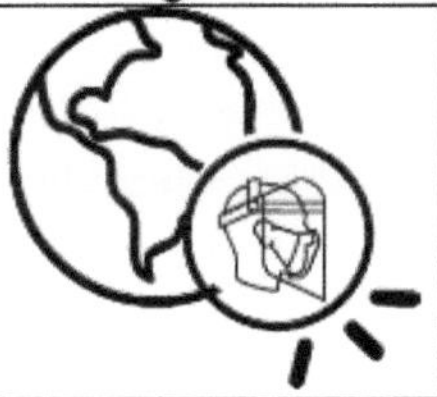	12	Sustainability: The need to transform oral health systems	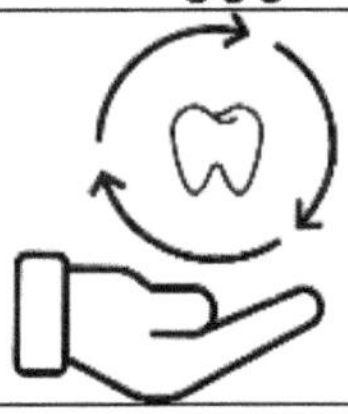

Fig. 1.3 A graphical representation of the book

The dental team, along with our medical and health partners, has an ethical responsibility to provide dental care with the least environmental footprint.

In the short time, since we wrote our BDJ papers in 2018 (published in 2019), much as changed in the landscape of sustainability; in general, the value given to sustainable health care in dentistry, and in the participation/research in this area.

We hope that by reading this textbook you will join us in improving the sustainability of dentistry and, by doing so, do your bit to improve planetary health.

1.3   How to Read This Book

This book highlights various environmental impacts, and the reader should understand what they mean for them to understand what we talk about within the chapters.

Being sustainable isn't just about reducing our carbon emissions. We need to look at a number of other important environmental impacts, such as air quality, water quality, and the effect of a product or system on carcinogenesis. In this chapter, we explain what these terms mean and how they will be used within dentistry.

We want readers of the book to understand what difference we can all make by changing things in our practice.

Life cycle assessment (LCA) is used both in industry and in health care to understand the environmental impacts of a particular service or product. In health care, LCA studies have been undertaken to compare sterile gloves with non-sterile gloves, and handwashing with the use of hand sanitiser [15, 25, 26]. In dentistry, LCA has been used to measure the impact of a dental examination and products such as toothbrushes [16].

As an example if we consider the life cycle of alcohol hand gel, the manufacturer can look at individual ingredients (e.g. ethanol, glycerol, distilled water), how these are processed, packaging both primary [27] [in direct contact with the product, for example, the hand gel container] and secondary/tertiary [28] [—the box in which the hand gel containers are marketed/transported] (e.g. paper/cardboard, plastic, or some sort of compostable material) see Fig. 1.4. We can also consider how consumers use the product (frequency, quantity), and how consumers dispose of the product in the waste stream.

In a number of our sustainability papers, we provide three different values, for example, in our recent hand gel and glove papers [26, 29]. Firstly, we present environmental impact values for each measure of sustainability (e.g. energy values and their overall environmental footprints). Secondly, we present the human health consequences of the environmental damage in DALYs (disability-adjusted life years). Finally, we present the results in normalised values. We explain each of these terms here.

1.3.1   Environmental Impact Categories

There are 16 measures of environmental impact you will see reported throughout this book, covering ecosystem health, human health, and resource use. These specific measures, called impact categories, are taken from European Union guidance on LCA. Each impact category has different units of measurement, for example, climate change is measured in kg's of carbon dioxide equivalence, whereas fossil fuel use is measured in MJ. Normalised results, explained below, allow for comparisons between the impact categories.

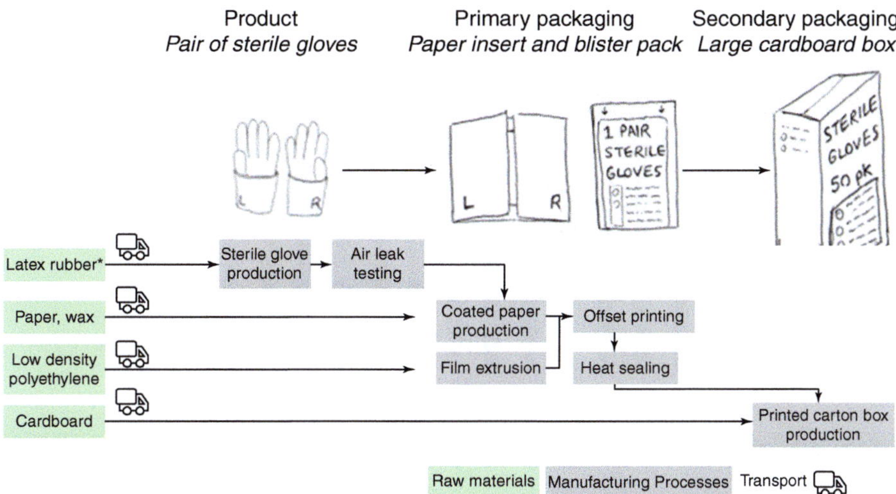

Fig. 1.4 Primary packaging and secondary packaging. An example showing the primary and secondary packaging for surgical gloves

A contribution analysis can be done for each impact category. This can identify what aspects of the life cycle contributed the most (or least) for each impact category. For example, Fig. 1.5 shows the contribution analysis for water fluoridation. You can see that land transport is the greatest contributor for most impact categories, including climate change (CC), but sulphuric acid was the biggest contributor for dissipated water (RDW). The big contributors are going to be the best areas to focus on when it comes to planning how to reduce the impact of a product or service. You can also see that some aspects of the life cycle barely contributed to any of the categories and are therefore less important (e.g. silica quartz).

1.3.1.1 Climate Change: Climate Change Total

The most obvious environmental effect is probably climate change. Climate change is usually measured as global warming potential—the ability of greenhouse gases (GHGs) to trap heat into the atmosphere over a selected time span. The three main GHGs (along with water vapour) are carbon dioxide, methane, and nitrous oxide [31]. In the same way that a nutritional label on a product purchased in a supermarket doesn't just provide fat content or energy content, consumers need to be careful not to consider climate change in isolation but think about the overall impact of a product across a number of other environmental impacts.

1.3.1.2 Ecosystem Quality: Freshwater Ecotoxicity

This category refers to the harmful effects of toxic substances—such as mercury and arsenic—on freshwater organisms [32]. Like the human health toxicity categories, it is measured in Comparative Toxic Units of Ecotoxicity (CTUe), which estimates the proportion of aquatic species in a body of freshwater that would get

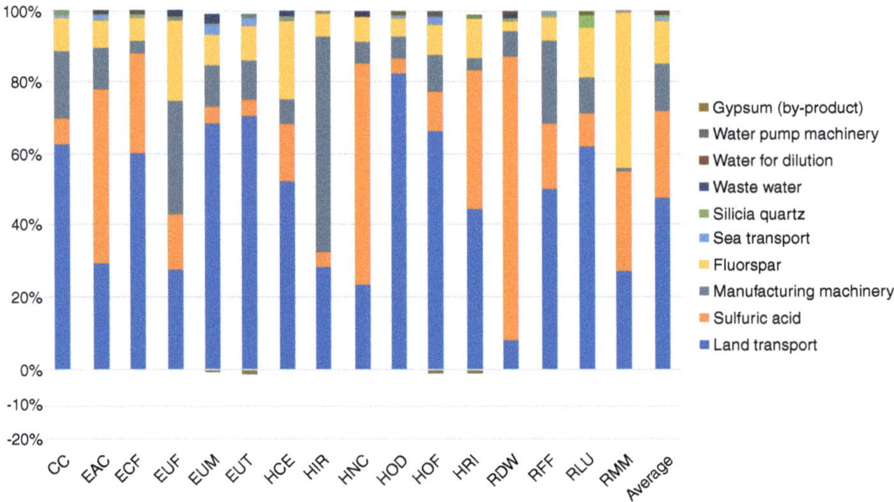

Fig. 1.5 Graph showing the contribution analysis for water fluoridation [30]

negative health effects. For example, in dentistry, using a manual plastic toothbrush for 5 years produced 13.5 CTUe, compared to an electric toothbrush which produced 139 CTUe, over ten times more. It should be noted, however, that at the time of writing, the EU recommended methodology for calculating CTUe in LCA is under review, and so results for freshwater and human toxicity should be interpreted with caution.

1.3.1.3 Ecosystem Quality: Freshwater Eutrophication

This category refers to the release of excess nutrients—such as phosphate and nitrogen—in freshwater systems. This causes excessive algal propagation, leading to hypoxia and death of the existing flora and fauna [33]. For example, using a pair of sterile surgical gloves produces the equivalent of 0.32 g of nitrogen, compared to just 0.01 g for a pair of non-sterile examination gloves.

1.3.1.4 Resources: Dissipated Water

This category measures the deprivation potential if more water was to be used in a defined area watershed [34].

1.3.1.5 Human Health: Respiratory Effects, Inorganics

This is the harm to human health caused by particulate matter emissions (respiratory disease). Particulate matter is a common product associated with travel and also from heating (e.g. use of internal wood burners). There been serious concerns raised that travel and heating can cause significant damage to respiratory health. We discuss these issues in the energy and travel chapters (Chaps. 3 and 4).

1.3.1.6 Resources: Land Use

This category assesses several land capacities: erosion resistance, mechanical filtration, physicochemical filtration, groundwater replenishment, and biotic production, which altogether provide an indication of the extent in which a portion of land is exploited and preserved [35].

1.3.1.7 Human Health: Photochemical Ozone Creation (POC)

This is the harm done to human health from gas emissions that contribute to smog in the lower atmosphere. Van Zelm (2016) has calculated the effect in respiratory mortality due to ozone exposure. POC can also cause changes in forest and grassland species due to changes in ground level ozone exposure [36].

In a publication, Duane demonstrated that significant POC resulted from the use of hand gel/sanitiser [29].

1.3.1.8 Human Health: Ozone Layer Depletion

This impact category refers to the negative effects on human health resulting from the damage of the ozone layer from anthropogenic sources. A depleted ozone layer causes the carcinogenic ultraviolet (UV) rays to enter more readily the atmosphere. The reaction of chlorofluorocarbons, halons, and hydrochlorofluorocarbons with UV light from the sun releases free chlorine amongst other compounds, which in turn interferes with the ozone layer, depleting it [37].

1.3.1.9 Human Health: Non-carcinogenic Effects

This category refers to be harmful to human health that is not related to cancer due to the release of toxic chemicals into the environment, such as mercury and cadmium. These compounds are released because of the use of fossil fuels, for example [32].

1.3.1.10　Human Health: Ionising Radiation

This category refers to the potential damage to human DNA resulting from the release of high energy particles, which ionise atoms and molecules. Ionising radiation can cause both direct tissue damage and cancer. Direct tissue damage (e.g. radiation burns) can happen when enough molecules are broken apart so the cells no longer function. In extreme cases, this can result in radiation sickness, organ failure, and death [38].

1.3.1.11　Resources: Fossils

This category represents the depletion of natural fossil fuels due to extraction of energy or transport, for example. Fossil fuels are products from ancient biomass transformed into energy-rich fuels [39, 40].

1.3.1.12　Human Health: Carcinogenic Effects

This category refers to the same phenomenon as the category "human health—carcinogenic effects", except that the effects in this classification are carcinogenic ones, such as chromium and nickel. The actual risk depends on the severity of the carcinogen, the amount of exposure, or the person's individual genetic make-up.

1.3.1.13 Ecosystem Quality: Marine Eutrophication

This category refers to nutrient pollution reaching marine ecosystems. This is due to the release of excess nutrients—such as Phosphorus (P) and Nitrogen (N)—in water systems, causing excessive algal propagation, hypoxia, and death of the existing flora and fauna [40].

1.3.1.14 Ecosystem Quality: Terrestrial Eutrophication

This category refers to nutrient pollution reaching terrestrial ecosystems. This is due to the release of excess nutrients—such as P and N—in water systems, causing excessive algal propagation, hypoxia, and death of the existing flora and fauna [40].

1.3.1.15 Ecosystem Quality: Freshwater and Terrestrial Acidification

This category refers to a pH reduction resulting from the reaction of acidic gases with atmospheric water. This phenomenon causes acid rain, which releases soil aluminium, making a hostile environment for certain fauna and flora [41].

1.3.1.16 Resources: Minerals and Metals

This category refers to the depletion of minerals and metals. Producing lithium batteries, solar panels or cellular phones are responsible for a high burden across this category.

1.3.2 DALYs (Disability-Adjusted Life Years)

The environmental impact factors discussed in this chapter will inevitably cause some personal health harm. The midpoint impact categories discussed above can cause damages to human health pathways with overall human health damage (see Fig. 1.6).

The impact assessment method recommended by the PEF guidelines provides burdens across a number of different environmental impact categories, for example, climate change, ozone depletion, ionising radiation, respiratory effects, photochemical ozone formation, human health (non-carcinogenic effects), human health (carcinogenic effects), and water consumption [42].

These impact assessments can be converted into endpoint assessments using recognised conversion factors [36].

DALYs for a disease or health condition are the sum of the years of life lost due to premature mortality (YLLs) and the years lived with a disability (YLDs) due to prevalent cases of the disease or health condition in a population [43].

Using DALYs, the burden of diseases that cause premature death but little disability (such as drowning or measles) can be compared to that of diseases that do not cause death but do cause disability (such as cataract causing blindness) [44]. In environmental terms, therefore DALYs can be useful as one can calculate not only loss of life from environmental catastrophes related to for example global warming,

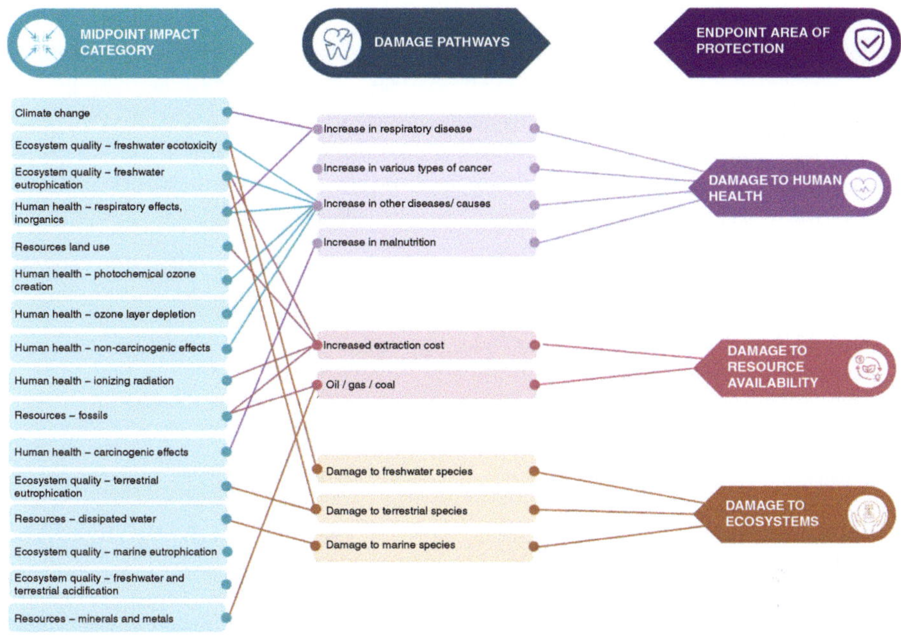

Fig. 1.6 Human health harm related to midpoint and endpoint environmental factors

but also calculate the burden of disease associated with, for example, loss of air quality.

The study undertaken on the electric toothbrush by Lyne highlighted its significant DALYs [45]. This is due to the fact that the electric toothbrush scored highly in water scarcity, ozone depletion, resource use, respiratory disease, POC, land use, human health (cancer/non-cancer), all eutrophication impacts measured, acidification, climate change, and ecotoxicity freshwater. Transforming these figures into DALYS, it was calculated that an electric toothbrush accounts over 5 years of use for 10 h of DALY loss, compared with a bamboo toothbrush which was just 44 min [46]. In a further paper, we calculated that recycling a toothbrush would reduce this loss by more than half [46]. In all of the toothbrush models studied, the most significant contributing factor to the DALY result was the water used to produce electricity, which is in turn used in the manufacturing processes (responsible for 50–90% of the total DALY result, depending on the model).

1.3.3 Normalised Figures

In this book, we also refer to normalised results. Normalising the results allows you to compare between impact categories, and you can visualise which impact categories are the most important or the most relevant for each LCA study. At the time of

Table 1.1 Normalised figures

Impact category	Normal annual impact of the Average Joe[a]	Impact of fluoridating the national water supply for 1 individual for 1 year
Climate change total	1	0.00006
Ecosystem quality—freshwater and terrestrial acidification	1	0.00010
Ecosystem quality—freshwater eutrophication	1	0.00004
Ecosystem quality—marine eutrophication	1	0.00003
Ecosystem quality—terrestrial eutrophication	1	0.00006
Human health—photochemical ozone creation	1	0.00007
Human health—ozone layer depletion	1	0.00003
Human health—respiratory effects, inorganics	1	0.00007
Human health—ionising radiation	1	0.00002
Resources—minerals and metals	1	0.00011
Resources—dissipated water	1	0.00003
Resources—fossil use	1	<0.00000
Resources—land use	1	<0.00000

[a]For the sake of Gender Equality "Joe" could be female, male, or non-binary

writing, EU guidance recommends that the three toxicity categories (freshwater ecotoxicity, carcinogenic effects, and non-carcinogenic effects) are excluded from normalisation while they review the robustness of the methodology.

Normalised results compare the raw data for each impact category against a reference figure—which is an individual's (the "average Joe's") annual share of all emission and resource use from living their daily life. The "normal" annual impact of 1 person is given a reference value of 1. For example, using a pair of sterile surgical gloves has a normalised climate change impact of 0.0001, or 0.01% of the average Joe's annual impact. If you were an "average Joe", your impact would look like this (see Table 1.1).

References

1. IPCC. Climate change widespread, rapid and intensifying—IPCC. https://www.ipcc. ch/2021/08/09/ar6-wg1-20210809-pr/.
2. Infoplease. World population. https://www.infoplease.com/world/population/ world-population-milestones.
3. NOAA. Climate change: atmospheric carbon dioxide. https://www.climate.gov/news-features/ understanding-climate/climate-change-atmospheric-carbon-dioxide. Accessed Aug 2021.

4. Mercator Research Institute on Global Commons and Climate Change. That's how fast the carbon clock is ticking. https://www.mcc-berlin.net/en/research/co2-budget.html. Accessed Aug 2021.

5. Whitmee S, Haines A, Beyrer C, Boltz F, Capon AG, de Souza Dias BF, Ezeh A, Frumkin H, Gong P, Head P, Horton R, Mace GM, Marten R, Myers SS, Nishtar S, Osofsky SA, Pattanayak SK, Pongsiri MJ, Romanelli C, Soucat A, Vega J, Yach D. Safeguarding human health in the Anthropocene epoch: report of The Rockefeller Foundation-Lancet Commission on planetary health. Lancet. 2015;386(10007):1973–2028. https://doi.org/10.1016/S0140-6736(15)60901-1. Epub 2015 Jul 15. Erratum in: Lancet. 2015 Nov 14;386(10007):1944.

6. WHO. World Health Assembly resolution grounds oral health and sustainable oral healthcare in the UN 2030 Agenda for Sustainable Development. 2021. https://www.who.int/news/item/27-05-2021-world-health-assembly-resolution-paves-the-way-for-better-oral-health-care.

7. Donkin A, Goldblatt P, Allen J, Nathanson V, Marmot M. Global action on the social determinants of health. BMJ Glob Health. 2017;3(Suppl 1):e000603. https://doi.org/10.1136/bmjgh-2017-000603. Erratum in: BMJ Glob Health. 2018 Jan 7;3(1):e000603corr1.

8. World Health Organisation. Climate Change. https://www.who.int/health-topics/climate-change#tab=tab_1. Accessed Aug 2021.

9. WHO Commission on Health and Environment & World Health Organization. Our planet, our health: report of the WHO Commission on Health and Environment. 1992. https://apps.who.int/iris/handle/10665/37933.

10. WHO global strategy on health, environment and climate change: the transformation needed to improve lives and wellbeing sustainably through healthy environments. World Health Organization. https://apps.who.int/iris/handle/10665/331959.

11. World Health Organization. WHO global strategy on health, environment and climate change: the transformation needed to improve lives and wellbeing sustainably through healthy environments. 2020. https://apps.who.int/iris/handle/10665/331959. License: CC BY-NC-SA 3.0 IGO.

12. World Health Organisation. One Health. https://www.who.int/news-room/q-a-detail/one-health. Accessed Aug 2021.

13. World Health Organisation. Social Determinants of Health. https://apps.who.int/gb/ebwha/pdf_files/EB148/B148_R2-en.pdf. Accessed Aug 2021.

14. United Nations. Sustainable development goals. https://www.un.org/sustainabledevelopment/development-agenda/

15. IPCC. AR6 Climate change 2021: the physical science basis. https://www.ipcc.ch/report/ar6/wg1/#FullReport.

16. NHS carbon footprint. Measuring carbon footprint. NHS requirements. Sustainable development unit. https://www.england.nhs.uk/greenernhs/. Accessed May 2021.

17. Malik A, Lenzen M, McAlister S, McGain F. The carbon footprint of Australian health care. Lancet Planet Heal. 2018;2(1):e2–3. https://doi.org/10.1016/S2542-5196(17)30180-8.

18. Pichler P-P, Jaccard IS, Weisz U, Weisz H. International comparison of health care carbon footprints. Environ Res Lett. 2019;14(6):064004. https://doi.org/10.1088/1748-9326/ab19e1.

19. Hung M, Lipsky MS, Moffat R, et al. Health and dental care expenditures in the United States from 1996 to 2016. PLoS One. 2020;15(6):e0234459. https://doi.org/10.1371/journal.pone.0234459.

20. Duane B, Hyland J, Rowan JS, Archibald B. Taking a bite out of Scotland's dental carbon emissions in the transition to a low carbon future. Public Health. 2012;126(9):770–7.

21. Duane B, Dixon J, Ambibola G, Aldana C, Couglan J, Henao D, Daniela T, Veiga N, Martin N, Darragh JH, Ramasubbu D, Perez F, Schwendicke F, Correia M, Quinteros M, Van Harten M, Paganelli C, Vos P, Moreno Lopez R, Field J. Embedding environmental sustainability within the modern dental curriculum—exploring current practice and developing a shared understanding. Eur J Dent Educ. 2021;25(3):541–9. https://doi.org/10.1111/eje.12631. Epub 2021 Mar 6.

22. FDI Sustainability in Dentistry. https://www.fdiworlddental.org/sustainability-dentistry.
23. Duane B, Stancliffe R, Miller FA, Sherman J, Pasdeki-Clewer E. Sustainability in dentistry: a multifaceted approach needed. J Dent Res. 2020;99(9):998–1003. https://doi.org/10.1177/0022034520919391.
24. World Health Organisation. Oral health. Achieving better oral health as part of the universal health coverage and noncommunicable disease agendas towards 2030. Report by the Director-General. https://apps.who.int/gb/ebwha/pdf_files/EB148/B148_8-en.pdf. Accessed Aug 2021.
25. Duane B, Pilling J, Saget S, Ashley P, Pinhas A, Lyne A. Hand hygiene with hand sanitizer versus handwashing. What are the planetary health consequences? Environ Sci Pollut Res. 2022;29:48736–47.
26. Jamal H, Lyne A, Ashley P, Duane B. Non-sterile examination gloves and sterile surgical gloves: which are more sustainable? J Hosp Infect. 2021;118:87–95. https://doi.org/10.1016/j.jhin.2021.10.001. Epub ahead of print.
27. Primary packaging. Difference between primary, secondary and tertiary packaging. https://www.saxonpackaging.co.uk/difference-between-primary-secondary-tertiary-packaging/#:~:text=Primary%20packaging%20is%20the%20packaging,contain%20and%20inform%20the%20consumer.&text=EXAMPLE%3A%20For%20beer%20the%20primary,be%20a%20can%20or%20bottle. Accessed 16 Sept 2021.
28. Saxon packaging. Difference between primary, secondary and tertiary packaging. https://www.saxonpackaging.co.uk/difference-between-primary-secondary-tertiary-packaging/#:~:text=Primary%20packaging%20is%20the%20packaging,contain%20and%20inform%20the%20consumer.&text=EXAMPLE%3A%20For%20beer%20the%20primary,be%20a%20can%20or%20bottle. Accessed 16 Sept 2021.
29. Duane B, Pilling J, Saget S, Ashley P, Pinhas A, Lyne A. Hand hygiene with hand sanitizer versus handwashing: what are the planetary health consequences? Environ Sci Pollut Res Int. 2022;29(32):48736–47.
30. Duane B, Lyne A, Parle R. et al. The environmental impact of community caries prevention - part 3: water fluoridation. Br Dent J. 2022;233:303–7. https://doi.org/10.1038/s41415-022-4251-5.
31. IPCC. Fifth Assessment Report—IPCC [WWW Document]. 2013. https://www.ipcc.ch/report/ar5/wg1/.
32. Rosenbaum RK, Bachmann TM, Gold LS, Huijbregts MAJ, Jolliet O, Juraske R, et al. USEtox—the UNEP-SETAC toxicity model: recommended characterisation factors for human toxicity and freshwater ecotoxicity in life cycle impact assessment. Int J Life Cycle Assess. 2008;13:532–46. https://doi.org/10.1007/s11367-008-0038-4.
33. Struijs J, Beusen A, Van Jaarsveld H, Huijbregts MAJ. Chapter 6: Aquatic eutrophication. In: Giedkoop, M., Heijungs, R., Huijbregts, MAJ, De Schryver, A., Struijs, J., Van Zelm, R editors. ReCiPe 2008 A life cycle impact assessment method which comprises harmonised category indicators at the midpoint and end. 2009.
34. UNEP. Global guidance for life cycle impact assessment indicators. 2016. https://www.life-cycleinitiative.org/training-resources/global-guidance-lcia-indicators-v-1/.
35. Beck T, Bos U, Wittstock B, Baitz M, Fischer M, Sedlbauer K. LANCA land use indicator value 4053 calculation in life cycle assessment—method report. Fraunhofer Institute for Building Physics; 2010.
36. Huijbregts MAJ, Steinmann ZJN, Elshout PMF, et al. ReCiPe2016: a harmonised life cycle impact assessment method at midpoint and endpoint level. Int J Life Cycle Assess. 2017;22:138–47. https://doi.org/10.1007/s11367-016-1246-y.
37. WMO. WMO/UNEP Scientific Assessment of Ozone Depletion: 1998. Geneva: WMO; 1999.
38. Frischknecht R, Braunschweig A, Hofstetter P, Suter P. Human health damages due to ionising radiation in life cycle impact assessment. Environ Impact Assess Rev. 2000;20:159–89. https://doi.org/10.1016/S0195-9255(99)00042-6.
39. Guinée JB, Gorrée M, Heijungs R, Huppes G, Kleijn R, de Koning A, et al. Handbook on life cycle assessment: operational guide to the ISO standards. Kluwer Academic Publishers; 2002.
40. van Oers L, de Koning A, Guinee J, Huppes G. Abiotic resource depletion in LCA. Amsterdam: Road and Hydraulic Engineering Institute, Ministry of Transport and Water; 2002.

41. Struijs J, Beusen A, Van Jaarsveld H, Huijbregts MAJ. Chapter 6: Aquatic eutrophication. In: Giedkoop M, Heijungs R, Huijbregts MAJ, De Schryver A, Struijs J, Van Zelm R, editors. ReCiPe 2008 A liife cycle impact assessment method which comprises harmonised category indicators at the midpoint and end. 2009.
42. European Commission. Product Environmental Footprint Guidance. https://ec.europa.eu/environment/eussd/smgp/pdf/PEFCR_guidance_v6.3.pdf.
43. Eufic. Measuring burden of disease: the concept of QALYs and DALYs. https://www.eufic.org/en/understanding-science/article/measuring-burden-of-disease-the-concept-of-qalys-and-dalys.
44. Rochmah TN, Wulandari A, Dahlui M, Ernawaty, Wulandari RD. Cost effectiveness analysis using disability-adjusted life years for cataract surgery. Int J Environ Res Public Health. 2020;17(16):6010. https://doi.org/10.3390/ijerph17166010.
45. Lyne A, Ashley P, Saget S, Porto Costa M, Underwood B, Duane B. Combining evidence-based healthcare with environmental sustainability: using the toothbrush as a model. Br Dent J. 2020;229(5):303–9. https://doi.org/10.1038/s41415-020-1981-0.
46. Duane B, Ashley P, Saget S, Richards D, Pasdeki-Clewer E, Lyne A. Incorporating sustainability into assessment of oral health interventions. Br Dent J. 2020;229(5). https://doi.org/10.1038/s41415-020-1993-9.

2 Building a Sustainable Dental Practice

Gavin Ballantyne, Clara Viviana, Carolina Valbuena, Nick Armstrong, and Brett Duane

2.1 Introduction

The greatest challenges we currently face as a society are the twin, interconnected threats of climate change and biodiversity loss. As dentists and academics, we want to highlight the industry's responsibility to integrate the principles of sustainability into our professional lives. This involves encouraging the use and development of more sustainable materials and technologies to develop replacements for single-use plastics, for example, ones that can instead be manufactured using biodegradable and/or recyclable materials (see Chap. 11). Just as important are considerations relating to how dental practice spaces, constructions, and wider habitats can be improved, either at the stage of construction or during a retrofit. All these aspects are integral to realising the new economic model of the circular economy and moving away from the current, obsolete linear economy to which the world has become accustomed [1]. It aims to redefine growth by reducing waste, lowering carbon impacts and shifting economic activity away from the consumption of finite resources. It encourages the transition to renewable energy sources, building economic, natural, and social capital in both urban and rural areas [2].

G. Ballantyne (✉)
Edinburgh Napier University, Edinburgh, UK
e-mail: G.Ballantyne@napier.ac.uk

C. Viviana · C. Valbuena
Javeriana University, Bogota, Colombia
e-mail: aldanac@javeriana.edu.co; valbuenas@javeriana.edu.co

N. Armstrong
Irish Dental Association Quality and Patient Safety Committee, Dublin, Ireland

B. Duane
Trinity College Dublin, Dublin, Ireland
e-mail: brettdu@tcd.ie

With the extreme effects of climate change causing more damage to human health each year [3], these concerns have never been more urgent. Construction and development in urban areas must be at the forefront of efforts to reduce the environmental impact of development and tackle the climate crisis. Many countries, regions, and cities have launched initiatives aiming to eliminate all carbon emissions associated with different professions and industries by 2050 (e.g. the UN Race to Zero campaign [4]).

With concerns over deforestation and loss of pollinators, more attention is now being given to the biodiversity crisis [5, 6]. To ensure the ecosystem services that we rely on are provided by natural habitats—and also for the huge advantage this will give us in the fight against climate change—it is essential that we halt and reverse biodiversity loss around the world.

Although these challenges seem intimidating, they are not threats that can be ignored. The habitats and environments we live in are already being altered, sometimes in drastic ways. It is, therefore, essential that we improve our ability to adapt to the increasing pace of environmental change. Adaptation to environmental threats can take many forms, for example, planning drainage to deal with flood events and adapting air conditioning and greenspace planting to blunt the worst of extreme heatwaves [7].

Improvements to urban environments can help usher in a new era of global well-being, greatly improve safety, promote health benefits, and enrich the human experience. The climate and biodiversity crises will jeopardise our future if we go about business as usual without addressing the essential changes that need to be made. The coronavirus pandemic has helped us to realise that everything is interconnected, and that climate change and biodiversity loss are urgent issues that need to be resolved, and that these negative effects impact on everything: quality of life, national security, the economy and, especially, public health.

Healthcare professionals worldwide have an obligation and a unique opportunity to monitor the environmental impact of day-to-day living, improve the built environment and undertake research that promotes positive change.

In this chapter, we will focus on methods of dental practice construction that promote sustainability and improve the wider habitat around the dental practice, benefiting staff, patients, and the local ecosystem.

2.2 Environmental Impact

The environmental impact of any business, healthcare initiative, or construction project can be thought of as its impact on biodiversity in the immediate vicinity and further afield. The term biodiversity encompasses the abundance and diversity of life in any area and supports us by providing the ecosystem services we depend on, such as nutrient cycling (the movement of nitrogen, phosphorus, and other resources into and between organisms), carbon sequestration (the capture and storage of carbon from the atmosphere into organisms and the soil), water regulation, and pollination services [8, 9].

To conserve the biodiversity in and around a building site, and to avoid serious impacts on the habitat, the built environment must be managed in a sustainable manner. This is especially important at the initial planning stages, when design teams must work with ecological consultants to estimate the effect the project will have on the wider habitat. This can be measured using features such as water runoff, infiltration, and quality, biodiversity, air quality, soil pH levels, soil nutrient levels, and carbon sequestration capacity in the soil and vegetation [10]. This kind of evidence should ideally be incorporated into long-term datasets that take into account the wider geography, thus allowing us to simulate future climate change models for increasing temperatures and changes in precipitation and model flood and drought risks [11].

While we touch on mitigation methods for many of these variables and environmental concerns, we will focus on greenhouse gas (GHG) emissions produced by the building and day-to-day activities of a dental practice for much of this chapter. GHG emissions are only one aspect of the environmental impact to consider, but they are one that has received most attention and research effort in recent years.

In 2015 in Paris, the Framework Convention on Climate Change (FCCC) made decisions on the urgent need to take action against the incremental levels of greenhouse gas aggregate emissions and to maintain the increase in the average temperature worldwide to below 2 °C [12]. At this convention, environmental goals were set and agreed for the majority of participating countries with an emission reduction of 80–95% by 2050 compared to 1990 levels for developed countries, and a reduction of global emissions to at least half by 2050 compared to 1990 levels in other countries. The EU plan is for a 55% reduction in GHGs by 2030 and to have zero emissions by 2050. Within such mitigation goals there are some sectors and industrial processes that have significant environmental impact, specifically transportation and buildings, waste, burning of oil by the oil industry, solvents, and electrical energy. Most anticipated contributions cover emissions of carbon dioxide CO_2, methane CH_4, and nitrous oxide N_2O. However, the failure of the majority of countries and corporations to implement these goals and put GHG reduction promises into practice only makes the case for change now more urgent.

New buildings and retrofit projects for dental practices must achieve carbon neutrality by eliminating a large percentage (or all) of the CO_2 emissions from the built environment. Therefore, construction must focus on minimising two primary sources: emissions related to the use of buildings (operating carbon) and those related to the manufacture of buildings (embodied carbon). To become carbon neutral, we need to eliminate or offset the impact of both operating and embodied energy. Embodied carbon refers to carbon dioxide emitted at all stages of a goods' manufacturing process, from the mining of raw materials through to the distribution process, to the final product provided to the consumer [13]. By conducting a life cycle assessment (LCA) for each component, and of the construction project as a whole, we can estimate some of the environmental impact involved and identify areas where improvements could be made.

Ideally, any construction or retrofit project should be accompanied by clear and achievable regenerative goals for the local habitat. Loss of biodiversity and ecosystem services at a construction site should be offset by measures that either restore habitat quality at the site following construction or invest in improving the environment at another location. The Vanga Blue Forest project provides an excellent example of how this can work well in practice, benefiting the environment and local communities [14]. In practice however, due to the long timescales required (and often superficial implementation by governments and corporations), biodiversity, and other environmental offsetting has a very poor record of success [15]. Instead, most efforts to reduce the resulting damage should be undertaken during the planning and construction stages.

While much of the effort of environmentalists is put into reducing the harm done to humans and the habitats we live in and exploit, our long-term goal should be more than just damage limitation. A shift in thinking towards a regenerative society is needed, one that helps to restore and recover what is being lost [16]. This change in mindset would promote regenerative building design by focusing on evidence-based re-wilding, enhancing biodiversity and steering away from the fundamentally flawed economic model of infinite growth.

To make this possible, the wider social and environmental context of the local area needs to be taken into account. While local regulations may limit the options available, it is possible to link new construction projects with pre-existing sustainable development schemes, working together to improve the area. Dental project developers should strive to engage with the local community, not just viewing them as potential patients, but as stakeholders in the project. By listening to the concerns and priorities of the community (and, as appropriate, acting on them), the project can help to empower marginalised people, promoting social equality, and identifying the most practical ways to enhance the built environment.

2.3   To Build or Not to Build (Retrofit)

The first key environmental and economic decision required when constructing or upgrading a dental practice is whether to build anew, or if retrofitting an existing structure is more appropriate. Clearly, the construction of a new building has a considerable environmental footprint when compared to the footprint of a retrofit. The extraction of raw materials, manufacturing of materials, transportation of the goods and the process of construction will be embedded in the environmental impact of the construction of a new building [17]. Planners, as a matter of course, must consider whether it is better to spend environmental resources on retrofitting an older building rather than building a new structure [18–22], Retrofits will be covered in more depth in Chap. 4 of this book.

While the construction of a new building—with high standards of energy efficiency—may at first seem desirable, it can take decades before the environmental advantages of a new building pay back the increased environmental impact of the construction, compared with retrofitting the old building with, for example, insulation. Health services should therefore think carefully before building a new healthcare structure. Indeed, it will often be a more environmentally friendly option to upgrade existing building stock, adapting them to better satisfy current and future needs. In addition to environmental considerations, for most practitioners, upgrading older premises is more practical from a fiscal and regulatory perspective than building new premises.

Where new builds are appropriate, it is essential that environmentally friendly construction methods are used. Technological strategies and knowledge to design and construct green buildings are well developed and available in most countries. Green building provides significant energy savings of up to 60% compared to typical 'non-green' buildings in various weather conditions at normal costs [23]. Savings can be achieved for new and refurbished buildings through simplicity in design, energy conservation, orientation, avoiding oversizing, native landscaping, lighting efficiency, waste management, design for flexibility, good air quality, water conservation, and reduction of emissions [24].

2.4   New Build Dental Surgery

If the decision is made to construct a new structure for a dental practice, then there are various issues the stakeholders (be they dentists, site owners, developers, or healthcare providers) need to consider, for example, the embedded energy in the new development. Embodied carbon emissions account for up to 75% of the total emissions for a building over its life span [25]. It is the responsibility of everyone involved in the building process to take whatever actions they can to address climate change and habitat loss by focusing on ecosystem conservation and reducing greenhouse gases through renewable energy and energy efficiency.

A new build may be a stand-alone building or part of a larger development. From a climate perspective, it is more efficient to densify urban areas [26]. While, in past decades, 'densification' was synonymous with high rise buildings, tall buildings generally require more energy for both their construction and operation. There has been an assumption that tall buildings are more efficient [27], but engineers who are aware of and concerned about climate change are questioning this belief. A recent study considered nine different building configurations from a 215-story building with 2000 residential units at one extreme to 2000 disbursed suburban homes at the other [28]. The authors concluded that, when rising from five stories and below to 21 stories and more the mean intensity of electricity and fossil fuel use increases by 137% and 42%, respectively. Single family houses and buildings are also not particularly energy efficient. Their dispersed heating and cooling infrastructure, and having four walls exposed to external weather conditions, increase carbon intensity. Research published concluded that a four-storey courtyard development was the most energy efficient [13].

More recently, 'densification' has now come to represent how we lay out a wider urban area. Ideally, new developments should be based on the 15 min town/neighbourhood [29]. This sort of planning would result in residents being able to meet their daily needs on foot within a 15 min radius of their homes. A new dental practice or a new health centre could be part of this type of more sustainable community but, where it is not logistically possible, construction can be integrated into other solutions, such as pioneering urban transport development and funding measures such as innovative mobility management schemes.

One of the most carbon-intensive aspects of dentistry is travel by staff and patients. As much as 64.5% of carbon emissions arise from dental-associated travel [30]. Locating the practice in a densely populated area near good public transport may reduce travel by car, and the availability of bicycle stands may encourage patients to cycle to the practice. There is a limit on how much the dentist can do to encourage patients to reduce their carbon footprint but making the right choices the easy ones may help. The new or refurbished practice should incorporate changing room facilities, showers, etc. for staff members who wish to shower/change after cycling and aim for treatment plans that reduce the number of patient visits needed to complete a course of treatment.

2.4.1 Energy Efficiency

Reducing the amount of energy required to operate different buildings and optimising their use is crucial to reducing the carbon footprint in the built environment when combined with clean and renewable energy strategies. The Institute of Civil Engineers calculates that the total embodied carbon emissions of new buildings and infrastructure in the UK account for around 49Mt CO_2 equivalent or over 10% of UK territorial emission [31]. Ideally, a new build or retrofit should aim to be a near zero energy building (NZEB) or have a 'passive house' standard of energy efficiency. An NZEB is one that has high energy efficiency and what energy is required in the running of the building comes from renewable sources and meets EU standards [32]. A passive house is a building for which thermal comfort can be achieved by the ventilation system alone rather than needing to use an additional heating system. Passive houses focus on energy savings rather than energy production and is also an enabler for the NZEB standard [33]. These houses have extremely low energy consumption as the fresh air coming into the house is warmed by a heat exchanger that removes some of the heat from the air being ventilated out of the building—thus mitigating the need for an additional heating system. However, dental surgeries need 6–12 air changes per hour and so passive house standard may need additional ventilation [34].

All properties built in the EU after 2020 must conform to the standards outlined in the EU Energy Performance of Buildings Directive (2010) [35] and the Energy Efficiency Directive [36] for NZEB design, with 'very high energy performance'. Relating to extensive retrofits of older buildings, if over 25% of 'surface envelope of the building undergoes renovation', the building should, where feasible, achieve a level of Building Energy Rating A2 (or equivalent).

While it is generally not practical to achieve the NZEB or passive house energy efficiency standard in a refurbished building, positive steps can still be taken. Insulation of walls, roof, draft proofing, and an efficient heating system can result in a significant improvement in the energy rating of the building (see Chap. 4 for more details on energy efficiency and retrofitting). Local regulations may vary from these EU examples, but the reader contemplating a new building should always aim for as high a standard of insulation and energy efficiency as possible.

2.4.2 Energy Production

If the roof of the building is facing south, it is worth considering the addition of photovoltaic cells (PVCs—solar panels) for solar electricity production, especially in lower latitudes. Solar electricity panels convert the sun's energy into electricity which can then be used to power a building. Solar PV cells are made from layers of semi-conducting material, usually silicon. Light shining on the PV cell results in electrons being knocked loose creating a flow of electricity. The cells do not need direct sunshine to function; they can work on cloudy days—but the stronger the sunshine, the more electricity is generated.

PV systems can be made of panels that fit on top of the roof or solar tiles. They can also be installed at ground level. The electricity generated is direct current (DC) and the electricity used in household and dental appliances is alternating current (AC). An inverter is incorporated into the PV system to convert DC electricity into AC. Such solar roof tiles are currently more expensive than solar panels.

In many countries, surplus electricity can be sold into the national grid. In the UK, for example, the EU's Smart Export Guarantee System allows owners of solar PV systems to earn a fixed amount of money from their surplus solar power. The UK government is beginning to provide financial support to households (and businesses) that store electricity in batteries/power banks [37].

New builds might also benefit from any existing or planned local community energy schemes. In the EU, the concept of energy communities has been introduced into its legislation [38]. The Directive on common rules for the internal energy market ((EU) 2019/444) includes new rules that enable consumer participation—either individually or through citizen energy communities—to participate in all markets either by generating, consuming, and selling electricity, or by providing services that increase flexibility through demand—response and storage. Demand response allows consumers to play a role in the operation of the electric grid by reducing or moving their electricity usage during peak times to cheaper time-based rates or other forms of financial incentive. These demand response programmes are being used by electrical system planners and operators as options for balancing supply and demand.

2.4.3 Heating System

A building with a very high level of insulation, such as a passive house, may not need any heating system. Many countries are planning to phase out gas and oil boilers (e.g. by mid-2030s in the UK), with the exceptions of boilers that use hydrogen gas. A 20% hydrogen mix across the network would work with most modern boilers.

The hydrogen used should be green hydrogen, made using renewable energy and electrolysis. Blue hydrogen is made from the conversion of natural gas and carbon capture. The blue hydrogen policies being considered by some countries—the UK being one [39]—will potentially have a bigger carbon footprint than green hydrogen.

Although not commonly found in healthcare settings in most parts of the world, wood burning stoves are obviously undesirable for various reasons. In the UK, wood burning stoves are the largest source of fine particulate matter of 2.5 μm ($PM_{2.5}$) and smaller, with emissions 2.5 times greater than those from road traffic [40]. A single log-burning stove used in a smokeless zone emits more $PM_{2.5}$ per year than 1000 petrol cars [41]. As well as contributing to greenhouse gas emissions, such particulate matter pollutants have serious implications for human health [42].

Heat pumps are a low carbon heating system which work by extracting heat from air or ground and transferring it into a building. These devices work best in buildings that are well insulated (with a building energy rating of at least B2 or equivalent) and have low temperature heating systems such as underfloor heating [43].

2.4.4 Ventilation

The Covid-19 pandemic, and risk of potential future pandemics, has serious implications for future dental surgery design. According to their recent report [44], the Intergovernmental Platform on Biodiversity and Ecosystem Services (IPBES) 'Pandemics have their origins in diverse microbes carried by animal reservoirs, but their emergence is entirely driven by human activities'. The main causes of pandemics are land use change, agriculture intensification and expansion, wildlife trade and consumption [45, 46]. Unless dramatic improvements are made in the way we manage ecosystems and produce our food, the Covid-19 pandemic is likely the first of many to come. This has resulted in an increased awareness of air quality in indoor environments, including dental facilities.

Ventilation is, therefore, a critical issue to consider when embarking on a new build or retrofitting an older property. It may not always be possible to install an air conditioning unit, but there are systems other than air conditioning that are less expensive and easier to install. Simple mechanical ventilations systems and natural ventilation (e.g. opening a window) can be used instead.

In well-sealed buildings, air quality is an important issue. In new builds, it is advisable to install an air conditioning system which can also control both temperature and humidity. Heating ventilation and air conditioning (HVAC) systems will filter the air while also controlling the humidity and temperature. By increasing the rate of air change, decreasing the recirculation of air and increasing the use of fresh outdoor air, HVAC systems may have a role to play in decreasing the spread of infection in indoor spaces. HEPA (high-efficiency particulate air) filters have shown performance with particles similar in size to SARS-CoV-2 virus (70–120 nm) [47]. It is likely that air quality in dental practices is going to be a critical issue in the very near future, and this may lead to a large increase in the use of these systems.

Unlike an HVAC system (which draws in fresh air and mixes it with the recirculated air before being filtered), air sterilisation and/or air disinfection units circulate air passing through filters of various types—some units use UV light as well. At the present time, we hesitate to recommend 'air sterilisation units' as they cannot be commissioned and periodically validated, therefore, there is doubt about their effectiveness. If these devices just recirculate air, but do not remove the bacteria and viruses contained therein, they may further enable the spread of these microorganisms.

An air extraction unit can be installed on an outside wall/window and such systems can be effective at circulating air and reducing infection risk. According to the UK Department of Health, 'Good standards can be achieved without resorting to unreasonably complex or expensive ventilation systems' [48]. The unit's instructions will specify the amount of air removed and, from this information, the number of air changes per hour can be calculated when the volume of the room is known. However, the environmental impact of ventilation and air conditioning systems must also be considered.

Typical air conditioners, depending on the season, consume 3000–5000 watts of electricity for every hour in use. The warmer the air, the more power they use to cool a building. As climate change increases global temperatures, the use of air conditioners in homes and offices is expected to be one of the main drivers behind global electricity demand over the next few decades (predicts the International Energy Agency (IEA) report 'The Future of Cooling') [49]. With global energy demand for A/C units expected to triple by the year 2050, the IEA is calling for urgent action to improve cooling efficiency. The report estimates that the global stock of A/C units will grow from the 1.6 billion in use today to 5.6 billion units.

Air conditioning units also use chemicals that damage the ozone layer. The Montreal Protocol of 1987 [50] banned the use of the most harmful CFCs (chlorofluorocarbons) to stop the destruction of the ozone layer; however, the CFCs permitted for use are still damaging. CFCs were banned in developed countries in 1995 and in 2010 in developing countries. They have now mostly been replaced by HCFCs (hydrochlorofluorocarbons). HCFCs (due to be phased out in 2020 in developed countries and 2030 in developing countries) are less damaging to the ozone layer as they more readily broken down in the troposphere. As current predictions estimate that by the year 2050, 27% of global warming will be caused by gases emitted from air conditioning, the American EPA (Environmental Protection Agency) has proposed the use of alternative gases that are less environmentally destructive [51].

Natural ventilation and other forms of mechanical ventilation use little energy. On warmer days, opening windows and doors can be effective, especially if more than one window is open which, consequently, allows a flow of air to go through the practice. A well-insulated building will stay warmer in cold weather and, if used correctly, also cooler in hot weather, reducing the need for air conditioning.

2.4.5 Water Management

Another important consideration for planners of new builds is the management of water use, both in and around the structure. As climate change/global warming progresses, extreme drought and flood events are becoming more common and many parts of the developed world already regulate restrictions on water use (e.g. in drought-stricken California and parts of Australia), while in parts of the developing world droughts are putting food security at risk and contributing to the displacement of people with increasing regularity.

As there will be increasingly heavy rain, which will result in increased flooding, it is important to avoid building within a floodplain and, when planning for the longer term, low-lying coastal areas. The IPCC Sixth Assessment Report (AR6) [52] has predicted a higher sea level rise than in their previous report. The new high-end risk scenario predicts a global rise in sea levels approaching 2 m by 2100 and by 5 m by 2150 using a very high greenhouse gas emissions scenario. Hopefully, this high emissions scenario will not happen, but sea levels continue to rise. This extremely important fact needs to be taken into consideration when building new premises or investing in retrofitting an older property near the coast.

To help combat drought, it is important that water efficiency is prioritised through the use of fixtures and design solutions that lower water consumption. It can also help to use captured rainwater or recycled grey water for non-potable (water that can be used for other purposes but not drinking) requirements.

Sustainable drainage systems (SuDS)—ones that make use of natural land contours and vegetation planting to slow and direct water runoff—are also recommended for new builds. They will help reduce both flood and drought conditions by preventing bottlenecks and the inflexible nature of traditional drainage systems, while also benefiting the wider habitat [53].

2.5 Habitat Level Considerations for Build Options

High quality greenspace habitat is vital for world-wide well-being as it provides a wide range of ecosystem services, including pollination services, pest control, waste management, and water regulation [54]. A clear relationship can be found between the provision of these services with higher biodiversity, the range of plants, animals, and other organisms sharing the habitats we live in [55]. Not only do these diverse species occupy different niches within the habitat (benefiting the living environment in various ways), biodiverse habitats also show greater resilience and robustness to adapt in the face of changing conditions and of being more capable of regenerating after a shock and, once again, to the benefit of local people [56]. Biodiversity also provides us with a rich source of cultural inspiration and, as previously mentioned in this chapter, emotional well-being [57].

While these benefits may at first seem a little abstract in relation to a dental practice, there's a great deal that a dental practice with access to outdoor space can do to improve local greenspace habitat, resulting in tangible benefits for dental staff, patients, and local residents.

Growing evidence suggests that incorporating natural elements in built environments can offer satisfying experiences and be beneficial for the health and well-being of both children and adults [58]. As well as contributing to the beneficial health service effects of the practice for patients [59], design that incorporates appropriate greenspace also improves employee emotional well-being and productivity [60].

2.5.1 Greenspace Area for Biodiversity

Where dental practices own or maintain land, a number of key management decisions can be considered. Some external space is likely to be paved or covered in asphalt for parking (and access). Ideally, this should be kept to a minimum, providing access for staff and patients (especially patients in wheelchairs who require smoothed paved access routes), without taking up excess space.

Asphalt and other artificial surfaces, like artificial grass, have a lower overall habitat quality and exacerbate urban heat island effect (UHI). UHI is especially affecting tropical regions but is becoming increasingly worrying in other parts of the world due to climate change. UHI exacerbates heat waves, with devastating health effects on urban populations, particularly on vulnerable and low-income inhabitants [61]. UHI has also been shown to lower air quality, leading to serious health concerns [62]. Plants have substantially lower temperatures in unshaded areas than all artificial materials that aren't specifically treated with a high albedo surface to reflect heat energy [63]. Urban green areas have a vital role in combating future urban heat waves [64].

Urban and rural gardens are hugely important in helping to increase the overall greenspace available in an area and also improve habitat connectivity [65, 66]. They can benefit birds, mammals (including at-risk groups like hedgehogs in the UK), and invertebrates, including pollinators. Higher diversity of plant species leads to more habitat heterogeneity, higher animal diversity, and improved provision of ecosystem services [67]. This can be encouraged with added shelter and structural diversity in the form of dead wood and stone.

Pollinator-friendly planting helps to provide a diverse range of nectar and pollen sources for flower visitors throughout the flowering season [68]. This should ideally make use of native wildflowers, shrubs, and perennials, avoiding heavily cultivated varieties that provide few resources for pollinators. Maintaining a few areas of bare ground and potentially installing 'bee hotels' also help pollinators by providing nesting sites for many species of solitary bees [69, 70].

With appropriate training and resources, on-site beehives may be a welcome addition in some countries (especially in sub-Saharan Africa) to promote local pollination and diversify revenue streams using hive products [71]. However, in many parts of the world, honeybees are not a native species and can outcompete native wild pollinators for resources [72] and so may not contribute to wider biodiversity in the area.

Supporting pollinators and other invertebrates necessitates restricted and careful use of pesticides, avoiding prophylactic use. Ideally, a thriving garden should enable natural integrated pest management by supporting its own community of pest controllers, for example, birds, beetles, spiders, and wasps [73].

2.5.2 Greenspace Areas That Facilitate Adaptation to Extreme Weather Events

With climate change increasing the frequency of extreme weather events, including the risks of stormwater flooding [74], renewed attention is being placed on methods of greenspace planting that can alleviate the risks to people, property, and the wider ecosystem. Rain gardens with high structural and taxonomic plant diversity have been shown to be particularly good at retaining rainfall, preventing it from becoming harmful runoff, and slowing the rate of any runoff that does occur [75]. While a forested area will be the most effective at this (especially on high ground), at the scale of most dental practice grounds, shrubs, and perennial seed mixes can create significant beneficial effects when compared to bare ground or grass lawns [76].

Where on-site tree planting is possible, this can hugely increase the habitat space within the site, provide natural shade, offset carbon emissions in the long term, and provide energy savings in the short term through shade and windbreak effects [77]. However, caution needs to be taken to ensure that planting is appropriate for the habitat and climate. This will involve obtaining advice from local horticulture groups and using native species that are well suited to the soil type on site.

2.5.3 Non-traditional Greenspace Areas

In recent years, we have seen an increased interest in the use of non-traditional greenspaces, to improve local habitat quality, aesthetic design, and the crop growing potential of a wide variety of urban spaces, for example, green roofs and green walls [78] (see Fig. 2.1).

Green roofs can generally be divided between extensive and intensive roofs. Extensive roofs are those with less than 200 mm of soil. They are capable of supporting fewer plant species, commonly being planted with sedum, but are also suitable for a wider range of buildings (including many retrofits). Intensive green roofs are those that can structurally support more weight of soil, increasing the options available for planting. This increases the diversity of wildlife the roofs can support and may also enable the space to be used as a garden or recreation area [79].

Green roofs and walls do present maintenance challenges, so drought-resistant planting is preferred in many areas. They also help mitigate urban heat island effect during the day. However, as green roofs may limit heat dissipation overnight, care should be taken to ensure planting is accompanied by other temperature control mechanisms [80]. With adequate training and preparation, these greenspace features provide huge potential benefits in increasing overall greenspace area and engaging people with the local habitat [32, 81].

While the full range of landscape modifications and strategies may involve a large amount of time and resources, a healthy and diverse habitat is not an all-or-nothing goal. Small improvements over time can contribute to a healthier environment for staff, patients, and the wider habitat. Dental practitioners do not need to tackle these challenges alone, local environmental charities, and university research groups are often keen to get involved and will help advise on changes and link them to citizen science and outreach programmes.

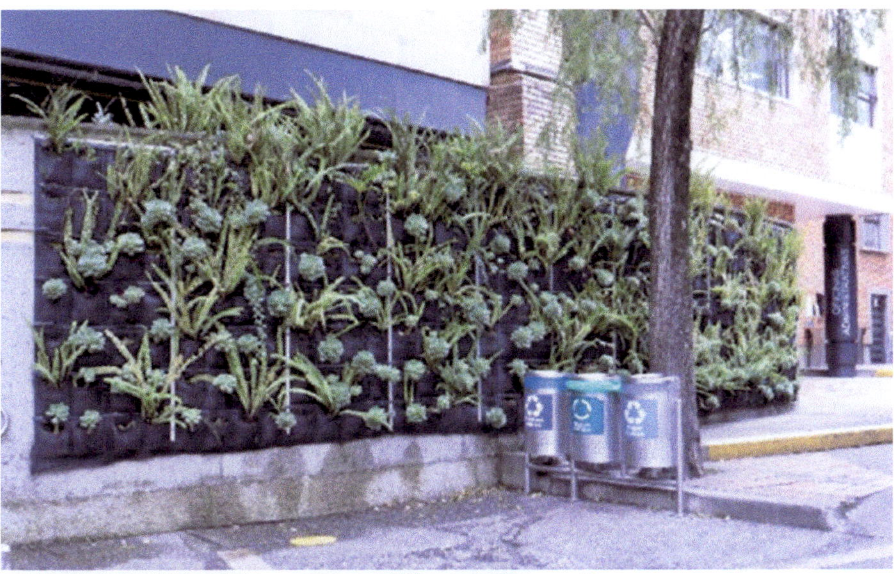

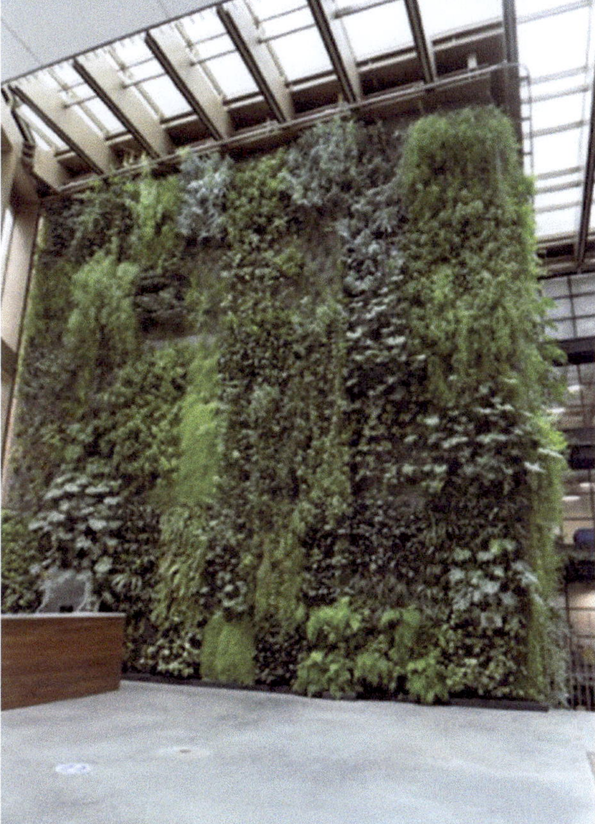

Fig. 2.1 Green wall, Universidad de Javeriana, Bogota

Take Home Points for the Dental Team

- Dental practice stakeholders share a responsibility for the environmental impact of that practice.
- As threats from climate change and biodiversity loss increase, in the form of extreme weather events and pandemics, successful adaptation to these changes is essential.
- Adaptation measures must be incorporated into both new builds and practice retrofits.
- Regardless of scale, proven measures are available to reduce energy expenditure and waste.
- Dental practices with greenspace can help to support local biodiversity through simple and sustainable measures.
- Improvements can lead to tangible benefits for the health and well-being of both staff and patients.

Box 2.1 Universidad de Javeriana, Bogota: Native Trees and Green Walls and Roofs

The Andean Forest has historically been subjected to land use change and degradation. At the nearby Javeriana University, in Bogotá, efforts are being made to contribute to the ecological rehabilitation of this ecosystem on the campus. In 2015, the university set out new environmental policy and institutional commitment to environmental responsibility, for the benefit of humans and the environment. This led to a dramatic redesign and expansion of the greenspace on campus.

The aims of the project were to:

1. Provide a representative sample of tree species typical of the Colombian Andean region and in particular species catalogued as 'rare, endangered, or of particular social interest'.
2. Offer opportunities to get closer to the ecosystem services of trees through the generation of recreational spaces and activities such as planting trees with the new students and the use of products obtained from them.
3. Explore options for green walls and green roofs based on new species and planting and management techniques.
4. Generate high quality spaces in terms of physical and mental health (with a large number of the species planted producing pleasing volatile scents).
5. To increase biodiversity by offering suitable habitat conditions on campus.

Project Outcomes

The project has led to the establishment of a botanical garden and initiated a cultural shift among the members of the PUJ community. The project has contributed to the conservation of tree species vulnerable to habitat change. It has carried out selective felling of non-native species and replaced them with ecologically important native species and others that have foliage and flowers that people find attractive. This has increased the number of trees of native species on campus by 65% and 13 plants species on the IUCN (The International Union for Conservation of Nature) red list can now be found growing on campus.

The project has been well received by both students and staff. To introduce students to these environmental goals, one of the first activities during induction of new students to the university is to plant a tree. This commitment to conservation and education has contributed to the PUJ receiving a number of awards for sustainability.

This case study illustrates what is possible within a campus-sized urban area, comparable to many hospitals, but also demonstrates the benefits that are possible at a smaller scale, especially when multiple small projects in an area can work together to support local socio-environmental goals.

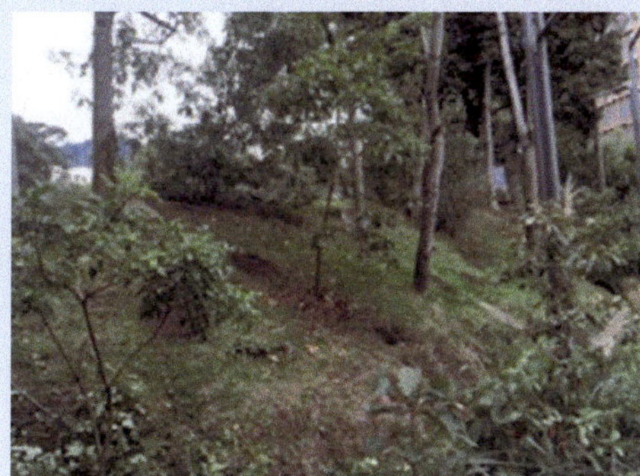
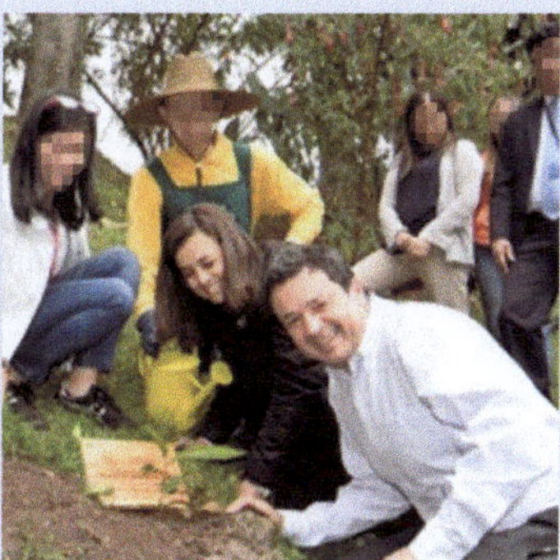
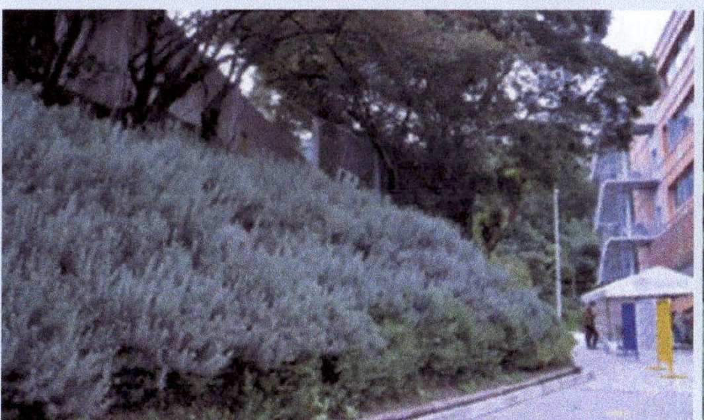
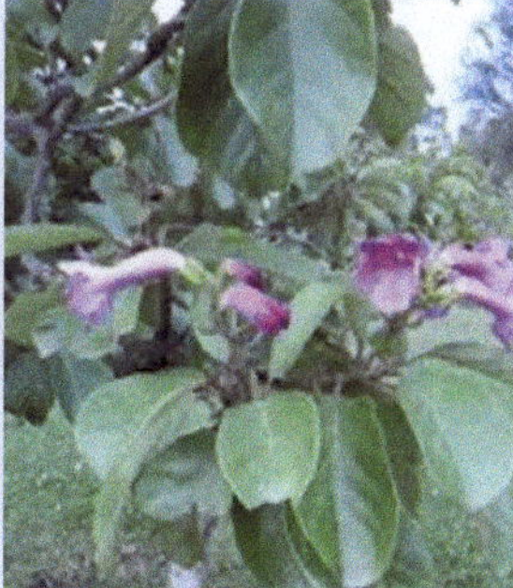

References

1. Pomponi F, Moncaster A. Circular economy research in the built environment: a theoretical contribution. In: Dastbaz M, Gorse C, Moncaster A, editors. Building information modelling, building performance, design and smart construction. Cham: Springer; 2017. p. 31–44.
2. United Nations Environment Programme, Ellen MacArthur Foundation. Global Commitment 2020 Progress Report. 2020.
3. Meierrieks D. Weather shocks, climate change and human health. World Dev. 2021;138:105228. https://doi.org/10.1016/j.worlddev.2020.105228.
4. UN Race to zero campaign. https://unfccc.int/climate-action/race-to-zero-campaign.
5. Grooten M, Peterson T, Almond R. Living planet report 2020—bending the curve of biodiversity loss. 2020; WWF, Gland, Switzerland.
6. UNEP-WCMC and IUCN. Protected planet report 2020: tracking progress towards global targets for protected and conserved areas. 2020.
7. Araos M, Berrang-Ford L, Ford JD, Austin SE, Biesbroek R, Lesnikowski A. Climate change adaptation planning in large cities: a systematic global assessment. Environ Sci Pol. 2016;66:375–82. https://doi.org/10.1016/j.envsci.2016.06.009.
8. Mace GM, Norris K, Fitter AH. Biodiversity and ecosystem services: a multilayered relationship. Trends Ecol Evol. 2012;27:19–26. https://doi.org/10.1016/j.tree.2011.08.006.
9. Food and Agriculture Organization of the United Nations. Ecosystem Services and Biodiversity. https://www.fao.org/ecosystem-services-biodiversity/en/.
10. Reyers B, Biggs R, Cumming GS, Elmqvist T, Hejnowicz AP, Polasky S. Getting the measure of ecosystem services: a social–ecological approach. Front Ecol Environ. 2013;11:268–73. https://doi.org/10.1890/120144.
11. Kumar P, Debele SE, Sahani J, Rawat N, Marti-Cardona B, Alfieri SM, et al. Nature-based solutions efficiency evaluation against natural hazards: modelling methods, advantages and limitations. Sci Total Environ. 2021;784:147058. https://doi.org/10.1016/j.scitotenv.2021.147058.
12. Framework Convention on Climate Change. https://unfccc.int/process-and-meetings/the-convention/what-is-the-united-nations-framework-convention-on-climate-change.
13. Drew C, et al. The environmental impact of tall vs small: a comparative study. Int J High Rise Build. 2015;4(2):109–16.
14. Plan Vivo. www.planvivo.org/vanga.
15. Bull JW, Suttle KB, Gordon A, Singh NJ. Biodiversity offsets in theory and practice. Oryx. 2013;47:369–80. https://doi.org/10.1017/S003060531200172X.
16. Mang P, Reed B. Designing from place: a regenerative framework and methodology. Build Res Inform. 2021;40:23–38. https://doi.org/10.1080/09613218.2012.621341.
17. Berg F, Fuglseth M. Life cycle assessment and historic buildings: energy-efficiency refurbishment versus new construction in Norway. J Archit Conserv. 2018;24(2):152–67. https://doi.org/10.1080/13556207.2018.1493664.
18. Troi A, Bastian Z. Energy efficiency solutions for historic buildings. Basel: Birkhäuser; 2014. p. 336.
19. Kohler N, Hassler U. Alternative scenarios for energy conservation in the building stock. Building Res Inform. 2012;40(4):401–16.
20. Norrström H. Sustainable and balanced energy efficiency and preservation in our built heritage. Sustainability. 2013;5(6):2623–43.
21. Moran F, Natarajan S, Nikolopoulou M. Developing a database of energy use for historic dwellings in Bath, UK. Energ Buildings. 2012;55:218–26.
22. Moran F, Blight T, Natarajan S, Shea A. The use of passive house planning package to reduce energy use and CO2 emissions in historic dwellings. Energ Buildings. 2014;75:216–27.
23. World Green Building Council. The benefits of green buildings. https://www.worldgbc.org/benefits-green-buildings.
24. Halliday S. Sustainable construction. London, UK: Butterworth Heinemann; 2008.

25. Akbarneznad A, et al. Estimation and minimisation of embodied carbon of buildings: a review. Buildings. 2017;7:5.
26. OECD. Rethinking Urban Sprawl. 2018. https://www.oecd.org/environment/tools-evaluation/Policy-Highlights-Rethinking-Urban-Sprawl.pdf.
27. Godoy-Shimizu D, et al. Energy use and height in office buildings. Build Res Inform. 2018;46(8):845–63.
28. Godoy-Shimizu D, Steadman P, Hamilton I, Donn M, Evans S, Moreno G, et al. Energy use and height in office buildings. Build Res Inform. 2018;46:845–63. https://doi.org/10.1080/09613218.2018.1479927.
29. Is your city a 15 minute city? https://www.15-minutes.city/.
30. Duane B, Steinbach I, Ramasubbu D, Stancliffe R, Croasdale K, Harford S, Lomax R. Environmental sustainability and travel within the dental practice. Br Dent J. 2019;226(7):525–30. https://doi.org/10.1038/s41415-019-0115-z.
31. Institute of Civil Engineers. Infrastructure carbon review 2020 data update. 2020. https://www.ice.org.uk/news-and-insight/the-civil-engineer/november-2020/carbon-in-infrastructure-where-and-how-much.
32. D'Agostino D, Mazzarella L. What is a nearly zero energy building? Overview, implementation and comparison of definitions. J Build Eng. 2019;21:200–12. https://doi.org/10.1016/j.jobe.2018.10.019.
33. NZEB. https://www.seai.ie/business-and-public-sector/standards/nearly-zero-energy-building-standard/.
34. Health Protection Scotland Infection Prevention and Control in Urgent Dental Care Settings during the period of COVID-19. ACPH CDC etc. 2020.
35. European Commission. Energy Efficient Buildings. https://ec.europa.eu/energy/topics/energy-efficiency/energy-efficient-buildings/energy-performance-buildings-directive_en.
36. European Parliament. Directive 2012/27/EU of the European Parliament. https://eurlex.europa.eu/LexUriServ/LexUriServ.do?uri=OJ:L:2012:315:0001:0056:en:PDF.
37. UK government. Domestic battery energy storage systems. https://www.gov.uk/government/publications/domestic-battery-energy-storage-systems.
38. European Commission. Energy communities. https://ec.europa.eu/energy/topics/markets-and-consumers/energy-communities_en.
39. United Kingdom Government. https://assets.publishing.service.gov.uk/government/uploads/system/uploads/attachment_data/file/1011283/UK-Hydrogen-Strategy_web.pdf.
40. DEFRA. Department for Environment Food & Rural Affairs. Statistics release: emissions of air pollutants in the UK, 1970 to 2014. https://www.gov.uk/government/statistics/emissions-of-air-pollutants.
41. AAQG. Health experts advise that current wood heater models are too polluting to be allowed. Australian Air Quality Group. 2015. http://woodsmoke.3sc.net/health.
42. Cohen AJ, Brauer M, Burnett R, Anderson HR, Frostad J, Estep K, et al. Estimates and 25-year trends of the global burden of disease attributable to ambient air pollution: an analysis of data from the Global Burden of Diseases Study 2015. Lancet. 2017;6736:1–12. https://doi.org/10.1016/S0140-6736(17)30505-6.
43. Energy Saving Trust. https://energysavingtrust.org.uk/advice/air-source-heat-pumps/.
44. IPBES. IPBES #PandemicsReport: escaping the 'era of pandemics'. https://ipbes.net/pandemics.
45. Keesing F, Belden LK, Daszak P, Dobson A, Harvell CD, Holt RD, et al. Impacts of biodiversity on the emergence and transmission of infectious diseases. Nature. 2010;468:647–52. https://doi.org/10.1038/nature09575.
46. Terraube J, Fernández-Llamazares A. Strengthening protected areas to halt biodiversity loss and mitigate pandemic risks. Curr Opin Environ Sustain. 2020;46:35–8.
47. ECDC. Heating and air conditioning systems in the context of COVID-19. 2020. https://www.ecdc.europa.eu/en/publications-data/heating-ventilation-air-conditioning-systems-covid-19.

48. Department of Health, UK. Decontamination in primary care dental practice (HTM 01–05). 2013.
49. The Future of Cooling. International Energy Agency. 2018.
50. Montreal Protocol, 1987. Montreal protocol on substances that deplete the ozone layer, Montreal. 1987, HMSO, London, Treaty Series No. 19. 1990.
51. EPA. U.S. Will Dramatically Cut Climate-Damaging Greenhouse Gases with New Program Aimed at Chemicals Used in Air Conditioning, Refrigeration. https://www.epa.gov/newsreleases/us-will-dramatically-cut-climate-damaging-greenhouse-gases-new-program-aimed-chemicals.
52. IPCC. Climate change 2021: the physical science basis. In Contribution of working group I to the sixth assessment report of the intergovernmental panel on climate change. Cambridge University Press; 2021.
53. Ashley R, Walker L, D'Arcy B, Wilson S, Illman S, Shaffer P, et al. UK sustainable drainage systems: past, present and future. Civ Eng. 2015;168:125–30. https://doi.org/10.1680/cien.15.00011.
54. Millennium Ecosystem Assessment. Ecosystems and human well-being: synthesis. Washington, DC: Island Press; 2005.
55. Cardinale BJ, Duffy JE, Gonzalez A, Hooper DU, Perrings C, Venail P, et al. Biodiversity loss and its impact on humanity. Nature. 2012;486:59–67. https://doi.org/10.1038/nature11148.
56. McPhearson T, Andersson E, Elmqvist T, Frantzeskaki N. Resilience of and through urban ecosystem services. Ecosyst Serv. 2015;12:152–6. https://doi.org/10.1016/j.ecoser.2014.07.012.
57. Dickinson DC, Hobbs RJ. Cultural ecosystem services: characteristics, challenges and lessons for urban green space research. Ecosyst Serv. 2017;25:179–94. https://doi.org/10.1016/j.ecoser.2017.04.014.
58. Kellert SR, Heerwagen J, Mador M. Biophilic design: the theory, science and practice of bringing buildings to life. Hoboken NJ: Wiley; 2008.
59. Markevych I, Schoierer J, Hartig T, Chudnovsky A, Hystad P, Dzhambov AM, de Vries S, Triguero-Mas M, Brauer M, Nieuwenhuijsen MJ, Lupp G, Richardson EA, Astell-Burt T, Dimitrova D, Feng X, Sadeh M, Standl M, Heinrich J, Fuertes E. Exploring pathways linking greenspace to health: theoretical and methodological guidance. Environ Res. 2017;158:301–17. https://doi.org/10.1016/j.envres.2017.06.028. Epub 2017 Jun 30.
60. Klotz AC, Bolino MC. Bringing the great outdoors into the workplace: the energizing effect of biophilic work design. Acad Manag Rev. 2021;46:231–51.
61. Santamouris M. Recent progress on urban overheating and heat island research. Integrated assessment of the energy, environmental, vulnerability and health impact. Synergies with the global climate change. Energy Build. 2020;207:109482.
62. Jacob DJ, Winner DA. Effect of climate change on air quality. Atmos Environ. 2009;43:51–63. https://doi.org/10.1016/j.atmosenv.2008.09.051.
63. Tan JKM, et al. The urban heat island mitigation potential of vegetation depends on local surface type and shade. Urban For Urban Green. 2021;62(2021):127128.
64. Carvalhoa D, Martinsa H, Marta-Almeidab M, Rochab A, Borregoa C. Urban resilience to future urban heat waves under a climate change scenario: a case study for Porto urban area (Portugal). Urban Clim. 2017;19:1–27.
65. Goddard MA, Dougill AJ, Benton TG. Scaling up from gardens: biodiversity conservation in urban environments. Trees. 2010;25:90–8. https://doi.org/10.1016/j.tree.2009.07.016.
66. Baldock KCR, Goddard MA, Hicks DM, Kunin WE, Mitschunas N, Osgathorpe LM, et al. Where is the UK's pollinator biodiversity? The importance of urban areas for flower-visiting insects. Proc Roy Soc B. 2015;282:2014284920142849. https://doi.org/10.1098/rspb.2014.2849.
67. Andersson E, Barthel S, Ahrné K. Measuring social-ecological dynamics behind the generation of ecosystem services. Ecol Appl. 2007;17:1267–78. https://doi.org/10.1890/06-1116.1.
68. Masierowska M, Stawiarz E, Rozwalka R. Perennial ground cover plants as floral resources for urban pollinators: a case of Geranium species. Urban For Urban Green. 2018;32:185–94. https://doi.org/10.1016/j.ufug.2018.03.018.

69. Bumblebee conservation. A brief guide to bee nest boxes. https://www.bumblebeeconservation.org/bee-nest-boxes/.
70. MacIvor JS. Cavity-nest boxes for solitary bees: a century of design and research. Apidologie. 2017;48:311–27. https://doi.org/10.1007/s13592-016-0477-z.
71. Tolera K, Ballantyne G. Insect pollination and sustainable agriculture in Sub-Saharan Africa. J Pollin Ecol. 2021;27:36–46.
72. Valido A, Rodríguez-Rodríguez MC, Jordano P. Honeybees disrupt the structure and functionality of plant-pollinator networks. Sci Rep. 2019;9:4711. https://doi.org/10.1038/s41598-019-41271-5.
73. Dara SK. The new integrated pest management paradigm for the modern age. J Integr Pest Manage. 2019;10(12):1–9. https://doi.org/10.1093/jipm/pmz010.
74. IPCC. Climate change 2013: the physical science basis. In: Stocker TF, Qin D, Plattner G-K, Tignor M, Allen SK, Boschung J, Nauels A, Xia Y, Bex V, Midgley PM, editors. Contribution of working group I to the fifth assessment report of the intergovernmental panel on climate change. Cambridge, UK and New York, NY: Cambridge University Press; 2013. p. 1535.
75. Krivtosov V, Birkinshaw S, Arthur S, Knott D, Monfries R, Wilson K, et al. Flood resilience, amenity and biodiversity benefits of an historic urban pond. Phil Trans A. 2020;378:20190389. https://doi.org/10.1098/rsta.2019.0389.
76. Yuan J, Dunnett N, Stovin V. The influence of vegetation on rain garden hydrological performance. Urban Water J. 2017;14:1083–9.
77. Ko Y. Trees and vegetation for residential energy conservation: a critical review for evidence-based urban greening in North America. Urban For Urban Green. 2018;34:318–35. https://doi.org/10.1016/j.ufug.2018.07.021.
78. Shafique M, Kim R, Rafiq M. Green roof benefits, opportunities and challenges—a review. Renew Sust Energ Rev. 2018;90:757–73. https://doi.org/10.1016/j.rser.2018.04.006.
79. Williams NSG, Lundholm J, MacIvor JS. Do green roofs help urban biodiversity conservation? J Appl Ecol. 2014;51:1643–9. https://doi.org/10.1111/1365-2664.12333.
80. Sailor DJ, Elley TB, Gibson M. Exploring the building energy impacts of green roof design decisions—a modeling study of buildings in four distinct climates. J Build Phys. 2012;35(4):372–91. https://doi.org/10.1177/1744259111420076.
81. Kaiser ML, Hand MD, Pence EK. Individual and community engagement in response to environmental challenges experienced in four low-income urban neighborhoods. Int J Env Res Public Health. 2020;17:1831. https://doi.org/10.3390/ijerph17061831.

Planning the Location, Skills Mix and Method of Delivery of Care, and Reducing Your Travel Emissions for Sustainable Dentistry

Brett Duane and Sharat Pani

3.1 Environmental Sustainability and Travel Within the Dental Practice

This chapter focuses on travel and transport. It considers how the dental team can both influence patient and staff travel patterns and also purchase goods with reduced travel emissions. See Fig. 3.1.

We know that poor air quality is a serious problem—both for personal health and environmental reasons. From a health perspective, the main problems are particulate matter (PM) and nitrogen oxides (NOx) [1]. We also know that a significant reason for their high concentrations in urban populations is travel (see Chap. 3). During the initial lockdown period of the Covid 19 pandemic, the amounts of these particles were halved [2]. Particulate matter can be classified as PM2.5 or PM 10 depending on the size of the particles measured in micrometres and the smaller particles are more dangerous as they can penetrate into the lungs [3]. There is increasing evidence that exposure to particulate matter can exacerbate and/or cause asthma, chronic obstructive pulmonary disease (COPD), and cardiovascular toxicity with potential impacts in the UK of between 29,000 and 40,000 deaths [4, 5]. The actual level of exposure is complex and depends on population density and where people live and work [1].

B. Duane (✉)
Trinity College Dublin, Dublin, Ireland
e-mail: brettdu@tcd.ie

S. Pani
Schulich School of Medicine and Dentistry, London, ON, Canada

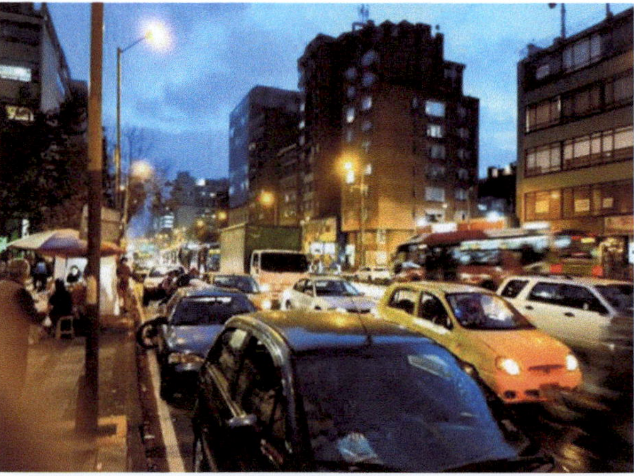

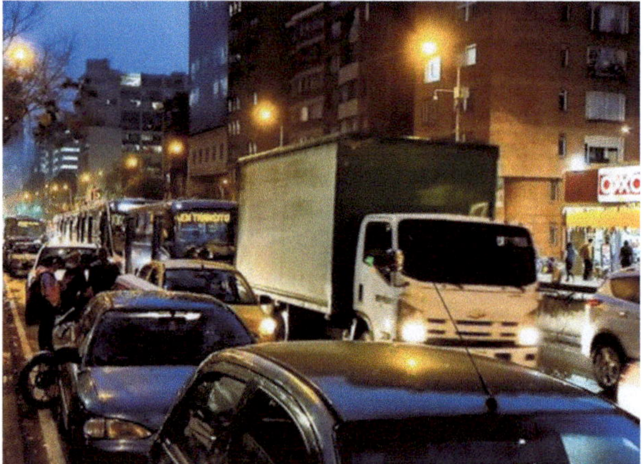

Fig. 3.1 Traffic in and around Universidad de Javeriana, Bogota Viviana

3.2 The Contribution of Dentistry to the Travel Footprint

We know from the Fife study and the PHE (Public Health England) study that travel gives rise to around 64.5% of the carbon footprint of the entire dental service [6, 7]. Interestingly within the PHE study total emissions of patient travel were similar to total staff travel.

The patient contribution to the carbon footprint of the dental appointment via their travel is 2.96 kg. The staff travel is considerably higher at 15.34 kg. This, according to both the Fife and English carbon footprinting studies [6, 7], is because staff generally live around five times further away from the practice than their patients.

This information is considered accurate for England since it was based on travel information from millions of mandatory patient claim forms. The staff travel data was based on a Scottish survey of approximately 100 community dental service staff but provides a similar picture. As travel emissions are high further research should be carried out to understand and reduce staff travel patterns.

Travel is a significant factor in dentistry as patients often travel for relatively long distances to receive dental care. In secondary care (or hospitals), patients spend a lot of time receiving care and use more non-travel-related resources [8]. The dental travel emissions are around five times the comparable travel component of secondary healthcare (10%).

The PHE study also showed the comparatively high carbon emissions associated with dental examinations since, apart from the use of an examination kit, the energy needed to run the dental practice for approximately a 5-min appointment is low, but the travel emissions are comparatively high [9].

As we explain in the prevention chapter (see Chap. 5), the travel component of a preventive appointment is significant which is why it is important to avoid bringing a patient in for a preventive visit only.

There are two methods for calculating a reduced quality of life in public health models:

1. Quality adjusted life years (QALYs) first originated in the 1970s and are a measure of the state of health of a person in which the benefits (in terms of life span) are adjusted to reflect the quality of life. One QALY is equal to 1 year of life in perfect health [10].
2. Disability adjusted life years (DALYs) were developed in the 1990s and are an alternative method of measuring the burden of disease. DALYs quantify the years of life lost (YLL) due to premature mortality and years lived with disability/disease (YLD) [11].

In our BDJ paper, we used the Health Outcomes of Travel Tool (HOTT) to calculate the impact travel had in environmental, financial. and health terms. We calculated that dental travel within England was 760 million miles. This travel released over 372 tonnes of nitrous oxide and 19 tonnes of PM2.5, with an economic cost of £17.5 million. This tool has unfortunately now been taken offline [12]. Within Table 3.1 the reader can see that dental travel causes loss of QALY and produces significant amounts of nitrous oxide and particulate matter.

Another method of assessing the harm caused by dental-associated travel is to use DALYs to calculate approximate harm to human populations from mid-level impact factors (such as fine particulate matter formation and global warming) [13]. By using industry agreed figures, we can calculate DALYs from each variable. The

Table 3.1 Illustrating the effect of dental travel emissions on population health using the HOTT tool (all travel)

	Staff business mileage by car	Patient travel	Staff commute	Total
Miles	41,261,174	476,471,033	241,134,752	758,866,959
QALY loss	19	195	111	325
Air pollution economic loss (£)	1,018,308	10,492,065	5,951,103	17,461,476
Tonnes of nitrous oxide	21.52	224.90	125.74	372
Tonnes of particulate matter (2.5)	1.2	11.01	7.03	19

Table 3.2 DALY for the NHS England dentistry-associated carbon footprint (all travel)

Travel	Impact factor	DALYs
Fine particulate matter formation	0.000629452	0.01
Global warming, human health	0.000000928	274.32
Ionising radiation	8.5E-09	0.18
Ozone formation, human health	8.76274E-07	0.99
Stratospheric ozone depletion	0.000531	0.03
Toxicity cancer	0.00000332	0.00
Toxicity human health	6.65E-09	0.00
Water consumption, human health	7.3518E-07	28.15
Total DALYS in years for the NHS England travel associated with dentistry		303.67

reader will see that the total NHS-associated footprint causes 304 DALYs, which equates to around 3.2 min lost per person living in England. In order to calculate travel, average community patterns were used, this included walking, cycling, car travel, bus travel, train etc. (Table 3.2) [14].

3.3 Improving Sustainable Travel

Dental teams need to consider innovative ways of reducing patient and staff travel. There are various ways this could be achieved:

3.3.1 Combining Appointments

Any practical way of minimising overall travel associated with appointments is important. This could involve, where practical, undertaking multiple procedures within one appointment (e.g. a scale and polish at the same time as a routine check-up appointment) or using scanning technology to reduce travel associated with prosthodontic care.

3.3.2 Only Undertaking Evidence-Based Dentistry

Another way of reducing travel is to ensure everything that you practice is evidence-based dentistry. Consider the scale and polish and the lack of evidence of its potential to improve oral health [15, 16].

3.3.3 Preventative Dentistry

This element is discussed in Chap. 5.

3.3.4 Appropriate Dental Examination Scheduling

It has been 15 years since NICE published their guidance on a risk assessment approach to scheduling dental examinations. There is no evidence base for the 6-month examinations currently performed by dental practitioners [17–19]. Reducing the frequency of examinations in an evidence-based manner will reduce travel-associated carbon emissions and the impact on air quality.

3.4 Using Information Technology

The number of physical dental appointments can also be reduced using information technology; a field that has come to be referred to as teledentistry. The American Dental Association describes teledentistry as the use of telehealth systems and methodologies in dentistry [20]. Telehealth is a broad term that refers to a variety of technology and tactics to deliver virtual medical, health, and education services. The idea of talking to your dentist or healthcare provider without having to go into the dental office is not new. Ever since the advent of the telephone patients have called their dental practice. Whether to book an appointment or to ask for instructions, the principle is that calling ahead reduces waiting times and facilitates a more efficient delivery of dental care. The rapid strides made in telecommunications (e.g. the internet and web-based platforms in the 1990s) led to the first studies exploring the reliability and accuracy of virtually transmitted dental information; a concept that is now termed teledentistry. In 1994, the US Army transmitted colour images from an intra-oral camera from Fort McPherson, Georgia to Fort Gordon, Georgia; a distance of 120 miles; over a 9600-band dial-up modem [21]. Even by the modest standards of the day, this would lay the foundations for the science of modern teledentistry. Although the next two decades would result in rapid strides being made in both the speed and availability of the internet, it was only during the COVID-19 pandemic in 2020 that dental regulators across the globe began issuing definite guidelines for the practice of teledentistry [22]. In this section, we look at the different aspects of teledentistry, their reliability, and the role each would play in reducing travel, eliminating waste and allowing for both efficient and sustainable dental care.

3.4.1 The Basics of Teledentistry

In its essence, teledentistry involves the capture of data, the storage of the data and the secure transmission of that data. Improved ability to capture and condense digital data, combined with higher bandwidth and the ability to transmit larger files, has seen the evolution of teledentistry into a reliable and safe method of providing not only consultations to patients but also to train fellow professionals, provide care and administer programs. Each of these steps reduces the time needed for travel and can, hypothetically, reduce the carbon footprint of these processes.

In order to understand how this could work, we must begin with a basic definition of the different aspects of telehealth. In 2017, Estai defined the different aspects of telehealth in a review of the topic. We have summarised the original definition with the current status in dentistry and potential impact on travel and/or carbon footprint in travel 3 (Table 3.3).

Table 3.3 Aspects of telehealth, their applicability in dentistry and potential impact on travel

Term	Interpretation	Stage of use in dentistry	Impact on travel and/or carbon footprint
Teleconsultation	The patient and/or the local health professional consult a specialist and obtain a treatment recommendation	Approved for use by dental organisations in several countries for routine dental screening	Elimination of a referral visit reduces travel costs (potential carbon based on UK data in grams
Tele-diagnosis	An outcome of the teleconsultation	Proof of reliability through several studies. Emergency use approved during the COVID-19 pandemic in several countries	Not yet ascertained
Tele-treatment	Treatment carried out through teledentistry when applicable	Approved for emergency prescription of pain medication during the pandemic	Potential to eliminate travel for emergency dental visits
Tele-education	Continuing professional development	Has been adopted across specialties in dentistry	Eliminates travel to conferences = significant environmental savings (see Duane 2020 for examples) [23]
Tele-training	Tele-training for oral health professionals	Has been implemented at different levels in dental schools	Not yet ascertained
Tele-monitoring	Regular monitoring of vital signs and/or biochemical variables in patients	Has been validated as an effective method of follow-up visit. Approved as an emergency measure during the pandemic	Elimination of physical follow-up visits
Tele-support	Support to remote health facilities located in isolated areas, remote places or in areas affected by natural disasters or armed conflict	In practice in many countries—effectiveness has been validated in the United States and Australia	Replaces the cost and environmental footprint of flying out a specialist and allows for a multiplication of the existing workforce

Table 3.3 (continued)

Term	Interpretation	Stage of use in dentistry	Impact on travel and/or carbon footprint
Tele-administration	Use of communications technology for purely administrative work (e.g. scheduling and managing appointments)	In practice at different levels in hospitals and clinics	Replaces the environmental/financial cost of travelling to work

3.4.2 Capturing the Data

The capture of accurate data is the bedrock upon which teledentistry is built. Early experiments in teledentistry had relied on the use of expensive intra-oral cameras. In this form, teledentistry was designed to be a method of communication between the general dentist and the specialist [24]. By the 2010s the practice of teledentistry between the dentist and the patient became a feasible concept with improvements both in internet bandwidth and in mobile phone technology, making the capture, transmission, and storage of digital images easier [25]. The improvements in the quality of images by mobile phone cameras led to the ability of patients and dentists alike to be able to capture relatively high-quality images at little or no extra cost. These images were found to be a valid measure of detecting and diagnosing oral diseases from dental caries to oral cancer [26–28]. Despite improvements in the quality of the images, for teledentistry to be practical these images need to be securely stored and transmitted.

3.4.3 Store and Forward Teledentistry

As the term suggests, store and forward teledentistry is the storage and secure transmission of captured images online. The advent of e-mail in the 1990s was the first time that data could be encrypted, transmitted, and decrypted over distances for non-military purposes. As early as 1999, Scheylar and Dasari suggested that the security mechanisms of web-based records could ensure the integrity and confidentiality of the patient information as well as that web-based records would make cumulative, longitudinal patient records possible thus enabling cost-effective teledentistry [28]. The launch and spread of several free email providers such as Hotmail™, Gmail™, and Yahoo™ meant that scanned images could be transmitted between persons without the need for expensive specialised equipment [29–32]. However, the biggest limitation of this type of communication was the need for the compression of images prior to transmission, resulting in the reduction of quality of the transmitted images.

The advent of cloud storage offered a solution to the issue of the secure storage of large files. Although initially developed in the 1960s, commercial cloud computing only became popular in the 2000s. The 2010s saw the emergence of many cloud storage platforms, each offering increasing amounts of storage space. Estai et al. (2016) documented this surge in cloud storage to suggest a proof of concept for a cloud-based telemedicine and teledentistry system [33]. There have been several studies since then that have shown the reliability of cloud-based store and forward teledentistry in the detection of dental caries, orthodontics, initial screening of oral cancer and oral medicine [34].

3.4.4   Security, Accuracy, and Acceptance

While teledentistry as a viable concept has been around since the early 2000s, the concept has faced several obstacles to acceptance by dentists and, perhaps more importantly, dental regulators. Even with the increasing evidence in literature regarding the accuracy of teledentistry, the principal objection to teledentistry has been the security of stored and transmitted data. While different countries have allowed different levels of data transmission over secure channels, concerns about ensuring the protection of confidential patient data have meant that, prior to 2020, most dental regulators were hesitant to accept teledentistry as a safe way to provide dental consultations. The global COVID-19 pandemic resulted in the acceptance of teledentistry by several countries though few have only provided permission for the use of teledentistry during the pandemic.

One way of overcoming security concerns and gaining greater acceptance of teledentistry has been the use of secure hospital servers for the storage and transmission of data. While the initial application of these servers was to allow for secure communication between specialists, there have been reports from England, Wales, Ireland, and Australia of the use of data transmitted across such servers for patient consultations [35]. Teleconferencing between the dentist and patient, for the purpose of consultation, using commercial platforms has also received permission (albeit only for the duration of the pandemic) [36].

3.4.5   Cost-Effectiveness of Teledentistry

Given the time and resources invested in the early development of telehealth by the US Armed Forces, it is not surprising that the first studies on the cost-effectiveness of teledentistry were conducted by the United States Armed Forces. The Total Dental Access (TDA), of the United States Department of Defense established the cost-effectiveness of teledentistry in patient care, continuing education and dentist-laboratory communications [21]. As the accuracy of diagnoses made using teledentistry has improved, teledentistry has shown to be an effective tool in the early detection of dental caries, thus greatly improving both the quality and cost-effectiveness of care [29]. The combination of telecommunications and teledentistry involving the exchange of clinical information and images over remote distances for dental consultation and treatment planning not only improves access to and delivery of oral healthcare; it also lowers its costs [37, 38]. A 2017 study on children in Australia, also found that the use of teledentistry can reduce the need for hospitalisation in children with early childhood caries who had limited access to dental care [39]. Data from Australia also showed that using teledentistry as an alternative to routine dental screening was a cost-effective and reliable method of providing dental care [40]. Data that has emerged from the pandemic-related lockdowns has only reinforced this thinking [41].

3.5 Mode of Travel

The mode or choice of travel is important. Active travel—walking or cycling—has negligible carbon emissions (although one does need to consider the manufacture of the bike within any environmental impact equations.) These environmental calculations are also highly variable depending on the hypothesised expected longevity of the vehicle, the number of people in the vehicle. Fuel source, and geography are just some factors.

Looking at the BEIS/Defra Greenhouse conversion factors it can be seen that for every kilometre of travel a train produces between 6 and 41 g of carbon; a bus between 27 and 104 g. A car with four passengers has a relatively low carbon emissions of 43 g per person, increasing to 171 g of emissions per person if the car only has one passenger [42].

3.5.1 Active Travel

Like most employers, dental practices should encourage their employees to use active travel to get to work [43]. There are numerous reasons for this including health benefits, reducing physical multi-morbidity [44] and economic benefits [45]. There are a number of ways staff can be incentivised to walk to work. For example, King's College, London, offered incentives such as pedometers and guided walks to staff [46].

For NHS England, it was calculated using HOTT that, as well as the health benefits of walking and cycling, even a 5% change towards walking and cycling would reduce air pollution by six tonnes of NOx and 0.4 tonnes of PM 2.5, thus saving an estimated £300,000 in financial costs to health and society [47]. In order to facilitate this however, practices need to consider the expense of cycles for staff (possibly overcome in some countries with cycle to work schemes), the need for cycle storage, and suitable changing and cleaning facilities [48].

3.5.2 Public Transport or Car Sharing

Patients and staff should be encouraged to lift share and make use of public transport [47]. It would be useful for staff to be familiar with popular bus routes. This would help them to support patients who have opted for more sustainable forms of travel. Information on bus routes could be included on practice websites, notice boards, and induction manuals. Staff could consider lift sharing to reduce costs and, in turn, this will also reduce environmental emissions. There are organisations which can help match people who require similar journeys such as Liftshare [49].

3.5.3 Rent a Car and Use It only When You Need It

Another way to reduce your overall environmental footprint is, rather than buy a car for your own personal use, to simply rent one and use it only when necessary [50]. Even if the car was used only once a week, its environmental footprint would be significantly lower as your planetary share of the environmental footprint-related construction of the car is a lot lower.

3.5.4 Electric Vehicles

In our BDJ papers, we highlighted the environmental advantages of electric cars [47].

However, in the same year that we wrote this paper, newer evidence was produced by Pero [50]. There are two aspects here: (1) the carbon emissions/other environmental emissions and (2) the health emissions. A significant part of the footprint of a car relates not to its use of fossil fuel (or, better, electricity) but to its manufacture. In Pero's later study comparing the carbon footprint of a fossil fuel car with an electric car, the electric car produced around two third of the carbon emissions. 16.3% of the carbon emissions (30,000 K tonnes) of the internal combustion/ fossil fuel car related to its manufacture; in an electric car, 46.3% of the carbon emissions (almost 20,000 K tonnes) related to its manufacture. The main reason for the other portion of the carbon emissions of the electric car was related to the high use of coal to produce the electricity [50]. As many countries are steadily increasing their proportion of electricity generated from renewable sources, electric cars are expected to become even more environmentally friendly with further reduced carbon emissions. Pero also demonstrates, however, that an electric car scores worse in every other impact factor such as resource depletion, photochemical formation, acidification, human toxicity, and particulate matter.

From a health perspective, electric vehicles (EV) used in the city will have a much lower air pollution impact; our BDJ paper showed that if 25% of all dental-related travel was by electric vehicle society would avoid over 68 tonnes NOx and 1.6 tonnes PM2.5 a year and reduce health impact costs by over £3.6 m a year [47].

3.5.5 Improving the Sustainability of Conventional Car Travel

There are a number of ways the environmental sustainability of conventional car travel can be improved. Firstly, purchase the smallest car possible that meets your needs [51]. Secondly, remove non-essential items within the car to reduce the weight; thirdly, check the car is tuned correctly, and finally ensure that the wheels have appropriate tyre pressure. Some government organisations in the UK save money by requiring their employees to undertake driver efficiency courses [52]. Some would even argue that colder coloured cars (e.g. a white car) traps less heat and require less air conditioning [53].

3.6   Travel Policies

Every dental practice should be encouraged to have a travel policy and there is guidance to do this [54]. Effective NHS travel plans can improve access to dental care and delivery of services (e.g. how outreach services are provided), support people in undertaking active travel and improve overall quality of life by reducing traffic congestion and improving air quality. The travel plan should consider ways of improving availability of information on travel modes and also look at changing current processes and systems within the dental practice. Staff, for example, might be allowed to adjust their work patterns to arrive and leave 10 min later to accommodate more sustainable ways of travel, e.g. public transport. Incentives could also be introduced to encourage more sustainable staff and patient travel.

Take Home Points for the Dental Team

- A significant amount of dentistry's carbon emissions originates from travel (64.5%).
- Travel affects air quality, nitrogen oxides, and particulate matter which, in turn, impacts on overall health. Dental travel causes the loss of 325 QALYs, at a cost to health and society of around £17.5 million.
- The dental team needs to increase their focus prevention of dental disease, decrease the number of physical appointments, and encourage active travel and use of public transport.

References

1. European Environmental Authority. Explaining road transport emissions. A non-technical guide. https://www.eea.europa.eu/publications/explaining-road-transport-emissions/at_download/file.
2. Irish Times. Air pollution falls dramatically in parts of Ireland following travel restrictions. https://www.irishtimes.com/news/ireland/irish-news/air-pollution-falls-dramatically-in-parts-of-ireland-following-travel-restrictions-1.4225401.
3. DEFRA. Air pollution in the UK. 2016. p. 21–22. https://uk-air.defra.gov.uk/assets/documents/annualreport/air_pollution_uk_2016_issue_1.pdf. Accessed July 2018.
4. The Royal College of Physicians 2016 report. Every Breath We Take. https://www.rcplondon.ac.uk/projects/outputs/every-breath-we-take-lifelong-impact-air-pollution. Accessed July 2018.
5. Zhao T, Qi W, Yang P, Yang L, Shi Y, Zhou L, Ye L, et al. Mechanisms of cardiovascular toxicity induced by PM2.5 a review. Environ Sci Pollut Res Int. 2021; https://doi.org/10.1007/s11356-021-16735-9. Epub ahead of print.

6. Public Health England. Carbon modelling within dentistry. https://assets.publishing.service. gov.uk/government/uploads/system/uploads/attachment_data/file/724777/Carbon_modelling_within_dentistry.pdf. Accessed 30 June 2021.

7. Duane B, Hyland J, Rowan JS, Archibald B. Taking a bite out of Scotland's dental carbon emissions in the transition to a low carbon future. Public Health. 2012;126(9):770–7.

8. Tennison I, Roschnik S, Ashby B, Boyd R, Hamilton I, Oreszczyn T, Owen A, Romanello M, Ruyssevelt P, Sherman JD, Smith AZP, Steele K, Watts N, Eckelman MJ. Health care's response to climate change: a carbon footprint assessment of the NHS in England. Lancet Planet Health. 2021;5(2):e84–92. https://doi.org/10.1016/S2542-5196(20)30271-0.

9. Byrne—awaiting acceptance—contact BDJ for more information.

10. National Institute for Health and Care Excellence. Glossary. https://www.nice.org.uk/ glossary?letter=q. Accessed July 2018.

11. Eufic. Measuring burden of disease: the concept of QALYs and DALYs. https://www.eufic.org/en/ understanding-science/article/measuring-burden-of-disease-the-concept-of-qalys-and-dalys.

12. Sustainable Development Unit. Health Outcomes of Travel Tool. Full guide. Available on request at https://www.england.nhs.uk/greenernhs/. Accessed May 2021.

13. Huijbregts MAJ, Steinmann ZJN, Elshout PMF, Stam G, Verones F, Vieira MDM, Hollander A, Van Zelm R. ReCiPe2016: a harmonized life cycle impact assessment method at midpoint and endpoint level. RIVM Report 2016–0104, Bilthoven, The Netherlands; 2016.

14. UK government. National Travel survey. https://www.gov.uk/government/collections/ national-travel-survey-statistics.

15. Jones C, Macfarlane TV, Milsom KM, et al. Patient perceptions regarding benefits of single visit scale and polish: a randomised controlled trial. BMC Oral Health. 2013;13:50. https://doi. org/10.1186/1472-6831-13-50.

16. Lamont T, Worthington HV, Clarkson JE. Beirne PV Routine scale and polish for periodontal health in adults. Cochrane Database Syst Rev. 2018;12(12):CD004625. https://doi. org/10.1002/14651858.CD004625.pub5.

17. SIGN Guideline 138. Dental interventions to prevent caries in children—a national clinical guideline. Scottish Intercollegiate Guidelines Network. 2014 www.sign.ac.uk/assets/sign138. pdf. Accessed July 2018.

18. Department of Health and British Association for the Study of Community Dentistry. Delivering better oral health: an evidence based toolkit for prevention. London: Department of Health. PHE gateway number: 2014126; 2014.

19. NICE Clinical Guideline 19. Dental recall—recall interval between routine dental examinations. National Institute for Health and Clinical Excellence. 2004. https://www.nice. org.uk/guidance/cg19/resources/dental-checks-intervals-between-oral-health-reviews-pdf-975274023877. Accessed July 2018.

20. ADA Policy on Teledentistry. https://www.ada.org/en/about-the-ada/ada-positions-policies-and-statements/statement-on-teledentistry#:~:text=Teledentistry%20refers%20to%20the%20use%20of%20telehealth%20systems%20and%20methodologies%20in%20dentistry.&-text=The%20ADA%20believes%20that%20examinations,of%20distance%20barriers%20to%20care.

21. Rocca MA, Kudryk VL, Pajak JC, Morris T. The evolution of a teledentistry system within the Department of Defense. Proc AMIA Symp. 1999:921–4.

22. Estai M, Kanagasingam Y, Xiao D, Vignarajan J, Huang B, Kruger E, Tennant M. A proof-of-concept evaluation of a cloud-based store-and-forward telemedicine app for screening for oral diseases. J Telemed Telecare. 2016;22(6):319–25. https://doi.org/10.117 7/1357633X15604554. Epub 2015 Sep 16.

23. Duane B, Lyne A, Faulkner T, Windram JD, Redington AN, Saget S, Tretter JT, McMahon CJ. Webinars reduce the environmental footprint of pediatric cardiology conferences. Cardiol Young. 2021:1–8. https://doi.org/10.1017/S1047951121000718. Epub ahead of print.

24. Chang SW, Plotkin DR, Mulligan R, Polido JC, Mah JK, Meara JG. Teledentistry in rural California: a USC initiative. J Calif Dent Assoc. 2003;31:601–8.

25. Khan SA, Omar H. Teledentistry in practice: literature review. Telemed J E Health. 2013;19:565–7.
26. Morosini Ide A, de Oliveira DC, Ferreira Fde M, Fraiz FC, Torres-Pereira CC. Performance of distant diagnosis of dental caries by teledentistry in juvenile offenders. Telemed J E Health. 2014;20(6):584–9. https://doi.org/10.1089/tmj.2013.0202. Epub 2014 Apr 2.
27. Estai M, Bunt S, Kanagasingam Y, Kruger E, Tennant M. Diagnostic accuracy of teledentistry in the detection of dental caries: a systematic review. J Evid Based Dent Pract. 2016a;16:161–72.
28. Schleyer TK, Dasari VR. Computer-based oral health records on the world wide web. Quintessence Int. 1999;30:451–60.
29. Kopycka-Kedzierawski DT, Bell CH, Billings RJ. Prevalence of dental caries in early head start children as diagnosed using teledentistry. Pediatr Dent. 2008;30:329–33.
30. Torres-Pereira C, Possebon RS, Simoes A, Bortoluzzi MC, Leao JC, Giovanini AF, Piazetta C. Email for distance diagnosis of oral diseases: a preliminary study of teledentistry. J Telemed Telecare. 2008;14:435–8.
31. Amavel R, Cruz-Correia R, Frias-Bulhosa J. Remote diagnosis of children dental problems based on non-invasive photographs—a valid proceeding? Stud Health Technol Inform. 2009;150:458–62.
32. Bradley M, Black P, Noble S, Thompson R, Lamey PJ. Application of teledentistry in oral medicine in a community dental service. N Ireland Br Dent J. 2010;209(8):399–404. https://doi.org/10.1038/sj.bdj.2010.928.
33. Estai M, Bunt S, Kanagasingam Y, Tennant M. Cost savings from a teledentistry model for school dental screening: an Australian health system perspective. Aust Health Rev. 2017a;42(5):482–90. https://doi.org/10.1071/Ah16119.
34. Fernández CE, Maturana CA, Coloma SI, Carrasco-Labra A, Giacaman RA. Teledentistry and mHealth for promotion and prevention of oral health: a systematic review and meta-analysis. J Dent Res. 2021;100(9):914–27. https://doi.org/10.1177/00220345211003828. Epub 2021 Mar 26.
35. Murthy V, Herbert C, Bains D, Escudier M, Carey B, Ormond M. Patient experience of virtual consultations in Oral Medicine during the COVID-19 pandemic. Oral Dis. 2021; https://doi.org/10.1111/odi.14006. Epub ahead of print.
36. Royal College of Dental Surgeons of Ontario. COVID-19: guidance for the use of teledentistry. https://www.rcdso.org/en-ca/rcdso-members/2019-novel-coronavirus/covid-19%2D%2D-emergency-screening-of-dental-patients-using-teledentistry. Accessed 30 Nov 2021.
37. Jampani ND, Nutalapati R, Dontula BS, Boyapati R. Applications of teledentistry: a literature review and update. J Int Soc Prev Commun Dent. 2011;1:37–44.
38. Daniel SJ, Wu L, Kumar S. Teledentistry: a systematic review of clinical outcomes, utilization and costs. J Dent Hyg. 2013;87:345–52.
39. Caffery L, Bradford N, Meurer M, Smith A. Association between patient age, geographical location, indigenous status and hospitalisation for oral and dental conditions in Queensland, Australia. Aust J Prim Health. 2017;23:46–52.
40. Estai M, Kanagasingam Y, Mehdizadeh M, Vignarajan J, Norman R, Huang B, Spallek H, Irving M, Arora A, Kruger E, Tennant M. Teledentistry as a novel pathway to improve dental health in school children: a research protocol for a randomised controlled trial. BMC Oral Health. 2020;20(1):11. https://doi.org/10.1186/s12903-019-0992-1.
41. Samaranayake L, Fakhruddin KS. Pandemics past, present, and future: their impact on oral health care. J Am Dent Assoc. 2021;152(12):972–80. https://doi.org/10.1016/j.adaj.2021.09.008. Epub 2021 Nov 6.
42. UK Government. Research and analysis Greenhouse gas reporting: conversion factors 2020. https://www.gov.uk/government/publications/greenhouse-gas-reporting-conversion-factors-2020.
43. National Institute of Clinical Excellence guidance—physical activity in the workplace. https://www.nice.org.uk/guidance/ph13. Accessed Apr 2018.
44. Vancampfort D, Smith L, Stubbs B, et al. Associations between active travel and physical multi-morbidity in six low- and middle-income countries among community-dwelling older

adults: a cross-sectional study. PLoS One. 2018;13(8):e0203277. https://doi.org/10.1371/journal.pone.0203277.

45. Department of Transport Research: cost benefits of active travel. https://www.gov.uk/government/publications/economic-case-for-active-travel-the-health-benefits.

46. Mapping Greener Healthcare. Walking incentives. http://map.sustainablehealthcare.org.uk/walking-incentives. Accessed Apr 2018.

47. Duane B, Steinbach I, Ramasubbu D, Stancliffe R, Croasdale K, Harford S, Lomax R. Environmental sustainability and travel within the dental practice. Br Dent J. 2019;226(7):525–30. https://doi.org/10.1038/s41415-019-0115-z.

48. Cycling UK. We are cycling UK. Overcoming the barriers to riding to work. https://www.cyclinguk.org/article/cycling-guide/overcoming-barriers-riding-work. Accessed Apr 2018.

49. Liftshare. https://www.liftshare.com/uk/lLiftShare. Accessed Apr 2018.

50. Pero FD, Delogu M, Pierini M. Life Cycle Assessment in the automotive sector: a comparative case study of Internal Combustion Engine (ICE) and electric car. Procedia Struct Integr. 2018;12:521–37.

51. DEEP Logo Connecticut Department of Energy and Environmental Protection. Available: https://portal.ct.gov/DEEP/P2/Individual/Reducing-Your-Environmental-Footprint. Accessed Apr 2021.

52. Kingdom FM. Driver efficiency course saves council thousands on fuel. https://www.kingdomfm.co.uk/news/local-news/driver-efficiency-course-saves-council-thousands-on-fuel/. Accessed Apr 2018.

53. DEEP Logo Connecticut Department of Energy and Environmental Protection. https://portal.ct.gov/DEEP/P2/Individual/Reducing-Your-Environmental-Footprint. Accessed Apr 2021.

54. Transport for London. Developing and implementing travel plans. A good practice guide for the NHS in London. http://www.eltis.org/sites/default/files/tool/nhs-travel-plan-guide-part-1.pdf. Accessed Apr 2018.

4 Reducing the Energy Needs of Your Dental Practice

Brett Duane, Ingeborg Steinbach, Sara Harford, and Nick Armstrong

4.1 Introduction to Energy and Water

Water and electricity have different environmental impacts. In our 2014 study, based on data from a small number of dental practices in Fife, we calculated that gas and electricity each contribute around 8% to the carbon footprint of a dental practice, adding up to around one sixth of the carbon equivalent emissions of a dental practice [1, 2]. In the same study, we calculated the carbon equivalent emissions of water at just 0.09% of the total footprint. The difference therefore between the amount of carbon equivalent emissions that are generated by the energy we use compared with the amount generated by the water we use is large.

However, the Fife study [2] and the study commissioned by Public Health England [1], only calculated carbon dioxide equivalent emissions rather than using a broad base of environmental impacts which would be more in keeping with a broader Life Cycle Assessment (LCA) approach.

In our waste chapter, we talked about the principles of waste reduction [3]— Reduce, Repair, Reuse, and Recycle. The reader should consider these principles in energy and water use too.

The most sustainable approach to planning energy and water use is to firstly consider how much of each utility is used in the dental practice and how this consumption demand can be minimised. Secondly, the most environmentally

B. Duane (✉)
Trinity College Dublin, Dublin, Ireland
e-mail: brettdu@tcd.ie

I. Steinbach · S. Harford
Centre for Sustainable Healthcare, Oxford, UK
e-mail: ingeborg.steinbach@sustainablehealthcare.org.uk

N. Armstrong
Irish Dental Association Quality and Patient Safety Committee, Dublin, Ireland

sustainable source of electricity needs to be considered. Thirdly, the dental team should explore whether the dental practice could generate its own energy.

4.2 Quantity of Each Utility Used in the Dental Practice

4.2.1 Quantity of Water Used in a Dental Practice

To clarify the previous paragraph, it is difficult to know the exact or average water use of a dental practice. In the Fife study [2], it was calculated that the average dental clinic used 41.55 m^3/year, whilst data from three practices in England showed usage of 24.33 m^3/year. North American data reports a much bigger amount of water usage equating annually to around 216 m^3 [4]. Based on the 24.33 m^3 rate and 15 patient visits per day [5] and 44 h of working week per year, the average patient visit uses 36.86 L of water.

Energy use was calculated using date from a number of dental practices where traditional coal-based electricity was used in combination with heating using natural gas. The calculation of disability-adjusted life years (DALYs) associated with energy use was based on the Fife study per average patient visit of 3.13 kWh electricity and 8.47 kWh of natural gas [2]. To further demonstrate the environmental impact, an LCA (life cycle assessment) was carried out using ecoinvent Version 3.6.1 and OpenLCA software [6].

4.2.2 Environmental Outcomes of Water

The water usage for dentistry per patient visit only contributes around 18.03 g of carbon dioxide equivalent emissions towards the overall carbon footprint and only 0.50 of a DALY. As this amount is comparatively small, the breakdown of this calculation is not shown here. Please see the PHE publication for more information [7].

4.2.3 Environmental Consequences of Energy Used in a Dental Practice

The energy use for dentistry per "average" patient visit to a dental practice contributes around 6 kg of carbon dioxide equivalent emissions (see Table 4.1).

The energy contribution to DALYs was around 3 min per patient visit, with the DALYs mostly originating from global warming (carbon dioxide equivalent emissions)

Environmental factor	DALYs	Percentage contributing to total
Global warming—human health	5.51024E-06	99.783
Stratospheric ozone depletion—human health	1.37E-10	0.002
Ionising radiation—human health	4.9997E-10	0.009

Environmental factor	DALYs	Percentage contributing to total
Fine particulate matter formation—human health	3.34E-11	0.001
Photochemical ozone formation—human health	1.12952E-08	0.205
Toxicity—human health (cancer)	2.02E-13	0.000[a]
Toxicity—human health (non-cancer)	4.09E-15	0.000[a]
Water consumption—human health	2.29986E-07	4.165
Total DALYs (years per patient visit)	5.52221E-06	100.00
Total DALYs of harm coming from travel (minutes per patient visit)	2.904459963	

[a]Negligible contribution

Table 4.1 Environmental outcomes from energy use; UK, per patient

Name	Impact result	Unit
Ecosystem quality—freshwater ecotoxicity	2.00968	CTU
Ecosystem quality—freshwater eutrophication	0.00209	Kg P-Eq
Ecosystem quality—terrestrial eutrophication	0.04438	Mol N-Eq
Resources—dissipated water	0.31283	M3 water-Eq
Human health—respiratory effects, inorganics	5.30E-08	Disease incidence
Resources—land use	10.56939	Points
Human health—photochemical ozone creation	0.01289	Kg NMVOC-Eq
Human health—ozone layer depletion	2.58E-07	Kg CFC-11-Eq
Human health—non-carcinogenic effects	6.14E-07	Ctuh
Human health—ionising radiation	0.05882	Kg U235-Eq
Resources—fossils	89.98716	MJ
Human health—carcinogenic effects	6.07E-08	Ctuh
Climate change—climate change total	5.93776	Kg CO2-Eq
Ecosystem quality—marine eutrophication	0.00434	Kg N-Eq
Ecosystem quality—freshwater and terrestrial acidification	0.03108	Mol H + -Eq
Resources—minerals and metals	9.43E-06	Kg Sb-Eq

4.3 How Demand Can Be Minimised

The first priority for dental practices should be minimising the demand for energy. The authors are aware however that some practices lease their practice space whilst others own it. Depending on the specific arrangement, some changes suggested below will require cooperation from the building owner.

4.3.1 Building Anew or Reconfiguring Existing Building

Firstly, newer buildings do not always have a lower environmental impact. The Fife study showed that the combined resource use of older clinics had a much better carbon footprint than newer clinics. This was put down to the fact that traditional dental clinics are smaller, with smaller clinics, smaller waiting rooms, and less energy consuming features such as air conditioning [2]. The newer, bigger purpose-built dental clinics had/have large staff and meeting rooms, which also need to be heated (see Sect. 4.3.2).

Secondly, and more crucially, the construction of new buildings creates a considerable environmental footprint. Earlier in this chapter, the use of an LCA to consider the life cycle of a product was discussed. The extraction of raw materials, manufacturing of materials, transportation of these, and the process of construction will be embedded in the environmental impact of the creation of a new building [8]. One also needs to consider the LCA consequences of demolishing and managing the waste of an old building.

Planners need to consider whether it is better to spend environmental resources on retrofitting an older building rather than building a new structure [9–13]. For example, when comparing the refurbishment of a 1930s residential building with the construction of a new building in Norway, researchers demonstrated that it would take more than 50 years before the environmental advantages (e.g. better energy efficiency) of a new building would pay back the increased environmental impact of constructing the new building compared with retrofitting the old building with insulation. Health services should therefore think carefully before undertaking the building of a new healthcare structure. It may be environmentally more beneficial to upgrade existing building stock instead.

One of the simplest ways of reducing carbon emissions is to become more energy efficient. This might involve, for example, insulation, better use of space (space utilisation), more efficient energy sources, or more efficient equipment.

4.3.2 Space Utilisation

Within dentistry, space utilisation is about how often and how much of dental space is used (a combination of a frequency and occupancy) [14]. In the carbon footprint study by Duane (2012), a number of the newer buildings used more energy per patient appointment than the older buildings that provided the same care [2]. Examples of inefficient space utilisation in dental practices are unnecessarily large waiting rooms and under-utilised meeting rooms, storage rooms, etc. [2] Since larger rooms require more heating, waiting rooms should be the optimal size for the practice.

Calculating optimal utilisation rates requires a structured approach to determine effective use of the dental surgery, reception, and waiting room areas [15]. An effectively run and sustainable dental practice would always have the dental chair in maximum use; the energy required to heat the building would therefore be optimal. Effective staff rota management would also assist with this process.

4.3.3 Energy Efficiency Can Be Improved in a Number of Ways in the Dental Practice

Insulation and draught proofing should probably be the first consideration. Good insulation will save money (as well as being good for the environment) and increase the energy efficiency of the practice. Insulation has been modelled in a study by Llantoy with the environmental payback of a structure insulated with mineral wool, polyurethane, and extruded polystyrene being 7 (12) years, 10 (15) years, and 12 (19) years, respectively, when evaluated with the ReCiPe (or GWP100a) indicator [16].

Insulation will also improve the energy performance certificate (EPC) and/or leadership in energy and environmental design (LEED) rating of the practice building. One of the most cost-effective ways to improve energy efficiency is to insulate the loft. The Energy Saving Trust estimates that 25% of heating is lost through uninsulated roof space [17]. All practices should increase their attic space insulation to a thickness of at least 270 mm. This will result in an improvement of 10–15 points in their EPC.

Insulating walls should be the next consideration. Cavity wall insulation is an expensive option with average annual savings in the region of £89 with possible cost of about £4282. Cavity wall insulation and solid wall insulation (dry lining or external wall insulation) increases the EPC rating by 5–10 points. Grants for insulation are available in many countries.

4.3.4   Sealing and Draught Proofing

Sealing and draught proofing windows and doors using products such as caulk and weather stripping is very cost-effective. There can be average savings of about £107 annually for a cost of about £12. This will also increase the EPC rating of the practice [18].

4.3.5   Double Glazing

Double or triple glazing will reduce heat loss and draughts resulting in lower air conditioning costs. This will also lead to an increase in the EPC rating by several points.

4.3.6   Blinds and Curtains

Other areas of improvements in sustainability could include the use of washable curtains and blinds to keep heat in or out as appropriate [19].

4.3.7   Timers and Thermostats

The use of timers will increase energy efficiency as they ensure optimum use of the heating system. Thermostats should be set at their most efficient setting and altered to suit the season. They should be positioned in seating areas but not close to radiators and clear of doors and draughts. Reducing the thermostat setting by one degree can save 8–10% of energy and result in an average saving £75 per year [20]. Radiators should be routinely cleaned and bled regularly.

4.3.8 Radiators and Closing Doors

Ideally only rooms that are being used should be heated and doors should be kept closed. Radiators in unused areas of the practice should be turned off [20]. Staff should report any over-heated areas to management. The use of automatic doors will reduce heat loss or gain [21].

4.3.9 Smart Meters

A survey of over 2000 people found that as well as having a high understanding, smart meter owners are generally more knowledgeable on energy use than those who have not yet had one installed [22]. However, the dental team should consider that each appliance they own (including a smart meter) will increase electricity use [23]. Moreover, from a sustainability perspective, it is concerning that annually 1.4 million smart meters are replacing functioning existing meters. These new meters require global resources to produce, with additional resources required to dispose of the old meter [24].

If dental practices intend to install smart meters, they should consider waiting for the second open protocol version, SMETS2 (smart metering equipment technical specifications), as these devices will enable a seamless change from provider to provider.

4.3.10 Boiler Efficiency

The efficiency of the boiler used to heat a property is important. Older boilers have an efficiency of about 60–70% compared to modern condensing boilers which, at around 95%, are much more efficient. All boilers should be serviced regularly in accordance with the manufacturers' advice. The use of room thermostats, timers, and thermostatic valves will increase energy efficiency and can save the average domestic user around £150 per annum and further reduce carbon emissions.

Many governments are banning the installation of fossil fuel boilers and moving to the use of heat pumps. Buildings need to be insulated to a good standard before installing a heat pump [25]. Heat pumps—which run on renewable electricity—have a very low carbon footprint compared to gas fired boilers.

4.3.11 Air Conditioning

Air conditioning systems may need to be installed in some poorly ventilated dental practices post Covid-19. Air conditioning is an energy intensive technology. In a 2012, UK study around 65% of office space was air-conditioned, and these systems used up about 10% of all UK electricity [26]. This would mean a bill of around £387.50 per year for a dental office of 100 m^2.

All doors and windows must be kept closed wherever possible in air-conditioned premises. Adjusting the thermostat setting can also lead to reduced costs, for example, natural ventilation such as open windows can be used during the warmer periods of the year. However, in light of the Covid-19 pandemic, air quality in dental surgeries may need to be improved. The recommended Air Changes per Hour (ACH) is 6–10 air changes per hour [27]. The effectiveness of natural ventilation will depend on the size of windows, the position of windows, the wind speed, and the temperature difference between the inside and outside environment. Mechanical ventilation, such as extraction fans, specify the amount of air removed and from this the ACH can be calculated [28].

Before installing an air conditioning system, alternative options should be considered, for example, use of insulation, reducing heat transfer through glass (e.g. blinds and curtains), and natural ventilation (strategically opening windows). Shading the outside of the building could also assist.

4.3.12 Water Heating

Heating water costs the average UK household about £140 per year [29]. The use of hot water in dental practice is less than that used domestically. The practice expenditure on water heating might be reduced by insulating the water tank and using a thermostat and timer [30]. A hot water recycling system, if not already installed, could also be considered for practices using a lot of hot water. Insulating a hot water tank could cost as little as £16 resulting in a potential annual saving of around £29 and improving the EPC rating of the building by a few points.

4.4   Choosing Sustainable Appliances

Table 4.2 shows the energy use of different appliances.

4.4.1   Energy Use of Different Appliances

Table 4.2 Energy use (electricity) within dentistry

Electrical appliance	Power (watts)	Hours per day	Electricity use per day (kWh per day)	Price per day (based on 14.4 pence per kWh)	Annual CO_2e if using supplier with coal-based energy
Amalgamator	70 [31]	0.07	0.00	0.00	0
Printer	40 [32]	0.25	0.01	0.01	1
Curing light	8 [33]	0.00	0.01	0.00	1
X-ray machine	100 [2]	0.17	0.02	0.01	2
Mobile phone charger	5 [34]	8.00	0.04	0.01	4
WiFi router	8 [35]	8.00	0.06	0.01	5
Laptop	25 [36]	8.00	0.20	0.03	21
Suction	950 [31]	0.3	0.29	0.04	31
Water cooler with timer	Energy use calculated from web page [37]		0.30	0.06	32
Dental chair	300 [38]	1.33	0.40	0.06	42
Computer monitor (20–24 inch)	50 [39]	8.00	0.40	0.06	42
Radio	5 [40]	8	0.04	0.01	59
Instant water	See [41]		0.57	0.08	60
Microwave	1200 [32]	0.50	0.60	0.09	63
Energy-efficient TV	40 [42]	8.00	0.32	0.05	68
Ultrasonic	1320 [43]	0.60	0.79	0.11	84
LED lights	10 [44]	80.00	0.80	0.12	85
Desktop computer	100 [45]	8.00	0.80	0.12	85
Kettle	1800 [35]	0.28	0.84	0.12	89
Ten compact fluorescent lamps	10*14 watts [46]	80.00	1.12	0.16	118
Overhead dental light	150 [47]	8	1.20	0.17	127
Refrigerator	Based on website [48]		1.50	0.22	159
One computer, monitor, and hard drive left overnight	125 [49]	16.00	2.00	2.9	211
Compressor	850 [31]	2.40	2.04	0.29	216
Energy TV	200 [49]	8	1.6	0.23	254
Ten incandescent light bulbs	60 watt [50]	80.00	4.8	0.69	507
Small electric heater	1000 [49]	4	4.00	0.576	634
Washer disinfector	2800	5.50	15.4	2.22	768
Air conditioner	1000 [51]	8.00	8.00	1.15	846
Autoclave	2220	7.33	16.27	2.34	1023

4.4.2 High Energy Appliances

4.4.2.1 Computers

Computers differ in their energy consumption. A laptop computer, such as a 13 -inch

Table 4.3 Energy savings in laptop use

Action	Watts used	Percentage of power used compared with fully on
Adaptor plugged in	0.03	0.075%
Laptop plugged in and off	0.3	0.75%
Laptop plugged in and asleep	1.1	2.75%
Laptop plugged in and idle	12	30%
Laptop plugged in and working	40	100%

MacBook, can use between 12 and 40 watts (up to £23 if paying 19.5 pence per kWh) of energy annually if used for 8 h a day, or up to £68 if used continuously/not powered down over the course of a year [52]. For a laptop, Energy Star calculated that having the power adapter plugged in and not in use uses 0.03 watts per hour having the laptop plugged in but off drains 0.3 watts per hour, having the laptop plugged in and asleep 1.1 watts per hour and plugged in and idle uses 8–12 watts per hour. The recommendation from this is that practices should ensure computers are turned off, not just put to sleep. Using the above figures, energy use for leaving a MacBook computer laptop on for 16 h overnight could cost £46 annually (see Table 4.3) [53].

Software is available to force computers and monitors into standby or sleep mode thus enabling computer over-night energy consumption to reduce to around 2% and monitor use to 35% [54].

4.4.2.2 Water Coolers

Water coolers are regarded as energy efficient if they use less than 160 watts per hour and the US Environmental Protection Agency, Energy Star, certifies them if they do not use more than 0.16 kilowatt hours (kWh) per day [55]. Figures calculated by reduction revolution showed a 50% drop in power if a timer is used to turn the cooler off and on as appropriate [56].

4.4.2.3 Televisions

Many dental practices have televisions in the patient' waiting room, and it is worth noting that older models often consume a significantly higher amount of energy than newer models. However, as has been discussed previously, the environmental cost embedded in the manufacture and retail of the television also needs to be considered—it is not always beneficial to simply purchase a new television to save energy. The dental team should check the wattage of any replacement television. LED (light-emitting diode) televisions are more energy efficient than alternatives. OLED televisions (98Watt), the next step up from LED, unfortunately use significantly more energy. Practices should check efficiency ratings [57–59].

4.4.2.4 Lighting

Dental practices can use a significant amount of power for lighting. Eight old-fashioned 60-watt incandescent light bulbs turned on for 10 h per day will cost the practice around £245 per annum [50].

The recent developments of LED light bulbs can reduce energy consumption even more, with the equivalent lighting lasting 15–25 times longer than the traditional incandescent bulbs they replace, producing one sixth of the carbon emissions, and 30% of the energy used by halogen incandescents [60].

An 8–10 W LED light bulb has the same intensity of lighting as a 60 W incandescent bulb [61]. Although LED bulbs are more expensive than incandescent, they last a lot longer and use much energy. Lighting costs and emissions can be further reduced by techniques such as daylight harvesting and automatic dimming controls with wireless sensors. Lights should be turned off when a room is not in use and bulbs should be dusted to ensure their intensity is not reduced. The dental team should always recycle light bulbs appropriately as some contain mercury (e.g. fluorescent bulbs).

To ensure critical appliances are not turned off either during the day or at night it may be wise to label switches.

Light sensors have been used in areas such as store rooms but, according to saveonenergy.com, with the use of energy-efficient bulbs the financial outlay of installing sensors is not warranted [62].

For outside lighting, practices could consider solar powered options.

4.4.2.5 Fridges

The motor of a fridge generally runs at around 30% of actual use, costing about £46 to run per year. The actual energy consumption depends on various factors including its size, the temperature of the fridge's location, how often the fridge door is opened, how full it is and the thermostat setting [63]. Dental practices can reduce the fridge's power consumption by ensuring it is not sited near a heat source, is around 75% full, has a low thermostat setting and has space around the appliance to allow cooling [30].

4.4.2.6 Dental Suction

The dental suction uses relatively little power at around £7 a year. Although the power consumption is relatively low, of more concern is the water consumption of potentially 750,000 L per year of water. The dental practice should consider switching to newer dry vacuum systems when the old system needs to be replaced. In addition, manufacturers should consider the resource use of these types of products [64].

4.4.2.7 Autoclaves, Washer Disinfectors, and Ultrasonic Cleaners

These devices are high energy users. For the purpose of simplicity, we discuss their use within the decontamination chapter.

4.4.3 Moderate Energy Appliances

Kettles, coffee makers, lighting (including overhead dental lights), radios, fridges, and microwaves are higher energy users. These appliances each consume an average of around £48 of electricity per year. Always consider buying the most energy-efficient products, especially in the case of the highest energy-consuming products (see Table 4.2).

Many electrical devices have an energy appliance rating. Upgrading less efficient products with more energy efficient ones before the end of their useful life may result in the consumption of more resources and energy to manufacture and have an overall bigger impact on resource use that may outweigh any efficiency gain. Purchasers should consider getting the longest cost-effective warranty to ensure that the piece of equipment lasts a long time resulting in the manufacturing emissions being extended over as long a time as possible. This is complicated however as it depends on who "owns" the extended warranty. If the manufacturer is responsible, you would hope they would do as much as possible to ensure longevity in the product, if it is a third-party insurance provider this may not be the case; the warranty just may result in the need for a replacement product thus requiring more resource!

If there is a high demand for hot water, instant water heating devices are generally more efficient than boiling a kettle. On average, it costs £26 per annum to boil 12 cups of water daily using a kettle compared to around £17.65 using an instant water device [65]. Kettles usually have a minimum water level that must be used (500 ml or so), and this is the main reason for the difference in efficiency. However, there is a large price difference between installing an instant water heater and buying a kettle, usually in the region of £400 [66]. It would possibly make more sense for the practice to buy an efficient kettle—especially one that can boil smaller quantities of water.

4.4.4   Low Energy Appliances

Much of the equipment used in dental practice (such as printers, Wi-Fi routers, x-ray machines, phone chargers, and curing lights) use very little energy. New curing lights use LED (light-emitting diode) which results in energy savings. Most of the environmental impact of these low energy appliances comes from their life cycle and includes the resources required to produce and dispose of them. More information on this can be found the procurement chapter in this book.

4.4.5   Turning Off Appliances

The Energy Saving Trust advises on the benefits of turning appliances off, with a potential energy saving of £35 per year by turning off all appliances every evening and before a period of closure, for example, at the end of the working week [67]. This should not involve just putting equipment into standby as appliances still draw power in standby mode. The Energy Saving Trust calculated £40 is wasted annually using standby mode [68]. One way of verifying this energy waste is to feel the warmth emanating from appliances or transformers [69].

One suggestion for eliminating energy waste, and therefore also financial waste, is to create a checklist of all the appliances that could be shut down to save money, for example, ensure television is turned off at the wall, power down non-essential computer devices, etc.

Table 4.4 Average fuel source mix of UK electricity [70]

Fuel	Fuel mix electricity supplied 2017 fourth quarter (%)	Fuel mix electricity supplied 2020 fourth quarter (%)
Oil	0.36%	0.33%
Imports	1.88%	6.20%
Hydro	2.21%	2.46%
Bioenergy	7.25%	10.08%
Coal	9.02%	1.42%
Nuclear	17.18%	15.23%
Wind/solar	20.77%	26.09%
Gas	40.15%	36.33%
Other	1.46%	2.02%
Pumped storage and net imports	−0.28%	−0.16%
		100%

Table 4.5 Environmental impact of different electricity sources from LCA

Name	Electricity from wind	Heat from wood	Electricity from coal	Electricity from solar	Heat from natural gas	Electricity from incineration	Unit
Ecosystem quality - freshwater ecotoxicity	0.09828	0.28386	0.40023	0.10151	0.02745	0.01136	CTU
Ecosystem quality - freshwater eutrophication	8.25E-06	1.19E-05	0.00065	1.05E-05	4.14E-06	1.84E-06	kg P-Eq
Ecosystem quality - terrestrial eutrophication	0.00019	0.00713	0.01289	0.00067	0.0011	1.82E-05	mol N-Eq
Resources - dissipated water	0.00636	0.0348	0.08811	0.01196	0.02821	0.00031	m3 water-Eq
Human health - respiratory effects, inorganics	1.09E-09	1.98E-08	1.38E-08	2.24E-09	5.75E-10	6.55E-11	disease incidence
Resources - land use	0.39478	123.22031	3.09423	1.99446	0.06755	0.02055	points
Human health - photochemical ozone creation	6.41E-05	0.00121	0.00349	0.0002	0.00031	4.17E-06	kg NMVOC-Eq
Human health - ozone layer depletion	1.11E-09	6.10E-09	1.27E-08	5.17E-09	3.33E-08	3.55E-11	kg CFC-11-Eq
Human health - non-carcinogenic effects	5.46E-09	2.36E-07	1.83E-07	5.02E-09	4.26E-09	1.41E-09	CTUh
Human health - ionising radiation	0.00101	0.00236	0.01121	0.00135	0.01197	3.81E-05	kg U235-Eq
Resources - fossils	0.20784	0.53533	18.57338	0.80242	6.81783	0.00738	MJ
Human health - carcinogenic effects	7.91E-09	8.45E-09	1.30E-08	5.67E-09	1.86E-09	6.87E-10	CTUh
Climate change - climate change total	0.01538	0.04655	1.19233	0.05748	0.39326	0.00202	kg CO2-Eq
Ecosystem quality - marine eutrophication	1.94E-05	0.00044	0.00127	6.53E-05	0.0001	1.37E-06	kg N-Eq
Ecosystem quality - freshwater and terrestrial acidification	7.92E-05	0.00149	0.00924	0.00026	0.00023	8.25E-06	mol H+-Eq
Resources - minerals and metals	1.28E-06	7.35E-07	9.38E-07	9.49E-07	6.88E-07	5.58E-07	kg Sb-Eq

4.5 The Environmental Impact of Energy Sources: Buying Appropriate Sustainable Energy and/or Generating Energy In-House

The fuel mix of UK electricity is listed below. Since, in the study commissioned by Public Health England (PHE) in 2017, the UK mix has shown a dramatic reduction in coal consumption, with an increase in the use of natural gas, wind/solar energy (see Table 4.4).

In our British Dental Journal (BDJ) paper [71], we ranked energy emissions via their carbon equivalent emission. Although knowledge of carbon dioxide equivalent emissions on a product-by-product basis is useful, solely concentrating on carbon dioxide equivalent emissions can be problematic. Table 4.5 shows the environmental impact of the equivalent of 1 kWh of energy.

4.5.1 Transmission of Energy and Embodied Environmental Impact

Readers need to be aware that, although the carbon emissions are close to zero to produce the energy, there are a number of other environmental costs that need to be considered. Firstly, any product that is created to generate power requires substantial resource investment. Secondly, there is a transmission cost to move the energy from where it is produced (e.g. an offshore wind farm) to where it is needed, with a loss in this travel of between 2 and 19% [72, 73]. This transmission cost is therefore negligible when renewable energy is generated onsite.

There are a number of green electricity providers (i.e. only use energy produced from wind or solar energy), which have very low carbon emissions and information on these emission levels can be found on energy comparison sites [74]. As more consumers choose to purchase green energy, this will also influence markets.

4.5.1.1 Wood Pellets

If you consider heat which is generated from wood pellets, you can see that the climate change total is low at around 2 g/kWh. The reason for this value is that wood pellets both emit carbon emissions when being burnt but remove carbon from the air when being cultivated. Biomass, such as wood, can only be considered sustainable when the waste wood used cannot be used for another more sustainable purpose (e.g. building) [75]. The use of biomass as an energy source also scores poorly in the area of land use (although solid wood is worse in this area than wood pellets which traditionally come from more waste wood) [75]. The other issue with the burning of wood pellets is its damage to human health, particularly respiratory effects, non/actual carcinogenic effects. A recent study highlighted the issue caused with high PM 2.5 and PM 1 in buildings where people are using a residential stove [76]. In fact, residential combustion of fuels within the UK—from wood burning stoves—contributes a similar amount of particulate matter to the environment as car use [77]. The World Health Organization has calculated that internationally more than 1.6 million deaths and over 38.5 million disability-adjusted life years can be attributed to indoor smoke from solid fuels.

4.5.1.2 Energy from Incineration

Energy from incineration seems the best from an environmental perspective because it is serving a dual function of removing waste and generating energy. It does not require land use and has a comparatively low impact across all the other categories included in an LCA. However, incineration has its flaws. As well as wasting potentially valuable resources by conversion into energy, incineration does cause pollutants such as acid gases, nitrogen oxides, metals, particulate matter, and sulphur; with consequential human health effects [78, 79].

As discussed in our waste chapter, a lot of the energy that comes from incineration is from waste which should be recycled. The vast majority of plastics, 79% for example is not recycled [80].

4.5.1.3 Solar Power

The obvious choices today are energy made from solar panels or wind. Looking at Table 4.5 solar panels do have some environmental impact particularly in the

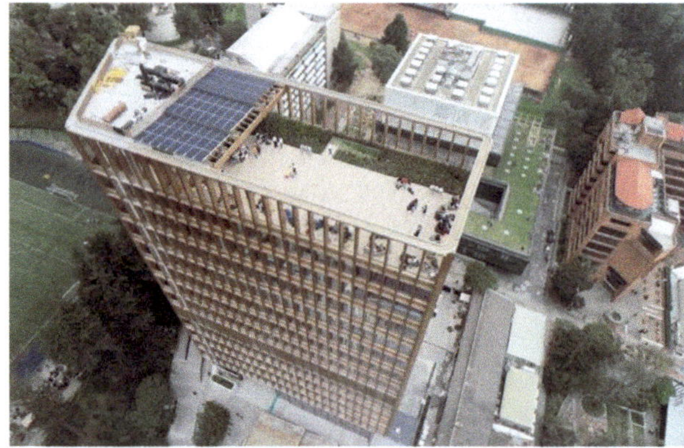

Fig. 4.1 Solar panels. Faculty of Engineering, University Javeriana, Bogotá

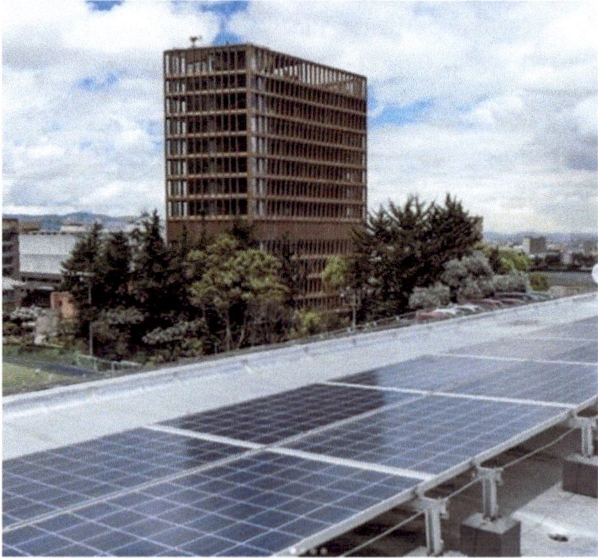

use of minerals and metals. The main metals used in solar panels include aluminium, copper, indium, iron, lead, molybdenum, nickel, silver, and zinc [81]. Increasingly common are solar photovoltaic systems. Dental practices would generally use a 3–4 kW generation capacity which would cost between £4750 and £8350 [82, 83]. Some countries continue to provide financial assistance for solar panels; without assistance the payback period is around 10–12 years [50]. There are some concerns that up to 40% of the UK's solar farms were built using panels manufactured by China's biggest solar panel companies, including Jinko Solar, JA Solar, and Trina Solar using panels linked to Xinjiang forced labour (see Fig. 4.1) [84].

4.5.1.4 Wind Energy

Although comparatively less harmful to the environment than solar energy, wind energy can have adverse environmental impacts, including the potential to reduce, fragment, or degrade habitat for wildlife, fish, and plants. Furthermore, spinning turbine blades can pose a threat to flying wildlife such as birds and bats. Wind turbines need a reasonable space, particularly noticeable in large-scale wind farms. It is important that it does not limit the availability of land for other purposes, for example, growing food, or maintaining, enriching biodiversity [85].

Wind turbines have a high environmental impact especially at the early stages of their life cycle, during construction [86]. For wind turbines sited in shallow water, it is the material extraction and processing to build the turbine which accounts for nearly 60% of the total life cycle impact, with installation requiring around one fourth of the environmental impact. For turbines sited in deeper water, there is a lot more material needed, with 4/5 of the life cycle impact used to manufacture a sufficiently robust product [86].

4.5.2 Comparison of Fuel Types, Cost, and Carbon Dioxide Emissions (CO₂e)

Table 4.6 Energy prices (as at 2021) clarifies the different types of fuel which can be considered by a dental practice.

4.5.2.1 Heating the Practice with Non-renewable Energy

There are also other systems dental practices could use to heat their practices.

Table 4.6 Energy prices (as at 2021)

Fuel type	Equivalent cost per kWh (UK pence)
Wood pellets	6.9 [87]
Natural gas	4.16 [87]
LPG	7.55 [87]
Coal	6.88 [87]
Electricity (average mix)	14.4 [88] to 19.88 [87]

4.5.2.2 Heat Pumps

There are two types of heat pumps. Ground source heat pumps (costing between £11,000 and £15,000) are an option for larger dental practices with larger back yards, or the space to place a bore hole. Working in the opposite way to a refrigerator, a heat pump transfers heat from the ground into the dental practice. This would require a practice building which was fairly airtight [89].

Alternatively, air source heat pumps take air from outside and remove the heat from it, releasing heat into the dental practice for use with hot water and heating [90] Air source heat pumps can cost between £5000 and £8000 [91] and should only be considered efficient if the building is insulated to a good standard [92].

4.5.2.3 Solar Thermal Systems

Solar thermal systems, usually running on the roof, use solar energy to heat water, and/or contribute to underfloor heating. However, in countries with a climate similar to that of the UK, this heating system may prove unreliable due to the lack of sunshine, especially during the winter months. In addition, hot water use is not a big part of most dental practice's energy usage.

4.5.2.4 Recycling of Hot Water Systems

These systems extract the heat from the hot water that might be used in the surgery. Once it enters the drainage system it is then used to warm new water which is in turn used in the clinic. The system often consists of a vertical copper pipe, where the water runs alongside the colder mains water to exchange the heat. The costs can be £1000, which may be prohibitive for some dental practices, but it all depends on how much water they use.

Take Home Points for the Dental Team

- One seventh of the carbon footprint in dentistry comes from the way the profession uses energy.
- In an ideal world, the team should consider how they can use energy more efficiency.
- The dental team should consider renewable energy sources for their electricity supply.
- There are financial and sustainable savings to be made with the use of efficient heating systems, lighting, appropriate insulation, and by regulating use of larger appliances, for example, computer monitors, autoclaves, washer, and disinfectors.
- Health services should therefore think carefully before undertaking the building of a new healthcare structure. It may be environmentally more beneficial to upgrade existing building stock instead.

References

1. Duane B, Berners Lee M, White S, Stancliffe R, Steinbach I. An estimated carbon footprint of NHS primary dental care within England. How can dentistry be more environmentally sustainable? BDJ. 2017;223:589–93.
2. Duane B, Hyland J, Rowan JS, Archibald B. Taking a bite out of Scotland's dental carbon emissions in the transition to a low carbon future. Public Health. 2012;126(9):770–7.
3. Conserve Energy Future. https://www.conserve-energy-future.com/reduce-reuse-recycle.php. Accessed 11 July 2021.
4. Ecodentistry. https://ecodentistry.org/green-dentistry/what-is-green-dentistry/save-water/conventional-suction-systems/. Accessed 11 July 2021.
5. Brunton P, Sharif M, Creanor S, et al. Contemporary dental practice in the UK in 2008: indirect restorations and fixed prosthodontics. BDJ. 2012;212:115–9. https://doi.org/10.1038/sj.bdj.2012.92.
6. Open LCA. https://www.openlca.org/. Accessed 11 July 2021.
7. Public Health England. Carbon modelling within dentistry. https://assets.publishing.service.gov.uk/government/uploads/system/uploads/attachment_data/file/724777/Carbon_modelling_within_dentistry.pdf. Accessed 30 June 2021.
8. Berg F, Fuglseth M. Life cycle assessment and historic buildings: energy-efficiency refurbishment versus new construction in Norway. J Archit Conserv. 2018;24(2):152–67. https://doi.org/10.1080/13556207.2018.1493664.
9. Kohler N, Hassler U. Alternative scenarios for energy conservation in the building stock. Build Res Inform. 2012;40(4):401–16.
10. Moran F, Blight T, Natarajan S, Shea A. The use of passive house planning package to reduce energy use and CO^2 emissions in historic dwellings. Energ Buildings. 2014;75:216–27.
11. Moran F, Natarajan S, Nikolopoulou M. Developing a database of energy use for historic dwellings in Bath, UK. Energ Buildings. 2012;55:218–26.
12. Norrström H. Sustainable and balanced energy efficiency and preservation in our built heritage. Sustainability. 2013;5(6):2623–43.
13. Troi A and Bastian Z. Energy efficiency solutions for historic buildings. Basel: Birkhäuser, 2014, 336 p. 3. https://issuu.com/birkhauser.ch/docs/birkhauser_eurac_energy_efficiency_.
14. Space Management Group. Implementing SMG Guidance. http://www.smg.ac.uk/documents/Implementing%20SMG%20Guidance%202007.pdf. Accessed 11 July 2021.
15. REoptimizer. How to determine the best utilization rate for your building. http://www.reoptimizer.com/real-estate-optimization-blog/real-estate-optimization-blog/bid/188410/how-to-determine-the-best-utilization-rate-for-your-building. Accessed 11 July 2021.
16. Zsembinszki G, Llantoy N, Palomba V, Frazzica A, Dallapiccola M, Trentin F, Cabeza LF. Life Cycle Assessment (LCA) of an innovative compact hybrid electrical-thermal storage system for residential buildings in Mediterranean climate. Sustainability. 2021;13(9):5322. https://doi.org/10.3390/su13095322.
17. Energy Saving Trust. Roof and Loft. Online information available at http://www.energysavingtrust.org.uk/home-insulation/roof-and-loft. Accessed 11 July 2021.
18. The Greenage. Top ten tips for improving your domestic EPC rating. https://www.thegreenage.co.uk/top-10-tips-improving-domestic-epc-rating/.
19. National Residential Landlords Association. Minimum energy efficiency for listed buildings. https://www.nrla.org.uk/resources/energy-efficiency/minimum-energy-efficiency-standards-listed-buildings.
20. Duane B, Harford S, Steinbach I, Stancliffe R, Swan J, Lomax R, Pasdeki-Clewer E, Ramasubbu D. Environmentally sustainable dentistry: energy use within the dental practice. Br Dent J. 2019;226(5):367–73. https://doi.org/10.1038/s41415-019-0044-x.
21. Energy Education. Door. https://energyeducation.ca/encyclopedia/Door. Accessed 11 July 2021.
22. Smart Energy. Smart meters offer the key to changing energy behaviour at home. https://www.smartenergygb.org/en/resources/press-centre/press-releases-folder/usage-tracker-may-2019.

23. Smart meters. Smart meters offer the key to changing energy behaviour at home. https://www.smartenergygb.org/en/resources/press-centre/press-releases-folder/usage-tracker-may-2019.

24. The Guardian. National Grid—keeping millions from landfill. https://www.theguardian.com/sustainable-business/keeping-millions-metres-landfill. Accessed 11 July 2021.

25. Specialty Air. 5 Essential factors to consider when buying a heat pump. https://www.specialtyairinc.com/5-essential-factors-to-consider-when-buying-a-heat-pump/.

26. Department of Energy and Climate change. Study on Energy use by Air conditioning. https://www.bre.co.uk/filelibrary/pdf/projects/aircon-energy-use/DECC-AC-summary-page.pdf. Accessed May 2018.

27. WHO. Consideration s for the provision of essential oral health services in the WHO. Consideration s for the provision of essential oral health services in the context of Covid-19 Interim Guidance. 2020.

28. Armstrong/O'Connor IDJ 2021;66(6).

29. Inteb Managed Services. How much does your water contribute to your energy bill? http://intebms.co.uk/2017/03/23/how-much-does-your-water-use-contribute-to-your-energy-bill/. Accessed May 2018.

30. Residential Landlords Association. Minimum energy efficient standards. https://www.rla.org.uk/landlord/guides/minimum-energy-efficiency-standards.shtml. Accessed July 2018.

31. Duane B, Taylor T, Stahl-Timmins W, Hyland J, Mackie P, Pollard A. Carbon mitigation, patient choice and cost reduction—triple bottom line optimisation for health care planning. Public Health. 2014;128(10):920–4.

32. Energy Use Calculator. https://www.energyusecalculator.com/. Accessed 11 July 2021.

33. Woodpecker. Curing light LED-B manual. https://www.woodpecker.cz/Documents/LED-B_manualEN.pdf. Accessed July 2021.

34. Energy Use Calculator: Electricity usage of a cell phone charger. http://energyusecalculator.com/electricity_cellphone.htm. Accessed July 2021.

35. Frequency cast. How many watts? Power consumption explained. https://www.frequencycast.co.uk/howmanywatts.html. Accessed July 2021.

36. Michael Blue Jay. Saving electricity. http://michaelbluejay.com/electricity/. Accessed July 2021.

37. Reduction Revolution. Water cooler energy consumption. https://reductionrevolution.com.au/blogs/news-reviews/57786245-water-cooler-water-boiler-energy-consumption-revealed. Accessed July 2021.

38. A-Dec. Product Information Brochure. http://a-dec.com/Products/Dental-Chairs/Dental-Chairs/A-dec-400. Accessed August 2018.

39. The home hacks diy. How Much Power (Watts) Does a Monitor Use? https://www.thehome-hacksdiy.com/how-much-power-watts-does-a-monitor-use/. Accessed July 2021.

40. Best radios. How much electricity does a radio use? https://bestradios.co.uk/how-much-electricity-does-a-radio-use/. Accessed July 2021.

41. The Telegraph. Instant boiling water tap will it cost more. https://www.telegraph.co.uk/money/ask-a-money-expert/i-want-an-instant-boiling-water-tap%2D%2Dwill-it-cost-more-than-usin/. Accessed August 2018.

42. The motherload. The Energy Consumption Of Your TV. https://the-motherload.co.uk/the-energy-consumption-of-your-tv. Accessed July 2021.

43. Ultrasonics Direct. www.ultrasonicsdirect.com. Accessed 11 July 2021.

44. Energy use calculator. Electricity use of a LED light bulb. https://energyusecalculator.com/electricity_ledlightbulb.htm. Accessed July 2021.

45. Energy use calculator. Electricity usage of a Desktop Computer. https://energyusecalculator.com/electricity_computer.htm. Accessed July 2021.

46. Energy use calculator. Electricity usage of a CFL Light Bulb. https://energyusecalculator.com/electricity_cfllightbulb.htm. Accessed July 2021.

47. Dentalcompare.com. Simplicity® Operatory Light from DentalEZ. www.dentalcompare.com. Accessed 11 July 2021.

48. Energuide. How much energy do my household appliances use. https://www.energuide.be/en/questions-answers/how-much-energy-do-my-household-appliances-use/71/. Accessed 11 July 2021.
49. Diverse Power. What uses watt. http://www.diversepower.com/energy-tools/watt-uses-watt/. Accessed 11 July 2021.
50. Energy use calculator. Electricity usage of an Incandescent Light Bulb. https://energyusecalculator.com/electricity_incandescent.htm. Accessed 11 July 2021.
51. Department of Energy and Climate change. Study on Energy use by Air conditioning. https://www.bre.co.uk/filelibrary/pdf/projects/aircon-energy-use/DECC-AC-summary-page.pdf. Accessed 11 July 2021.
52. Energy use calculator. Electricity usage of a Laptop, Notebook or Netbook. https://energyusecalculator.com/electricity_laptop.htm. Accessed 11 July 2021.
53. Energy Star. Activate power management on your computer. https://www.energystar.gov/products/low_carbon_it_campaign/power_management_computer. Accessed 11 July 2021.
54. Microsoft. Introduction to power management in System Center Configuration Manager. https://docs.microsoft.com/en-us/sccm/core/clients/manage/power/introduction-to-power-management. Accessed 11 July 2021.
55. Quench. https://quenchwater.ca/wp-content/uploads/2017/11/Energy_Star_Information_Sheet_05052017_LR.pdf. Accessed 11 July 2021.
56. Reduction revolution. Office Water Cooler Energy Consumption Revealed. https://reductionrevolution.com.au/blogs/news-reviews/57786245-water-cooler-water-boiler-energy-consumption-revealed. Accessed 11 July 2021.
57. The Energy Community. What's the difference #1: TVs. http://www.theenergycommunity.com/information/energy-use-tv-types/. Accessed 11 July 2021.
58. The Guardian. How to reduce your carbon footprint. https://www.theguardian.com/environment/2017/jan/19/how-to-reduce-carbon-footprint. Accessed 11 July 2021.
59. Rtings. OLED and LED TV Power Consumption and Electricity Cost. https://www.rtings.com/tv/learn/led-oled-power-consumption-and-electricity-cost 57Watt.
60. Energy gov. Lighting Choices to Save You Money. https://www.energy.gov/energysaver/save-electricity-and-fuel/lighting-choices-save-you-money. Accessed 11 July 2021.
61. LED Hut. LED equivalent wattages against traditional lighting. https://ledhut.co.uk/blogs/news/led-equivalent-wattages-against-traditional-lighting.
62. Save on energy. How do energy saving light bulbs impact your energy bill and the environment. https://www.saveonenergy.com/uk/energy-saving/how-do-energy-saving-lightbulbs-impact-your-energy-bill-and-the-environment/.
63. Reduction Revolution. Fridge power consumption—can the star rating be trusted? https://reductionrevolution.com.au/blogs/news-reviews/57784517-fridge-power-consumption-can-the-star-rating-be-trusted. Accessed 11 July 2021.
64. Oral health group. A Buyers' guide to dental vacuum systems. https://www.oralhealthgroup.com/features/a-buyers-guide-to-dental-vacuum-systems/. Accessed 11 July 2021.
65. Which. Are instant hot water taps really cheaper than kettles? https://www.which.co.uk/news/2019/01/are-instant-hot-water-taps-really-cheaper-than-kettles/. Accessed 11 July 2021.
66. Victorian plumbing. Palma Instant Boiling Water Kitchen Tap (Includes Tap, Boiler + Filter). https://www.victorianplumbing.co.uk/palma-instant-boiling-water-tap-includes-tap-boiler-filter. Accessed 11 July 2021.
67. Energy Saving Trust. Quick tips to save energy. https://energysavingtrust.org.uk/hub/quick-tips-to-save-energy/. Accessed 11 July 2021.
68. The Greenage. Do standby savers really save you energy? https://www.thegreenage.co.uk/standby-savers-saving-you-energy-in-your-home/. Accessed 11 July 2021.
69. Harvard University. Green indicators. https://green.harvard.edu/tools-resources/poster/top-5-steps-reduce-your-energy-consumption. Accessed 11 July 2021.
70. Ofgem. Wholesale market indicators. https://www.ofgem.gov.uk/data-portal/electricity-generation-mix-quarter-and-fuel-source-gb. Accessed 11 July 2021.

71. Duane B, Harford S, Steinbach I. et al. Environmentally sustainable dentistry: energy use within the dental practice. Br Dent J 226, 367–373 (2019). https://doi.org/10.1038/s41415-019-0044-x.

72. IEA Electricity Information Statistics (OECD iLibrary, 2018); https://www.oecd-ilibrary.org/energy/data/iea-electricity-information-statistics_elect-data-en. Accessed 11 July 2021.

73. Surana K, Jordaan S. The climate mitigation opportunity behind global power transmission and distribution. Nat Clim Chang. 2019;9:660–5. https://doi.org/10.1038/s41558-019-0544-3.

74. Sust-it. UK Energy companies address and phone numbers. https://www.sust-it.net/switching-energy-electricity-gas/uk-providers-companies/. Accessed 11 July 2021.

75. Chatham House. The Impacts of the Demand for Woody Biomass for Power and Heat on Climate and Forests. https://www.chathamhouse.org/2017/02/impacts-demand-woody-biomass-power-and-heat-climate-and-forests. Accessed 11 July 2021.

76. Torres-Duque C, et al. Biomass fuels and respiratory diseases: a review of the evidence. Proc Am Thorac Soc. 2008;5(5):577–90.

77. Department for environmental food and rural affairs. National Statistics. Emissions of air pollutants in the UK—Particulate Matter (PM10 and PM2.5). https://www.gov.uk/government/statistics/emissions-of-air-pollutants/emissions-of-air-pollutants-in-the-uk-particulate-matter-pm10-and-pm25. Accessed 11 July 2021.

78. Sharma R, Sharma M, Sharma R, Sharma V. The impact of incinerators on human health and environment. Rev Envrion Health. 2013;28:67–72.

79. Darbre P. Overview of air pollution and endocrine disorders. Int J Gen Med. 2018;11:191–207.

80. National geographic. A whopping 91% of plastic isn't recycled. https://www.national-geographic.com/science/article/plastic-produced-recycling-waste-ocean-trash-debris-environment#:~:text=The%20vast%20majority%E2%80%9479%20percent,tons%20of%20plastic%20in%20landfills.

81. The World Bank. Climate-smart mining: minerals for climate action. https://www.worldbank.org/en/topic/extractiveindustries/brief/climate-smart-mining-minerals-for-climate-action. Accessed 11 July 2021.

82. Household quotes. https://householdquotes.co.uk/solar-panel-cost/. Accessed 11 July 2021.

83. Homebuilding & renovating. A guide to renewables. https://www.homebuilding.co.uk/renewable-technology-guide/. Accessed 11 July 2021.

84. The Guardian. Revealed: UK solar projects using panels from firms linked to Xinjiang forced labour. https://www.theguardian.com/environment/2021/apr/23/revealed-uk-solar-projects-using-panels-from-firms-linked-to-xinjiang-forced-labour. Accessed 11 July 2021.

85. Energy Sage. https://www.energysage.com/about-clean-energy/wind/environmental-impacts-wind-energy/. Accessed 11 July 2021.

86. Chipindula J, Botlaguduru VSV, Du H, Kommalapati RR, Huque Z. Life cycle environmental impact of onshore and offshore wind farms in Texas. Sustainability. 2018;10(6):2022. https://doi.org/10.3390/su10062022.

87. Nottingham Energy Partnership. https://nottenergy.com/resources/energy-cost-comparison/. Accessed 11 July 2021.

88. Nottingham Energy Partnership. https://www.gov.uk/government/collections/domestic-energy-prices. Accessed 11 July 2021.

89. Centre for Sustainable Energy. https://www.cse.org.uk/advice/renewable-energy/ground-source-heat-pumps. Accessed 11 July 2021.

90. Latent Heat. Heat pump. https://www.latentheat.co.uk/air-source-heat-pumps/?gclid=CjwKCAjwtpGGBhBJEiwAyRZX2lf9d-4HWGUcwbk8XkTyCiacrkJ5-f0aK6cegamle8BnDMJ-fuxhNxoCGAsQAvD_BwE. Accessed 11 July 2021.

91. The Renewable Energy Hub UK. https://www.renewableenergyhub.co.uk/main/heat-pumps-information/a-guide-to-heat-pump-prices-in-2019/. Accessed 11 July 2021.

92. Specialty Airinc. 5 Essential factors to consider when buying a heat pump. https://www.specialtyairinc.com/5-essential-factors-to-consider-when-buying-a-heat-pump/.

Prevention: The Sustainable Practice Initiative

5

Alexandra Lyne, Brett Duane, John Crotty, Sheryl Wilmott, Agi Tarnowski, and Paul Ashley

5.1 Introduction

Oral diseases are highly prevalent in humans and have significant health and economic burdens for society. They impact across all communities with disadvantaged groups being affected disproportionately [1]. Oral diseases can be categorised as dental caries, periodontal disease, oral cancer, and non-carious tooth tissue loss. Strategies to prevent these diseases are well known and well evidenced. Prevention of these diseases will greatly reduce their societal impacts and mitigate against the inequity of access to care. A preventive approach is fundamental to the development of more environmentally sustainable healthcare systems [2].

In this chapter, we will consider the sustainability of key preventive therapies for each of the oral diseases described therein. We will focus on preventive approaches with good evidence of effectiveness selected from strategies recommended for use in England. For each therapy, we will consider its use at an individual level (e.g. delivered by a dentist as part of a treatment episode) and interventions that are recommended for use in communities with high caries risk.

A. Lyne (✉) · P. Ashley
University College London, London, UK
e-mail: alexandra.lyne@nhs.net; p.ashley@ucl.ac.uk

B. Duane · J. Crotty
Trinity College Dublin, Dublin, Ireland
e-mail: Brett.Duane@dental.tcd.ie; John.Crotty@dental.tcd.ie

S. Wilmott
Leeds Teaching Hospitals NHS Trust, Leeds, UK
e-mail: sheryl.wilmott@nhs.net

A. Tarnowski
NHS England, Horley, UK
e-mail: a.tarnowski@nhs.net

  73
B. Duane (ed.), *Sustainable Dentistry*, BDJ Clinician's Guides,
https://doi.org/10.1007/978-3-031-07999-3_5

5.2 Caries

Dental caries is one of the most common communicable diseases in humans affecting children and adults alike [1]. The global burden has remained largely unchanged over the last 30 years. Where reductions in prevalence have occurred, they tend to be in higher income countries [1]. In common with other oral diseases, increased prevalence of dental caries is associated with higher levels of deprivation.

Management of the carious lesion (e.g. restoration or extraction) is expensive to deliver. It is often unaffordable in many lower income countries and is not usually part of universal health coverage in higher income countries [2]. This condition is completely preventable with a range of therapies available supported by a high-quality evidence base. Each patient appointment for the treatment of caries will have an associated environmental burden, i.e. from the patient and staff travel to the clinic, the equipment and materials needed, and the energy use and cleaning of the clinic.

Delivery of preventive therapies makes economic sense and leads to improved outcomes for patients. Public health programmes, such as water fluoridation, will be discussed as a key population-level caries prevention used globally.

There are various international documents recommending therapies for caries prevention. The Public Health England document is Delivering Better Oral Health [3] which provides dentists and associated professionals with evidence-based recommendations for caries prevention. Evidence supporting these therapies is ranked by quality. In this section we will only be considering those interventions supported by evidence at level I (strong evidence from at least one systematic review of multiple well-designed randomised control trial/s). These are:

- Toothbrushing with a fluoride toothpaste
- Fluoride varnish
- Fissure sealants
- Fluoride mouth rinses

Diet advice will also be briefly discussed, despite its low evidence base.

5.2.1 Public Health Measures to Prevent Caries

Dental public health programmes aimed at reducing caries can target an entire population (e.g. adjusting the level of fluoride in the domestic water supply) or can target-specific groups of at-risk patients. General dental practices should have a working knowledge of the dental public health schemes in their area.

Water fluoridation programmes are commonly used and benefit more than 35% of the world's population [4]. Studies have found that water fluoridation is effective and will result in a reduction of caries at a population level [5].

As of 2021, approximately 10% of the UK population live in areas with a water fluoridation programme. Professional bodies, such as the Department of Health, recognise the benefits of water fluoridation in not only reducing the decay experience in children, but also reducing the number of dental general anaesthetics [6]. Furthermore, as it is a population-level intervention, children from both affluent and deprived regions benefit.

Recent life cycle assessment (LCA) data found that the process of fluoridating water for one person produces the equivalent of just 0.443 kg carbon per year [7–9]. This study was based on water fluoridation processes in the Republic of Ireland, it is assumed that similar processes would generate comparable results internationally. When compared to LCA data from other forms of community-level programmes aimed at children's oral health (fluoride varnish application in schools, provision of toothpaste and toothbrush provision to young children, supervised toothbrushing in schools), water fluoridation was found to have the lowest environmental impact (see Table 5.1).

Given the benefits of water fluoridation for dental public health, and the associated low environmental emissions, there are compelling reasons why this intervention should be supported by dental practices, dental professional groups and trade organisations. In many countries (e.g. England, Scotland, and Wales), targeted dental public health programmes have been introduced to reach populations who are most at risk. This includes supervised toothbrushing and the application of fluoride

Table 5.1 LCA data for community dental caries prevention methods

Impact category	Water fluoridation	Fluoride varnish application in schools	Targeted provision of toothbrushes and toothpaste	Supervised toothbrushing in schools
climate change (kg CO2 eq)	4.43E-01	3.31E+00	2.89E+00	1.95E+00
acidification (mol H+ eq)	5.83E-03	1.14E-02	1.36E-02	8.11E-03
freshwater ecotoxicity (CTU)	8.70E-01	7.04E+00	5.28E+00	3.22E+00
freshwater eutrophication (kg P eq)	9.66E-05	6.70E-04	1.06E-03	5.30E-04
marine eutrophication (kg N eq)	9.30E-04	3.18E-03	3.70E-03	1.93E-03
terrestrial eutrophication (mol N eq)	9.84E-03	2.66E-02	2.80E-02	1.75E-02
carcinogenic effects (CTUh)	1.55E-08	2.99E-07	2.59E-07	1.04E-07
ionising radiation (kg U235 eq)	8.32E-02	1.40E-01	2.40E-01	1.41E-01
non-carcinogenic effects (CTUh)	1.47E-07	3.35E-07	4.51E-07	1.96E-07
ozone layer depletion (kg CFC-11 eq)	7.24E-08	3.12E-07	3.33E-07	3.92E-07
photochemical ozone creation (kg NMVOC eq)	2.89E-03	8.14E-03	9.24E-03	5.97E-03
respiratory inorganics effects (disease inc)	4.58E-08	1.32E-07	2.28E-07	9.02E-08
dissipated water (m3 water eq)	2.96E-01	1.22E+00	8.37E+00	2.43E+00
fossil use (MJ)	8.32E+00	3.57E+01	5.19E+01	3.19E+01
land use (pts)	4.50E+00	2.01E+01	2.08E+01	1.17E+01
mineral/metal use (kg Sb eq)	6.62E-06	2.64E-05	1.87E-05	1.79E-05

varnish in schools, and the provision of oral health kits to children at risk. As shown in Table 5.1, all these targeted interventions have a higher environmental impact than water fluoridation. The provision of toothbrushes and toothpaste for at-risk children to use at home had the greatest environmental impact in 11 out of the 16 impact categories. The same study found the disability adjusted life years (DALY) impact was just 20 s for water fluoridation, compared to 57 s for supervised toothbrushing in schools, 85 s for provision of toothbrushes and toothpaste, and 97 s for fluoride varnish application in schools.

Most dental practices would not provide these community-level programmes in schools; however, any staff involved in such a service should look for ways to reduce its environmental impact. The notable contributing factors to these targeted public health programmes included staff travel to work, plastic toothbrushes, and the use of single-use instruments. General dental practitioners should be aware of any schemes in their area; in particular, check if young children are part of a fluoride varnish application scheme at their school. This may influence the clinician's decision on whether to apply fluoride to that child's teeth.

Table 5.1 illustrates the environmental consequences of the resources used to provide different preventive modalities to one 5-year-old child for 1 year.

5.2.2 Diet Advice

Whilst the relationship between diet and dental caries is well evidenced, interventions to modify diet in relation to dental caries are not. Although it is important for patients to understand the aetiology of their disease, dental professionals giving diet advice is not an evidence-based intervention for caries prevention.

The environmental impact of giving diet advice in dental practice can be assumed to be relatively low, providing the patient does not attend solely for this purpose. The environmental cost of giving diet advice would come from the time spent in the dental chair (the associated energy use of the practice, and a portion of the patient and staff travel into the practice), and any physical leaflets or diet sheets given to the patient. Finding alternative ways to provide this information, for example, directing patients to good online resources, or using tele-dentistry may help make diet advice more sustainable (see Chap. 3). However, in terms of evidence-based methods for prevention, interventions such as fluoride toothpaste, varnishes, or mouth rinses are likely to be more effective.

5.2.3 Toothbrushing with a Fluoride Toothpaste

Toothbrushing with a fluoridated toothpaste is often viewed as one of the most effective oral health strategies introduced worldwide in recent years and is considered to be the cornerstone of prevention. Fluoride is added to toothpaste in a variety of different forms (sodium fluoride, sodium monofluorophosphate, amine fluoride, stannous fluoride) with formulations containing sodium fluoride or sodium monofluorophosphate most widely available. The effect of fluoride in the toothpaste is thought to be dose dependent with strengths of 1000 ppm usually recommended as a minimum [10]. In common with other fluoride therapies, the main risk associated with use is dental fluorosis, however evidence of a direct link is weak [11]. Current UK caries prevention guidelines recommend prescribing higher dose fluoride toothpaste for children over 10 years of age (2800 ppm sodium fluoride, or 5000 ppm sodium fluoride for patients 16 years and over) [3].

Fluoride toothpaste is commonly used as a personal care product and is considered to be part of a 'normal' self-care routine. Community-wide interventions using fluoride toothpaste usually involve increasing the availability of fluoride toothpastes and brushes and/or promoting their use in schools.

The LCA data on fluoride toothpaste suggests that a single 100 mL tube of 1450 ppm sodium fluoride toothpaste has a relatively low carbon footprint (0.34 kg of carbon). For prescription strength toothpastes (e.g. 2800 ppm and 5000 ppm sodium fluoride), there is very little change in the environmental impact. In fact, assuming the additional weight of sodium fluoride is balanced by reducing the weight of sorbitol in the toothpaste, the climate change impact remains the same for 2800 ppm fluoride toothpaste, and actually decreases by 0.21% for the 5000 ppm fluoride toothpaste. Sorbitol (a humectant used in toothpaste to produce its gel-like consistency) is responsible for most of the environmental impact of a tube of toothpaste—most likely because it is the largest component ingredient in toothpaste accounting for between 50 and 70% of toothpaste composition by weight. Sorbitol contributed more than any other aspect of fluoride toothpaste in all but five measures of sustainability.

The DALY impact of different concentrations of toothpaste were similar (all within 18.26–18.32 s per tube of toothpaste). Given this data, there is no environmental consideration required when it comes to choosing a dose of toothpaste—instead the decision should be made based on the patient's age and risk factors.

Recently, toothpaste tablets have come on the market. Toothpaste tablets are often advertised as a 'zero-waste' alternative to toothpaste as the toothpaste comes packaged in recyclable glass containers and aluminium lids instead of a plastic or aluminium tube. Sorbitol (which is the greatest contributing factor to the environmental impact of normal fluoride toothpaste) is not an ingredient of toothpaste tablets as toothpaste tablets do not need the gel consistency. Additionally, tablets are lighter than gel toothpaste, which would in turn reduce the impact of product distribution. Although logically it follows that they would, therefore, have a reduced environmental impact, this has not been studied or quantified with LCA data. There is currently little evidence regarding the clinical effectiveness of toothpaste tablets; however, there is some data indicating that fluoride bio-availability in saliva after using a fluoridated-toothpaste tablet is comparable to traditional toothpaste. Therefore, it is considered likely they will have similar levels of effectiveness [12].

There is no evidence that the type of toothbrush being used to brush teeth has an impact on caries prevention. Toothbrushes, with regard to their periodontal benefit, are discussed in more detail in Sect. 5.3. Therefore, in the context of caries prevention, the recommendation to patients about what type of toothbrush they should use should be based on sustainable principles. Lyne et al. 2020 and Duane et al. 2020 found that alternative toothbrushes (e.g. manual toothbrushes with a bamboo handle, or manual plastic toothbrushes with replaceable plastic heads) performed better in all measures of sustainability compared to traditional manual and electric toothbrushes [13, 14]. We will not consider the effect of toothbrushing with a non-fluoride toothpaste on dental caries as there is no evidence this has any impact [15, 16].

5.2.4 Fluoride Mouth Rinse

The other commonly used method of fluoride delivery at home is fluoride mouth rinses (see Fig. 5.1) [17]. Increasingly available in alcohol-free formulations, these are commonly available in a strength of 0.05% fluoride and recommended for daily use. The active agent most commonly used is sodium fluoride. Stronger formulations (0.2%) are also available; however, these are for weekly rather than daily use.

Unlike toothpastes or varnishes, mouth rinses are not intended for use by young children as correct usage requires the ability to rinse and spit without swallowing

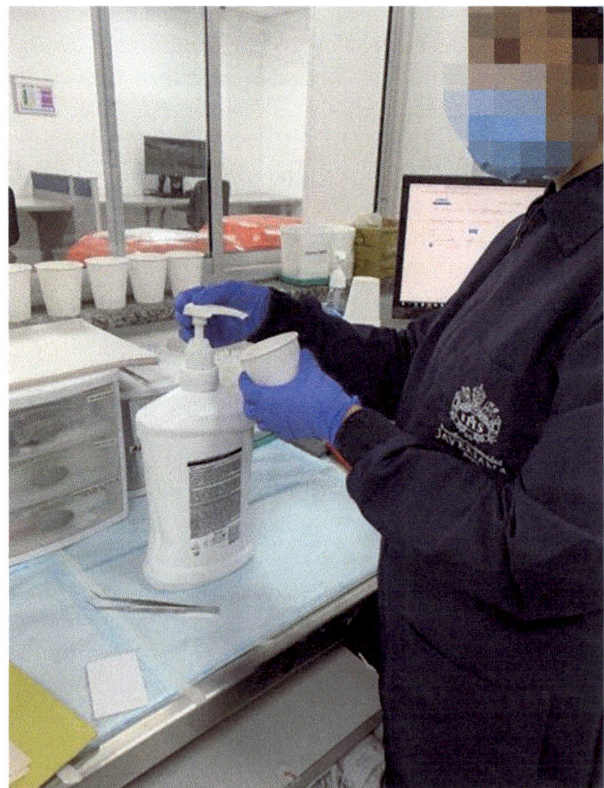

Fig. 5.1 Person dispensing fluoride mouth rinse, used in the clinics of the Faculty of Dentistry, Universidad de Javeriana, Bogota

the formulation. Evidence for both daily and weekly rinses is principally sourced from supervised use in a school setting and demonstrates the preventive effect against caries in permanent teeth [17]. The authors of this chapter (AL, PA, BD) calculated LCA data for an individual 10 mL of sodium fluoride mouth rinse for 5 years, comparing a 0.05% daily mouth rinse with a 0.2% weekly mouth rinse. Both mouth rinses were assumed to be packaged and transported in the same 500 mL plastic bottle to and from the same location and have the same ingredients (water, glycerine, propylene glycol, sorbitol, peppermint oil, sodium fluoride, sodium saccharine, and menthol) with only the sodium fluoride and water amounts varying between the two formulations. The results showed that the daily mouth rinse produced 148 kg of carbon, approximately seven times more than the 21.1 kg produced for the weekly mouth rinse (see Table 5.2). Clearly, this is because much less mouth rinse and plastic bottles need to be produced for the weekly mouth rinse (1/7th of the volume of mouthwash and weight of plastic). Similarly, the DALY impact of the daily mouth rinse was approximately seven times greater than that of the weekly mouth rinse (the equivalent of 100.3 and 14.3 DALY minutes, respectively).

The decision to recommend a fluoride mouth rinse should depend on the patient's caries risk. Clinicians should bear in mind that a daily mouth rinse has a greater environmental impact than a weekly rinse and balance this with patient preference. Daily mouth rinses are more widely available and may, therefore, be preferable/more convenient for patients' oral healthcare routines.

Table 5.2 LCA data for mouth rinse use by an individual over 5 years

Impact category	Daily mouth rinse	Weekly mouth rinse
Climate change (kg CO2 eq)	1.48E+02	2.11E+01
Acidification (mol H+ eq)	9.80E-01	1.40E-01
Freshwater ecotoxicity (CTU)	1.13E+02	1.61E+01
Freshwater eutrophication (kg P eq)	1.31E-01	1.87E-02
Marine eutrophication (kg N eq)	2.42E-01	3.46E-02
Terrestrial eutrophication (mol N eq)	1.71E+00	2.44E-01
Carcinogenic effects (ctuh)	2.70E-06	3.86E-07
Ionising radiation (kg U235 eq)	6.81E+00	9.73E-01
Non-carcinogenic effects (ctuh)	3.54E-05	5.05E-06
Ozone layer depletion (kg CFC-11 eq)	4.63E-05	6.61E-06
Photochemical ozone creation (kg NMVOC eq)	4.11E-01	5.87E-02
Respiratory inorganics effects (disease inc)	4.84E-06	6.92E-07
Dissipated water (m³ water eq)	7.25E+01	1.04E+01
Fossil use (MJ)	2.42E+03	3.45E+02
Land use (pts)	2.56E+03	3.65E+02
Mineral/metal use (kg Sb eq)	1.32E-03	1.90E-04

5.2.5　Fluoride Varnish Application

Fluoride varnishes (see Fig. 5.2) are a commonly used method for delivery of fluoride by dentists and/or dental care professionals. Unlike toothpastes they are not intended for home use. They are designed to be applied to teeth two to four times yearly by a dental professional and promote a slower release of fluoride than toothpaste. Formulations vary with Duraphat (5% NaF in a resin/alcohol solvent) and Fluor Protector (0.9% difluorosilane in a polyurethane-based varnish) most often cited or used [18]. It should be noted that fluoride varnish use is not normally associated with dental fluorosis [11]. Varnishes are often used as part of a preventive regime in dental practices but are also used as a community intervention commonly delivered in a school setting.

LCA data shown in Table 5.3 compares fluoride varnish application in schools with that in dental practice [7]. The data clearly demonstrates that applying fluoride varnish when a patient is already attending an appointment at the dental practice has the lowest impact in all measures of environmental sustainability. The reason for this is simple, patients already sitting in the dental chair for another appointment (e.g. routine recall appointment or an appointment for a specific dental procedure)

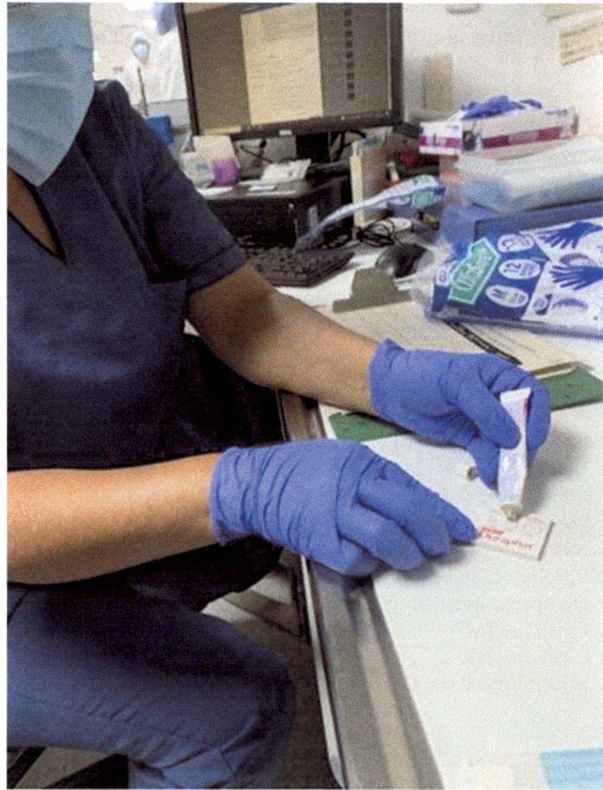

Fig. 5.2 Person dispensing fluoride varnish, used in the clinics of the Faculty of Dentistry, Universidad de Javeriana, Bogota

Table 5.3 LCA data for fluoride varnish application in schools, at an existing practice appointment, and at a separate practice appointment

Impact category (units)	In school	During existing practice appointment	At separate practice appointment
climate change (kg CO2 eq)	3.31E+00	1.09E+00	8.12E+00
acidification (mol H+ eq)	1.14E-02	2.51E-03	3.17E-02
freshwater ecotoxicity (CTU)	7.04E+00	2.09E+00	1.85E+01
freshwater eutrophication (kg P eq)	6.70E-04	2.10E-04	1.41E-03
marine eutrophication (kg N eq)	3.18E-03	1.27E-03	8.35E-03
terrestrial eutrophication (mol N eq)	2.66E-02	6.94E-03	8.25E-02
carcinogenic effects (CTUh)	2.99E-07	3.98E-08	3.64E-07
ionising radiation (kg U235 eq)	1.40E-01	3.92E-02	4.99E-01
non-carcinogenic effects (CTUh)	3.35E-07	7.33E-08	7.15E-07
ozone layer depletion (kg CFC-11 eq)	3.12E-07	1.13E-07	1.23E-06
photochemical ozone creation (kg NMVOC eq)	8.14E-03	1.92E-03	2.72E-02
respiratory inorganics effects (disease inc)	1.32E-07	2.45E-08	3.27E-07
dissipated water (m3 water eq)	1.22E+00	7.17E-01	1.75E+00
fossil use (MJ)	3.57E+01	7.52E+00	1.07E+02
land use (pts)	2.01E+01	5.88E+00	6.15E+01
mineral/metal use (kg Sb eq)	2.64E-05	4.95E-06	8.92E-05

have already travelled to the practice (as have the dental practice staff), the practice is already in use, the staff are already wearing PPE, and much of the equipment needed is already ready for use. In fact, the only additional resources needed at the end of the existing appointment is the fluoride varnish itself, some cotton rolls to dry the teeth (alternatively, compressed air could be used), and a dappens pot and micro-brush to apply the varnish.

This study suggests that sustainable dental practices should, as appropriate, use any opportunity where the patient is already sitting in the dental chair to apply fluoride varnish to the teeth. Fluoride varnish can be applied every 3–4 months for patients at a high caries risk [3]. The study also suggests that having separate 'prevention' appointments (where the patient comes back on another day just to have fluoride varnish applied) have a greater environmental impact and therefore are not recommended by the authors. Public health programmes, such as fluoride varnish application in schools, should still be supported. Dental services that provide fluoride varnish in schools can look at ways to reduce the environmental impact of their service, including their methods of travel, and using reusable instruments wherever possible.

In recent years, interest has grown in the use of silver diamine fluoride to prevent and arrest dental caries. Whilst the evidence base for this therapy is growing, it does not currently form part of UK prevention guidelines and therefore did not meet the threshold specified for inclusion in this chapter.

5.2.6 Fissure Sealants

Fissure sealants (see Fig. 5.3) are probably the single most effective non-fluoride therapy for caries prevention. Classically, the technique involves placement of a resin-based sealant material over the occlusal fissures of molar teeth; the rationale being that bacterial growth will be limited in these otherwise hard to clean areas. Other materials, such as glass ionomer-based sealants, have been used but most of the evidence recommends resin-based sealants for permanent teeth [19]. Placement of sealants is usually done in a practice-based setting as it is a technique-sensitive procedure. Community fissure sealant schemes do exist but can be challenging due to the difficulties of placing them correctly outside of a dental setting.

Fissure sealants can also be placed as part of a composite restoration. In a recent paper, Martin provided some commentary on the environmental impact of composites versus amalgams, but there is currently little information on composite type restorations including fissure sealants [20].

A carbon footprinting study in England found that a fissure sealant had a carbon footprint of 8.58 kg [21]. However, the data cannot be compared to any of the more recent LCAs carried out due to the age of the study (2014) and the fact that this modelling was carried out using a hybrid input output analysis rather than a more detailed life cycle assessment approach. Mulligan et al. (2018) described the potential environmental pollutants from resin-based composite but also conceded that no quantitative data has been collected on their environmental impacts [22].

We would envisage however that a fissure sealant's environmental footprint would be similar to that of the application of fluoride varnish with a large proportion of its environmental footprint not coming from the materials needed, but rather from the associated patient and staff travel, and from energy use, procurement, and waste.

The decision on whether or not to place fissure sealants for an individual patient should be based on the patient's caries risk. In line with English prevention

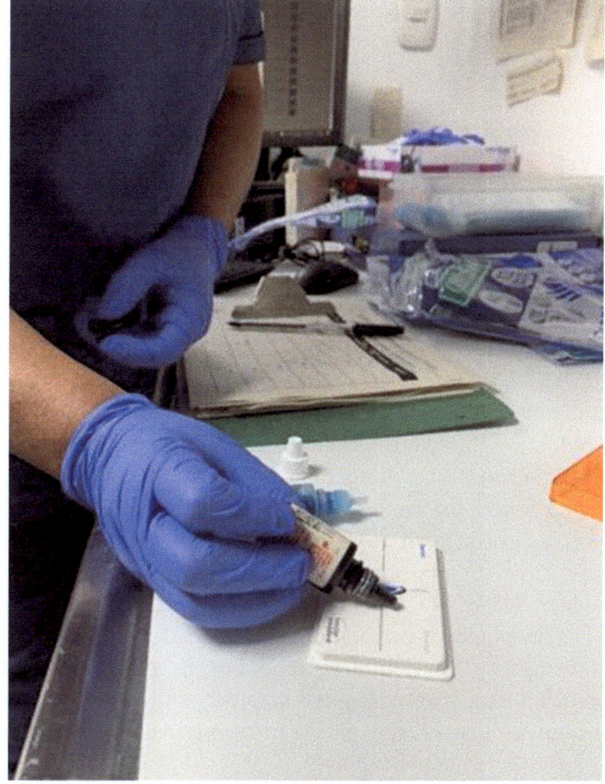

Fig. 5.3 Person dispensing light curing sealants, used in the clinics of the Faculty of Dentistry, Universidad de Javeriana, Bogota

guidelines, it is suggested that patients who are at risk of developing dental caries in their permanent molars should have them fissure sealed and maintained with resin-based sealants. The placement of fissure sealants can be planned with environmental concepts in mind, thus ensuring travel and the number of appointments are minimised. For example, apply as many fissure sealants as possible in one visit, combine procedures with a general recall appointment, or combine with other preventative measures (such as fluoride varnish).

5.3   Periodontal Disease

Periodontal disease is a common inflammatory condition that affects approximately 50% of the adult population [23]. Severe periodontal disease has an increased risk of tooth loss and affects approximately 10% of the adult population [24]. Severe periodontal disease is a hyper-inflammatory state that increases the risk of systemic diseases including diabetes and cardiovascular disease [25]. The prevalence of severe disease has remained relatively unchanged since 1990 [26] and is associated with local, modifiable, and non-modifiable risk factors, as displayed in Table 5.4. Significant non-modifiable risk factors include biological sex, ethnicity, and age

Table 5.4 Local, modifiable, and non-modifiable risk factors associated with the development of periodontitis

Local	Modifiable	Non-modifiable
Cemento-enamel projections	Diabetic control	Age
Open contacts	Obesity	Biological sex
Root grooves	Smoking	Ethnicity
Root proximity	Socio-economic status	Genetic susceptibility
Sub-gingival restorations	Stress	

[27]. Significant modifiable risk factors include smoking, medical conditions (e.g. diabetes), and socio-economic status [28].

Initial management of periodontal disease depends on the extent and severity of the disease and includes personalised oral hygiene instructions and smoking cessation advice. This is followed by extraction of teeth with a poor prognosis and supra- and sub-gingival debridement. Following initial therapy, lifelong maintenance programmes and surgery or extraction of non-responding teeth is required. Periodontal therapy is expensive to undertake, and periodontal disease has been ranked as the sixth most prevalent untreated disease in adults [29]. Delivery of therapy involves many patient visits, use of dental consumables and copious use of water. This will in turn have a significant environmental impact.

Prevention of periodontal disease is the simplest way to reduce the environmental impact of periodontal treatment. It is currently not possible to use clinical or biochemical markers to predict who will develop periodontal disease. Since periodontitis is always preceded by gingivitis [30], the primary target for prevention of periodontitis is the prevention or resolution of gingivitis [31]. Longitudinal studies have demonstrated that improvements in oral hygiene have reduced the prevalence of plaque, gingivitis, and periodontal pockets in populations [32, 33].

5.3.1 Toothbrushes

Plaque is not removed effectively from teeth by natural means [34]. Toothbrushing reduces the level of plaque in the mouth but residual levels of plaque covering up to 60% of the tooth surfaces have been recorded [35]. It is currently not known what level of plaque control is required to prevent the development of periodontitis [36].

To date, toothbrushing techniques have not been shown to directly relate to the efficacy of plaque removal [37, 38]; moreover, patients tend to revert to their original pattern of brushing following instruction [39]. A certain level of force is required to remove plaque but increasing force does not increase efficacy [40]. A brushing frequency of less than once a day has been reported to have an increased risk for the development of periodontitis [41] but the relationship between higher levels of frequency and the development of periodontitis is unclear. Most patients tend to spend between 30 and 60s brushing their teeth [42]. Plaque removal has been reported to increase from approximately 27% following 1 min of brushing to 41% following 2 min of brushing [43] with little improvement in plaque removal reported with additional time [43]. Video evidence indicates that the time spent brushing is distributed unevenly across surfaces and may account for reduced efficacy [44]. Given this, dental care professionals should keep their toothbrushing advice short and not waste clinical time attempting to change the patient's technique unless there is a clear clinical need for that individual patient.

A Cochrane Review comparing the efficacy of manual and powered toothbrushes has reported that powered toothbrushes may reduce plaque levels by an additional 11% within 3 months of use and by 21% over a longer period of time with associated reductions in gingivitis [45]. An 11-year follow-up of patients using powered toothbrushes has reported reductions in periodontal parameters and retention of more teeth than in the manual toothbrushing group [46].

However, LCA data comparing electric and manual toothbrush types suggests that manual toothbrushes in general have a lower environmental impact than electric toothbrushes (see Table 5.5). In particular, the bamboo and replaceable head manual toothbrushes performed well from an environmental perspective. The

Table 5.5 LCA data comparing different types of toothbrushes

Impact category	Plastic manual toothbrush	Bamboo manual toothbrush	Plastic manual toothbrush with replaceable heads	Electric toothbrush with replaceable heads
climate change (kg CO2 eq)	2.56E+01	4.26E+00	5.16E+00	4.79E+01
acidification (mol H+ eq)	1.12E-01	4.50E-02	2.26E-02	5.66E-01
freshwater ecotoxicity (CTU)	1.35E+01	4.53E+00	2.72E+00	1.39E+02
freshwater eutrophication (kg P eq)	1.42E-03	1.99E-03	2.87E-04	3.05E-02
marine eutrophication (kg N eq)	1.90E-02	6.60E-03	3.83E-03	8.54E-02
terrestrial eutrophication (mol N eq)	1.99E-01	7.70E-02	4.02E-02	9.47E-01
carcinogenic effects (CTUh)	3.69E-07	2.34E-07	7.46E-08	1.27E-06
ionising radiation (kg U235 eq)	3.26E-01	1.13E-01	6.58E-02	3.21E+00
non-carcinogenic effects (CTUh)	1.18E-06	1.14E-06	2.39E-07	4.15E-05
ozone layer depletion (kg CFC-11 eq)	1.33E-06	1.82E-07	2.69E-07	9.09E-06
photochemical ozone creation (kg NMVOC eq)	8.30E-02	1.59E-02	1.68E-02	2.65E-01
respiratory inorganics effects (disease inc)	9.51E-07	2.93E-07	1.92E-07	4.21E-06
dissipated water (m3 water eq)	2.36E+01	1.18E+01	4.78E+00	2.13E+01
fossil use (MJ)	5.68E+02	4.69E+01	1.15E+02	7.01E+02
land use (pts)	1.25E+02	2.22E+01	2.53E+01	8.14E+02
mineral/metal use (kg Sb eq)	4.04E-05	1.49E-05	8.16E-06	6.50E-03

environmental impact of the electric toothbrush originated not only from the additional components and materials needed for the charger/handle/replaceable heads, but also, the additional weight of all these items increased the impact of transporting the product from its manufacturing base to the UK.

A further LCA study looked at how to make a toothbrush as sustainable as possible (Duane et al. 2020) [14]. Several hypothetical toothbrushes were modelled based on new 'eco-friendly' products advertised in the UK market, including manual toothbrush handles made from bioplastic, aluminium, and recycled plastic. The research found that the most sustainable type of toothbrush was a manual toothbrush with a replaceable head, where the manufacturer recycles used polypropylene handles (the consumer sends the used toothbrush handle back to the manufacturer, where it is cleaned, autoclaved, and shredded for use in new toothbrush handles). This relies on the consumer and manufacturer reliably recycling 90% of the plastic. Although there are some schemes in place that recycle toothbrush products into other, non-dental-related recycled plastic products, there is no current toothbrush manufacturer that collects and recycles their plastic toothbrushes into more toothbrushes. It should be noted that, in order to do this effectively, either the consumer or the manufacturer will need to dismantle the toothbrush bristles from the toothbrush head; this is time consuming and perhaps unrealistic.

Interestingly, using a toothbrush made from 'bioplastic' did not have a significantly lower carbon footprint compared to normal plastic (climate change impact was reduced by only 6%). Bioplastics are produced from oil-producing crops, such as corn, and resources are needed to grow, cultivate, fertilise, and process the oil. Many products market themselves as 'eco-friendly' or 'sustainable' because they use bioplastic; this type of advertising should be ignored unless it is backed up with data. Plastic itself is not necessarily an unsustainable material—in fact, if it is properly recycled, it is more sustainable than a bioplastic that is thrown away after use. Focus should be on reducing the levels of waste materials and recycling materials that have been produced.

The recommendation on what type of toothbrush to recommend to a patient will therefore depend on the patient's periodontal disease risk, and what type of toothbrush they currently use. Figure 5.4 suggests a pathway for decision-making when it comes to recommending a specific toothbrush.

5.3.2 Interdental Cleaning Aids

The interproximal gingival tissue fills the shape afforded by the adjoining teeth and forms a papilla with a concave surface, known as a col. [47] These sites more readily trap plaque but have a non-keratinised epithelium [48], are more susceptible to disease and tend to respond less well to therapy [49]. The interproximal area in molars is relatively large and is harder to access and clean and, as a consequence, molar teeth are at a higher risk of loss through periodontal disease [50–52].

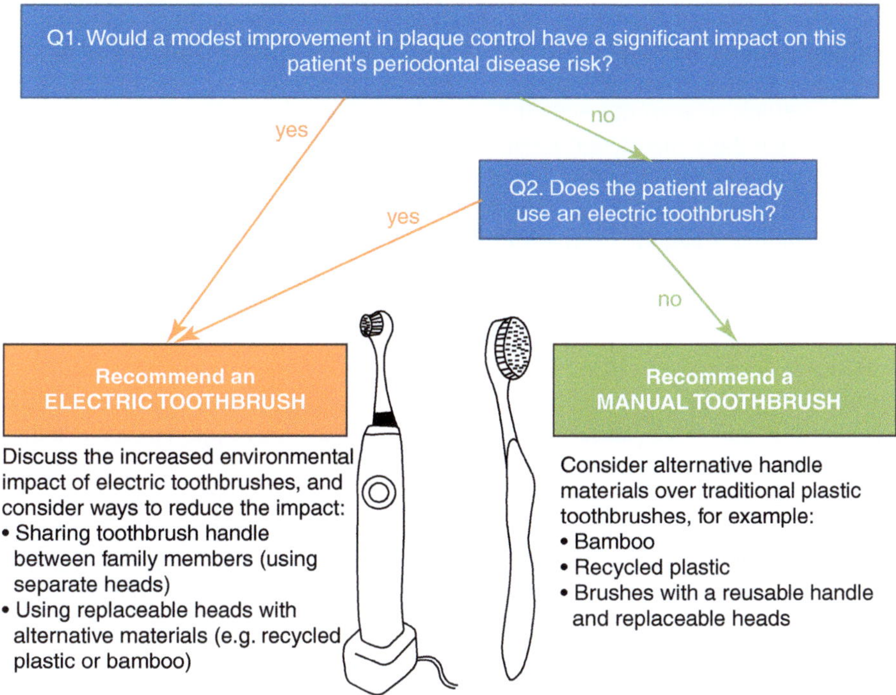

Fig. 5.4 Decision-making tool for toothbrush recommendations for patients

Toothbrushing alone cannot remove plaque interproximally [53] and interproximal aids, when used often enough and correctly, can reduce plaque more than brushing alone. US population-level data (NHANES) has reported that low-frequency interproximal aid users are significantly more likely to have severe disease than high-frequency interproximal aid users [54].

A wide variety of interproximal aids are available. All assist to some degree in the reduction of periodontal parameters such as bleeding [55]. The quality of evidence to recommend one tool in preference to another is poor, both in terms of the reduction of plaque and in the improvement of gingival parameters [56]. Floss has long been the mechanism of choice and still has uses where spaces are too small for other aids, especially in gingival health [31]. Interdental brushes have been shown to remove plaque up to 2 mm below the gingival margin [57] and are favoured over floss by European experts [31]. A recent Cochrane Review has also favoured interdental brushes, albeit with a low-quality evidence base [56]. Overall, it is best to form a tailored solution for patients based on their oral health status and risk profile.

LCA data suggests that there are differences in environmental impact between different types of floss and interdental brushes, as shown in Table 5.6. Some types of interdental cleaning aids had a greater environmental impact than others, for example, the floss picks (floss tape that is 'strung up' on a plastic handle) and the daily interdental brushes (often referred to as toothpicks—a silicone brush head on a plastic handle, for single use). All other types of floss/interdental brushes performed better than these two 'picks'.

For patients who would benefit from using an interdental brush, the LCA data suggests that daily interdental brushes (toothpicks) should be avoided in favour of the weekly interdental brushes. Interdental brushes with replaceable heads or made from bamboo may slightly improve their environmental impact. For patients who would clinically benefit from using floss (e.g. in areas too tight for interdental brushes, they should be advised to avoid the floss picks where possible and to consider alternative forms of floss, such as bamboo floss, which demonstrate a modest improvement in climate change impact compared to regular floss (reduction from 3.07 kg of carbon to 2.11 kg for use of floss over a 5-year period). There will be a small group of patients, for example, those with mobility or dexterity issues, where regular floss may not be feasible and floss picks are the only option to achieve their interdental cleaning.

When the LCA data in Table 5.6 compared to the LCA data for using a toothbrush over the same period of time, the impact of using a toothbrush over a 5-year period is significantly higher than that of any interdental cleaning aid. This supports the recommendation to tailor the interdental cleaning aid recommendations to the individual, based on their risk of periodontal disease and oral anatomy.

5.3.3　Systemic Disease and Periodontal Disease

The evidence for an association between periodontal disease and various systemic diseases is robust. In the last 10 years, consensus reports have been published that link periodontitis with non-communicable diseases (NCDs) such as cardiovascular disease, adverse pregnancy outcomes and diabetes [58–60]. The strongest evidence exists for a two-way relationship between diabetes and periodontitis. Periodontitis has been associated with raised HBA1C levels in non-diabetic people and a higher risk of developing type 2 diabetes. Patients with a diagnosis of type 2 diabetes have been shown to have poorer glycaemic control in the presence of periodontal disease [60].

Periodontitis has also been linked to an increased risk of coronary artery disease, cerebrovascular disease, and peripheral artery disease and has a modest association with low birth weight, pre-term labour, and pre-eclampsia in pregnant women [59, 61]. Rheumatoid arthritis and Alzheimer's disease may also be associated with poor oral health [62].

Two mechanisms have been proposed to account for the proposed association. The Direct Mechanism theorises that periodontal pathogens pass through the inflamed gingival epithelium and enter the systemic circulation causing a bacteraemia [63]. Bacteraemia has also been demonstrated after toothbrushing, flossing, chewing, and professional mechanical plaque removal. Oral bacteria have been identified in atherosclerotic plaques and thrombi, but their precise role is as yet unknown [64]. The Indirect Mechanism proposes that systematic disease is a result

Table 5.6 LCA data for different types of floss and interdental brush

Impact category	Floss				Interdental brushes			
	Normal floss	Floss picks	Super floss	Bamboo floss	Plastic weekly IDB	Plastic daily IDB	Plastic weekly IDB with replaceable heads	Bamboo weekly IDB
climate change (kg CO2 eq)	3.07E+00	1.14E+01	2.29E+00	2.11E+00	2.11E+00	6.53E+00	1.38E+00	1.31E+00
acidification (mol H+ eq)	8.75E-03	4.28E-02	8.31E-03	1.58E-02	8.45E-03	2.16E-02	5.46E-03	7.92E-03
freshwater ecotoxicity (CTU)	2.95E+00	1.05E+01	1.63E+00	4.60E+00	2.77E+00	8.59E+00	2.86E+00	2.62E+00
freshwater eutrophication (kg P eq)	1.10E-03	3.14E-03	4.80E-04	5.90E-04	6.80E-04	1.55E-03	4.40E-04	4.30E-04
marine eutrophication (kg N eq)	2.08E-03	1.06E-02	2.23E-03	4.27E-03	2.05E-03	5.12E-03	1.42E-03	3.08E-03
terrestrial eutrophication (mol N eq)	1.85E-02	9.02E-02	1.84E-02	4.28E-02	1.78E-02	4.37E-02	1.23E-02	2.12E-02
carcinogenic effects (CTUh)	3.97E-08	1.89E-07	3.44E-08	3.15E-07	1.17E-07	1.05E-07	1.06E-07	1.13E-07
ionising radiation (kg U235 eq)	3.05E-01	1.13E+00	1.26E-01	1.42E-01	2.57E-01	6.23E-01	1.56E-01	1.07E-01
non-carcinogenic effects (CTUh)	1.64E-07	8.08E-07	1.64E-07	3.38E-07	2.42E-07	4.17E-07	2.02E-07	2.54E-07
ozone layer depletion (kg CFC-11 eq)	1.16E-07	5.35E-07	8.63E-08	1.26E-07	1.24E-07	6.84E-06	1.86E-06	9.52E-08
photochemical ozone creation (kg NMVOC eq)	6.74E-03	3.34E-02	7.31E-03	1.07E-02	6.37E-03	1.61E-02	4.04E-03	6.00E-03
respiratory inorganics effects (disease inc)	6.37E-08	3.87E-07	9.25E-08	1.60E-07	9.71E-08	1.86E-07	7.70E-08	7.29E-08
dissipated water (m3 water eq)	9.38E-01	4.91E+00	9.25E-01	5.39E-01	3.38E+00	2.32E+00	3.08E+00	5.77E+00
fossil use (MJ)	5.86E+01	2.78E+02	5.25E+01	2.69E+01	4.74E+01	1.33E+02	2.23E+01	1.30E+01
land use (pts)	1.59E+01	1.71E+02	4.02E+01	6.40E+01	3.64E+01	4.69E+01	3.46E+01	1.10E+02
mineral/metal use (kg Sb eq)	1.04E-05	5.14E-05	1.04E-05	1.78E-05	1.25E-05	3.60E-05	9.98E-06	8.76E-06

of cytokines common to periodontitis and systemic disease that are released during the inflammatory response to oral bacteria [62].

Globally, NCDs kill approximately 41 million people each year (71% of all deaths). Cardiovascular disease and diabetes account for almost half of these deaths. They are recognised as a major global challenge in the United Nation's 2030 agenda for sustainable development, and prevention of the four major risk factors are seen as a cost-effective method for countries to reduce deaths from NCDs [65]. A patient with a chronic systemic NCD requires multiple clinic visits and medications and, in the case of uncontrolled or acute disease, may require surgery and inpatient hospital stays. All this management comes with significant environmental impact and, therefore preventing NCDs is important for any healthcare professional who is interested in sustainability.

Dentists have a responsibility not only to encourage behaviours that prevent oral disease, but also to promote the importance of systemic health. There is overlap between the common risk factors for periodontal disease and systemic disease and dentists can encourage patients to eat a healthy, low sugar diet, avoid smoking, and limit alcohol intake as well as encourage physical activity [66]. To maximise the benefit of a patient appointment, there may also be a role for dentists to screen for systemic disease. Research into chairside screening for signs such as raised blood glucose or hypertension have been shown to be feasible and acceptable to both the public and to dentists [67, 68]. However, barriers to implementation still exist and no published data on the additional environmental impact of such programmes exists. Questions about how this additional work will be funded, how dentists will be appropriately trained and the development of care pathways for the continued management of patients who show signs of disease, still need to be answered [69].

5.4   Non-carious Tooth Tissue Loss

Non-carious tooth tissue loss (NCTTL), often referred to simply as tooth surface loss (TSL) or tooth wear, is defined as the irreversible loss of hard tooth structure caused by factors other than those responsible for dental caries [70] and can be further described by cause and clinical appearance observed:

- Erosion: observed as smooth concave lesion on the tooth with preferential loss of dentine compared to enamel caused by the dissolution of hard tissues by acid not produced by bacteria. The source of the acid can be intrinsic (persistent or prolonged vomiting, eating disorders, gastroesophageal reflux disease [GERD]) or extrinsic (most commonly dietary acids or acidic medications). Erosion on teeth may also be more prolific when saliva function is reduced.
- Attrition: observed as flat occlusal surfaces caused by tooth-to-tooth contact, associated with excessive activity such as bruxism.
- Abrasion: observed as localised worn surfaces caused by contact from external objects or habits, for example, pen chewing.

- Abfraction: observed as class five lesions usually on the buccal surfaces of teeth caused by tensile stress generated from cyclic non-axial occlusal forces. Abfraction is not a common form of TSL and therefore will not be discussed in this chapter.
- Combination: observed as lesions which show a combination of the above characteristics from multiple aetiological factors.

According to the last Adult Dental Health survey (2009) [71], TSL in the UK is very common, with 77% of adults showing some tooth wear on anterior teeth. Although severe tooth wear is rare, a worrying trend from this survey was an increased prevalence of moderate tooth surface loss of 10–15% from the previous decade, specifically in the younger adult age group. As TSL is a progressive condition and is becoming more prevalent in younger populations, the environmental cost of managing these patients in dental practice is likely to increase. The environmental burden of managing TSL with restorative dentistry will arise from multiple dental practice visits (patient and staff travel, energy use of the practice, and the equipment and materials needed). Therefore, prevention of TSL in the first instance is the most obvious way to reduce the environmental impact of this disease.

Recognition and diagnosis of TSL in the early stages, with prompt implementation of an appropriate preventative regime, could halt or slow progression of the condition so that complex restorative intervention is not needed.

5.4.1 Erosion

In the UK, the Department of Health Prevention toolkit offers evidence-based guidance for prevention of erosion [3]. The basic erosive wear examination (BEWE) offers guidance to dental professionals on how to monitor and record erosion [72]. A summary of preventative recommendations is shown in Table 5.7.

Identifying the aetiological risk factors for erosion should be part of a routine medical and dental history taken or updated at every patient recall, as would giving tailored advice for patients. Ideally, giving preventative advice for erosion would not require any additional physical resources and therefore would

Table 5.7 Preventative recommendations for erosion

Advice for patients	Professional interventions
• Limit frequency of acidic food and drink intake • Use non-acidic forms of medication where possible	• Identify risk factors from medical and dental history (including diet and oral hygiene habits) and discuss factors with the patient • Record and monitor TSL, for example, using the BEWE index [73] • Seek medical advice for management of intrinsic acid sources (e.g. eating disorders, gastrointestinal reflux, acidic medications)

have a negligible environmental impact. Using existing resources, such as smart phone apps [74] and NHS resources that digitally support promotion of good diet [75] could support patients virtually as well as face to face. Rather than these being specific to erosion and tooth surface loss, it is more meaningful to make sure that advice is given to promote and support principles of good general health and diet.

For a diagnosis of erosion of an intrinsic nature, communication with the patient's medical team would equally have a negligible environmental impact. Ideally, an electronic method of a two-way relationship between the dental and medical team would allow a sustainable and clinically beneficial way for high-risk individuals to be identified in either setting and referred for support and increased prevention in the other [76].

Similarly, in cases of erosion, clinicians should consider targeting the underlying dietary or other factors and provide the relevant preventive interventions, for example, fluoride. Although there is no specific environmental impact data or studies on different interventions and preventative methods for erosion, it stands to reason that the environmental impact of using fluoride therapies to reduce erosion is less than the environmental impact of restoring lost dental tissue and maintaining those restorations during the patient's lifetime.

5.4.2 Attrition

Preventing attrition is challenging because parafunction has a psychological component for individual patients and their way of dealing with stress on a subconscious level.

Therefore, the best way to prevent this type of TSL and save the environmental burden of restoring teeth with attrition, is through early diagnosis, preventative advice, prompt liaison with mental health, and/or medical teams and provision of protective mouthguards (where appropriate).

Mouthguards and splints address the dental consequences of parafunctional activity and may offer some relief of symptoms, but they do not address the cause of the behaviour. Giving basic advice to high-risk patients on well-being and relaxation, or signposting to online resources, should be routine. Even very brief interventions have been found to prompt and support positive changes in health [77] and aligns with the principle of Making Every Contact Count [78].

Monitoring TSL using study casts has been suggested. The conventional production of study casts will have an environmental impact arising from the time and materials needed for impressions, transport of the materials to and from a dental laboratory, and the construction of the models themselves. Gypsum, used in the construction of some study cast models, falls under The Environmental Protection Act 1990, Controlled Waste Regulations 2012, and the Hazardous Waste Directive 2011 and needs to be separated from other dental waste to prevent production of hydrogen sulphide gas which could occur if disposed of in normal landfill [79]. To reduce this environmental burden, gypsum should be recycled; the derivatives can then be used in the textile, agriculture, and pharmaceutical industries among others

[80]. Alternatively, using a more modern approach to monitor TSL, such as clinical photographs taken digitally and stored in digital patient records, would not require these physical resources. Additional benefits of clinical photographs include easier storage, they are less prone to damage compared to study casts, and they can be used to track the progression of the condition with the patient or other healthcare professionals.

For patients who would benefit from a splint to prevent their TSL, consideration should be given to reducing the environmental impact of the splint's construction and maintenance. Digital scanning instead of conventional impressions (with splint construction carried out on three-dimensional plastic-printed models) may help reduce the environmental impact. Scans and printed models can be kept or given to the patient for reuse if repeat splints are needed/required. Another consideration could be the life span of the splint itself. A Michigan-type hard splint may last considerably longer than a soft biteguard; however, its initial construction is more costly—both in clinical time and laboratory costs. There is no strong clinical evidence that one type of splint is better than another and, to date, no studies have quantified the reduction in tooth wear by splint use [81].

5.4.3 Abrasion

For abrasion to be prevented, the abrasive factor needs to be identified and then advice given to mitigate its impact. A common cause of abrasion is the toothbrush being used and the environmental impact of different types of toothbrush has been discussed earlier in this chapter. For individual patients at a high risk of abrasion because of the way they use their toothbrush, the clinician may want to consider the toothbrushing advice being given. Ideally, patients would use a sustainable manual toothbrush type (e.g. bamboo or recycled plastic) with some professional toothbrushing technique instructions to prevent the abrasion. However, if this does not prove effective for individual high-risk patients, the clinician may want to recommend a specific toothbrush—even if this means the environmental impact is greater. For example, some electric toothbrushes have a pressure sensor to help the patient's technique. Other 'habits' that cause abrasion cannot be stopped, for instance, playing the saxophone/clarinets.

As no additional resources are used, the environmental impact of identifying these risk factors and discussing preventative measures with the patient should be negligible.

5.5   Oral Cancer

Oral and oropharyngeal cancers (OOPC) are the seventh most frequently occurring cancer and the nineth cause of cancer deaths globally [82]. In the UK, OOPC cost the NHS £213 million between 2006/07 and 2010/11; the highest cost being associated with inpatient care, and the lowest with chemotherapy and radiotherapy [83]. At the time of writing, there are no published data on the environmental impact of treating OOPC in any country. However, it is reasonable to assume the environmental cost is huge; the management of OOPC can involve surgery, inpatient stays, multiple outpatient appointments, dental surgery and implants, and radio- or chemotherapy. Operating theatres are generally the most resource-intensive areas of a hospital; with carbon emissions ranging from 146 to 232 kg CO2e per operation from the UK, the USA, and Canadian hospital data [84, 85]. In the UK, NHS acute care organisations, who are most likely to provide treatment for patients with OOPC, have the largest carbon footprint when compared to primary care, mental health, or community healthcare organisations [86].

Reducing the incidence of OOPC is the only way to avoid the environmental cost of treating this disease. OOPC are strongly associated with tobacco use, alcohol consumption, and human papilloma virus (HPV) infection [87]. The preventative dentist must therefore focus on the reduction or prevention of these factors in their patient population. Earlier diagnosis is embedded into the dental examination through routine oral soft tissue screening at every patient appointment.

5.5.1 Tobacco

Tobacco use is a preventable risk factor for various non-communicable diseases, including OOPC. A review of national guidelines from 22 countries for the treatment of tobacco dependence showed that all guidelines recommend that smokers who wish to stop should be offered assistance/behavioural support (evidence level A) and be given or encouraged to use pharmacotherapy such as nicotine replacement therapy (evidence level A) [88]. Twenty of the countries recommended that each patient's smoking status should be identified and recorded, and that brief advice be given to all smokers (evidence level A).

One quick intervention (recommended in the UK) that would have a negligible environmental impact is the 'Very Brief Advice Framework' (ask, advise, act), which is designed to be used opportunistically in less than 30s during any healthcare contact with a patient. Longer interventions have been shown to have no, or very small additional benefit [89].

5.5.2 Alcohol

Misuse of alcohol leads to 3.3 million preventable deaths a year globally, not just from OOPC [90].

Similar to tobacco use, guidelines in the UK recommend the Very Brief Advice Framework for discussions with patients regarding their alcohol consumption—evidence for this is graded as strong (level I) [3]. This type of opportunistic general health promotion is deemed to be feasible, accepted, and welcomed by dentists and their patients [91–95].

5.5.3 HPV Infection

Human papilloma virus (HPV) infection was implicated in 30% of oropharyngeal and 2% of oral cancers globally in 2012 [96]. Infection can be prevented through safer sex and vaccination [97, 98]. Dental professionals can support their patients HPV vaccination by discussing its benefits during routine recall visits. However, professionals have expressed reluctance about discussing the vaccine with younger patients and their parents, stating barriers such as the discussion being outside of their perceived role, confidence in their knowledge, and the possibility of parental opposition [99]. The recommended 'age' for HPV vaccination is adolescence [98] and healthcare professionals have also exhibited some discomfort regarding talking about sexual behaviour with patients in this age group [100]. Dental undergraduate and postgraduate training could improve understanding of the link between OOPC and HPV and help professionals feel more comfortable discussing vaccination with adolescents and their families or signposting them to pre-existing resources [101, 102].

5.6 Conclusion

Prevention and sustainability go hand in hand and the ability to prevent the burden of managing oral diseases will have positive impacts for both patients and the planet. The sustainable dental practice will address prevention in two ways:

1. Ensuring prevention is at the heart of every single patient contact and following evidence-based prevention guidelines.
2. Consider ways to deliver this prevention that will minimise the impact on the environment.

It essential to keep all members of the clinical team familiar with current evidence-based guidelines as they evolve and take any new evidence into account. However, implementing and following these guidelines is not always instinctual. For example, consider the caries prevention methods of diet advice vs applying fluoride varnish. The instinct of an ethical dental care professional is to spend clinical time discussing diet with the patient, help them to understand the aetiology of the disease, and encourage the individual to take ownership of their oral health. However there is very little evidence that this well-intentioned advice translates into reduced caries incidence. On the other hand, fluoride varnish has a stronger evidence base for caries reduction; but may not be applied routinely to patients at all levels of caries risk at every visit. The sustainable dental care professional will recognise the need to balance the two; communicating the key diet messages succinctly (e.g. following the format of very brief interventions discussed earlier in this chapter—ask, advise, act), whilst also prioritising clinical time for evidence-based interventions, such as fluoride varnish.

It is clear that patient travel to a dental practice, for any reason, will have an environmental burden. For this reason, every patient contact should be seen as an opportunity to screen and deliver prevention. Planning appointment diaries accordingly and using the full scope of the dental team could help facilitate this. Some prevention methods will have a greater environmental cost; for example, recommending patients use an electric toothbrush. These 'costly' methods of prevention should be reserved for patients who are at particularly high risk of developing a certain disease, for example, electric toothbrushes only for individuals with specific periodontal concerns, or providing mouthguards only for individuals with specific risk factors for tooth surface loss.

Beyond the individual dental practice itself, it is important for the dental profession to support community-level programmes such as water fluoridation and align with public health campaigns such as reducing sugar and smoking cessation.

Take Home Points for the Dental Team

- Preventing dental disease will always be more environmentally sustainable than treating established disease. A sustainable dental practice will prioritise prevention and continuingly screen patients at appropriate intervals to identify those at high risk of dental caries, periodontal disease, tooth surface loss, and oral cancer.
- Prevention should be delivered whilst the patient is already attending the practice, for example, for routine recall. It is not environmentally defensible for patients to travel to dental practices for additional prevention-only appointments.
- In an ideal world, time would be factored into all patient appointments for prevention and the scope of the full dental team would be used to facilitate this.
- If there is limited time available for prevention whilst the patient is sitting in the chair, then priority should be given to preventative measures with the greatest evidence base, for example, fluoride varnish for caries prevention.
- For prevention methods that involve giving advice to the patient, signposting to practice-specific or pre-existing electronic resources is advisable if time is limited.
- A sustainable dental practice should openly support community and population-level prevention regimes, such as water fluoridation and school-based prevention programmes, as well as public health campaigns for general health messages, such as reducing sugar intake and smoking cessation.
- Only patients at high risk of developing disease should be given environmentally 'costly' interventions. For example, only recommend electric toothbrushes to those at high risk of periodontal disease, or only provide mouthguards to patients at high risk of tooth surface loss from attrition.

References

1. Peres MA, Macpherson LMD, Weyant RJ, Daly B, Venturelli R, Mathur MR, Listl S, Celeste RK, Guarnizo-Herreno CC, Kearns C, Benzian H, Allison P, Watt RG. Oral diseases: a global public health challenge. Lancet. 2019;394(10194):249–60.

2. World Health Organisation. Environmentally sustainable health systems: a strategic document. https://www.euro.who.int/__data/assets/pdf_file/0004/341239/ESHS_Revised_WHO_web.pdf. Accessed May 2021.

3. UK Government. Delivering better oral health: an evidence-based toolkit for prevention. Delivering better oral health: an evidence-based toolkit for prevention—GOV. UK. www.gov.uk.

4. Tulchinsky T, Varavikova E. Chapter 7—Special community health needs, The new public health (3rd ed), Academic Press, 2014;381–418. https://doi.org/10.1016/B978-0-12-415766-8.00007-0.

5. Iheozor-Ejiofor Z, Worthington HV, Walsh T, O'Malley L, Clarkson JE, Macey R, Alam R, Tugwell P, Welch V, Glenny A. Water fluoridation for the prevention of dental caries. Cochrane Database Syst Rev. 2015;2015(6):CD010856. https://doi.org/10.1002/14651858.CD010856.pub2.

6. UK Government. Water Fluoridation Health Monitoring Report for England. https://assets.publishing.service.gov.uk/government/uploads/system/uploads/attachment_data/file/692754/Water_Fluoridation_Health_monitoring_report_for_England_2018_final.pdf. Accessed 30 June 2021.

7. Lyne A, Ashley P, Johnstone M, et al. The environmental impact of community caries prevention - part 1: fluoride varnish application. Br Dent J. 2022;233:287–94. https://doi.org/10.1038/s41415-022-4901-7.

8. Ashley P, Duane B, Johnstone M, et al. The environmental impact of community caries prevention - part 2: toothbrushing programmes. Br Dent J. 2022;233:295–302. https://doi.org/10.1038/s41415-022-4905-3.

9. Duane B, Lyne A, Parle R, et al. The environmental impact of community caries prevention - part 3: water fluoridation. Br Dent J. 2022;233:303–07. https://doi.org/10.1038/s41415-022-4251-5.

10. Walsh T, Worthington HV, Glenny AM, Marinho VCC, Jeroncic A. Fluoride toothpastes of different concentrations for preventing dental caries. Cochrane Database Syst Rev. 2019;3(3):CD007868. https://doi.org/10.1002/14651858.CD007868.pub3.

11. Wong MC, Glenny AM, Tsang BW, Lo EC, Worthington HV, Marinho VC. Topical fluoride as a cause of dental fluorosis in children. Cochrane Database Syst Rev. 2010;2010(1):CD007693. https://doi.org/10.1002/14651858.CD007693.pub2.

12. Naumova EA, Arnold WH, Gaengler P. Fluoride bioavailability in saliva using DENTTABS® compared to dentifrice. Cent Eur J Med. 2010;5:375–80. https://doi.org/10.2478/s11536-010-0002-0.

13. Lyne A, Ashley P, Saget S, Porto Costa M, Underwood B, Duane B. Combining evidence-based healthcare with environmental sustainability: using the toothbrush as a model. Br Dent J. 2020;229(5):303–9. https://doi.org/10.1038/s41415-020-1981-0.

14. Duane B, Ashley P, Saget S, Richards D, Pasdeki-Clewer E, Lyne A. Incorporating sustainability into assessment of oral health interventions. Br Dent J. 2020;229(5):310–4. https://doi.org/10.1038/s41415-020-1993-9.

15. Hujoel PP, Hujoel MLA, Kotsakis GA. Personal oral hygiene and dental caries: a systematic review of randomised controlled trials. Gerodontology. 2018;35:282–9. https://doi.org/10.1111/ger.12331.

16. Stein C, Santos NML, Hilgert JB, Hugo FN. Effectiveness of oral health education on oral hygiene and dental caries in schoolchildren: systematic review and meta-analysis. Community Dent Oral Epidemiol. 2018;46:30–7. https://doi.org/10.1111/cdoe.12325.

17. Marinho VCC, Chong L-Y, Worthington HV, Walsh T. Fluoride mouthrinses for preventing dental caries in children and adolescents. Cochrane Database Syst Rev. 2016;(7):CD002284. https://doi.org/10.1002/14651858.CD002284.pub2.

18. Marinho VCC, Worthington HV, Walsh T, Clarkson JE. Fluoride varnishes for preventing dental caries in children and adolescents. Cochrane Database Syst Rev. 2013;7:CD002279. https://doi.org/10.1002/14651858.CD002279.pub2.

19. Ahovuo-Saloranta A, Forss H, Walsh T, Nordblad A, Mäkelä M, Worthington HV. Pit and fissure sealants for preventing dental decay in permanent teeth. Cochrane Database Syst Rev. 2017;7(7):CD001830. https://doi.org/10.1002/14651858.CD001830.pub5.
20. Mulligan S, Kakonyi G, Moharamzadeh K, Thornton S, Martin N. The environmental impact of dental amalgam and resin-based composite materials. Br Dent J. 2018;224:542–8.
21. Public Health England. Carbon modelling within dentistry. https://assets.publishing.service.gov.uk/government/uploads/system/uploads/attachment_data/file/724777/Carbon_modelling_within_dentistry.pdf. Accessed 30 June 2021.
22. Mulligan S, Kakonyi G, Moharamzadeh K, et al. The environmental impact of dental amalgam and resin-based composite materials. Br Dent J. 2018;224:542–8. https://doi.org/10.1038/sj.bdj.2018.229.
23. Eke PI, Dye BA, Wei L, Slade GD, Thornton-Evans GO, Borgnakke WS, Taylor GW, Page RC, Beck JD, Genco RJ. Update on Prevalence of Periodontitis in Adults in the United States: NHANES 2009 to 2012. J Periodontol. 2015;86(5):611–22. https://doi.org/10.1902/jop.2015.140520. Epub 2015 Feb 17.
24. Van Dyke TE. Shifting the paradigm from inhibitors of inflammation to resolvers of inflammation in periodontitis. J Periodontol. 2020;91(Suppl 1):S19–25. https://doi.org/10.1002/JPER.20-0088. Epub 2020 Jun 20.
25. Sanz M, Del Castillo AM, Jepsen S, Gonzalez-Juanatey JR, D'Aiuto F, Bouchard P, Chapple I, Dietrich T, Gotsman I, Graziani F, Herrera D, Loos B, Madianos P, Michel JB, Perel P, Pieske B, Shapira L, Shechter M, Tonetti M, Vlachopoulos C, Wimmer G. Periodontitis and Cardiovascular Diseases. Consensus Report Glob Heart. 2020;15(1):1. https://doi.org/10.5334/gh.400.
26. Peres MA, Macpherson LMD, Weyant RJ, Daly B, Venturelli R, Mathur MR, Listl S, Celeste RK, Guarnizo-Herreño CC, Kearns C, Benzian H, Allison P, Watt RG. Oral diseases: a global public health challenge. Lancet. 2019;394(10194):249–60. https://doi.org/10.1016/S0140-6736(19)31146-8. Erratum in: Lancet. 2019 Sep 21;394(10203):1010.
27. Genco RJ, Borgnakke WS. Risk factors for periodontal disease. Periodontol 2000. 2013;62(1):59–94. https://doi.org/10.1111/j.1600-0757.2012.00457.x.
28. Schuch HS, Peres KG, Singh A, Peres MA, Do LG. Socioeconomic position during life and periodontitis in adulthood: a systematic review. Community Dent Oral Epidemiol. 2017;45(3):201–8. https://doi.org/10.1111/cdoe.12278. Epub 2016 Dec 29.
29. Genco R, Sanz M. Clinical and public health implications of periodontal and systemic diseases: an overview. Periodontol. 2020;83(1):7–13.
30. Loe H. Principles of aetiology and pathogenesis governing the treatment of periodontal disease. Int Dent J. 1983;33(2):119–26.
31. Chapple IL, Van der Weijden F, Doerfer C, Herrera D, Shapira L, Polak D, Madianos P, Louropoulou A, Machtei E, Donos N, Greenwell H, Van Winkelhoff AJ, Eren Kuru B, Arweiler N, Teughels W, Aimetti M, Molina A, Montero E, Graziani F. Primary prevention of periodontitis: managing gingivitis. J Clin Periodontol. 2015;42(Suppl 16):S71–6. https://doi.org/10.1111/jcpe.12366.
32. Axelsson P, Nyström B, Lindhe J. The long-term effect of a plaque control program on tooth mortality, caries and periodontal disease in adults. Results after 30 years of maintenance. J Clin Periodontol. 2004;31(9):749–57. https://doi.org/10.1111/j.1600-051X.2004.00563.x.
33. Hugoson A, Koch G, Göthberg C, Helkimo AN, Lundin SA, Norderyd O, Sjödin B, Sondell K. Oral health of individuals aged 3-80 years in Jönköping, Sweden during 30 years (1973-2003). II. Review of clinical and radiographic findings. Swed Dent J. 2005;29(4):139–55.
34. Loe H, Theilade E, Jensen S. Experimental gingivitis in man. J Periodontol. 1965;36:177–87. https://doi.org/10.1902/jop.1965.36.3.177.
35. De la Rosa M, Zacarias Guerra J, Johnston DA, Radike AW. Plaque growth and removal with daily toothbrushing. J Periodontol. 1979;50(12):661–4. https://doi.org/10.1902/jop.1979.50.12.661.

36. Sälzer S, Graetz C, Dörfer CE, Slot DE, Van der Weijden FA. Contemporary practices for mechanical oral hygiene to prevent periodontal disease. Periodontol 2000. 2020;84(1):35–44. https://doi.org/10.1111/prd.12332.
37. Gibson JA, Wade AB. Plaque removal by the Bass and Roll brushing techniques. J Periodontol. 1977;48(8):456–9. https://doi.org/10.1902/jop.1977.48.8.456.
38. Hansen F, Gjermo P. The plaque-removing effect of four toothbrushing methods. Scand J Dent Res. 1971;79(7):502–6.
39. Ganss C, Duran R, Winterfeld T, Schlueter N. Tooth brushing motion patterns with manual and powered toothbrushes-a randomised video observation study. Clin Oral Investig. 2018;22(2):715–20. https://doi.org/10.1007/s00784-017-2146-7. Epub 2017 Jun 16.
40. Van der Weijden GA, Timmerman MF, Danser MM, Van der Velden U. Relationship between the plaque removal efficacy of a manual toothbrush and brushing force. J Clin Periodontol. 1998;25(5):413–6. https://doi.org/10.1111/j.1600-051x.1998.tb02464.x.
41. Zimmermann H, Zimmermann N, Hagenfeld D, Veile A, Kim TS, Becher H. Is frequency of tooth brushing a risk factor for periodontitis? A systematic review and meta-analysis. Community Dent Oral Epidemiol. 2015;43(2):116–27. https://doi.org/10.1111/cdoe.12126. Epub 2014 Sep 26.
42. van der Weijden GA, Hioe KP. A systematic review of the effectiveness of self-performed mechanical plaque removal in adults with gingivitis using a manual toothbrush. J Clin Periodontol. 2005;32(Suppl 6):214–28. https://doi.org/10.1111/j.1600-051X.2005.00795.x.
43. Slot DE, Wiggelinkhuizen L, Rosema NA, Van der Weijden GA. The efficacy of manual toothbrushes following a brushing exercise: a systematic review. Int J Dent Hyg. 2012;10(3):187–97. https://doi.org/10.1111/j.1601-5037.2012.00557.x. Epub 2012 Jun 6.
44. Ebel S, Blättermann H, Weik U, Margraf-Stiksrud J, Deinzer R. High plaque levels after thorough toothbrushing: what impedes efficacy? JDR Clin Trans Res. 2019;4(2):135–42. https://doi.org/10.1177/2380084418813310. Epub 2018 Nov 14.
45. Yaacob M, Worthington HV, Deacon SA, Deery C, Walmsley AD, Robinson PG, Glenny AM. Powered versus manual toothbrushing for oral health. Cochrane Database Syst Rev. 2014;2014(6):CD002281. https://doi.org/10.1002/14651858.CD002281.pub3.
46. Pitchika V, Pink C, Völzke H, Welk A, Kocher T, Holtfreter B. Long-term impact of powered toothbrush on oral health: 11-year cohort study. J Clin Periodontol. 2019;46(7):713–22. https://doi.org/10.1111/jcpe.13126. Epub 2019 May 22.
47. Holmes CH. Morphology of the interdental papillae. J Periodontol. 1965;36(6):455–60.
48. Cohen B. Morphological factors in the pathogenesis of periodontal disease. Br Dent J. 1959;107:31–9.
49. Loos B, Nylund K, Claffey N, Egelberg J. Clinical effects of root debridement in molar and non-molar teeth. A 2-year follow-up. J Clin Periodontol. 1989;16(8):498–504. https://doi.org/10.1111/j.1600-051x.1989.tb02326.x.
50. Hirschfeld L, Wasserman B. A long-term survey of tooth loss in 600 treated periodontal patients. J Periodontol. 1978;49(5):225–37.
51. Matuliene G, et al. Influence of residual pockets on progression of periodontitis and tooth loss: results after 11 years of maintenance. J Clin Periodontol. 2008;35(8):685–95.
52. McFall WT Jr. Tooth loss in 100 treated patients with periodontal disease. A long-term study. J Periodontol. 1982;53(9):539–49. https://doi.org/10.1902/jop.1982.53.9.539.
53. Christou V, Timmerman MF, Van der Velden U, Van der Weijden FA. Comparison of different approaches of interdental oral hygiene: interdental brushes versus dental floss. J Periodontol. 1998;69(7):759–64. https://doi.org/10.1902/jop.1998.69.7.759.
54. Marchesan JT, Morelli T, Moss K, Preisser JS, Zandona AF, Offenbacher S, Beck J. Interdental cleaning is associated with decreased oral disease prevalence. J Dent Res. 2018;97(7):773–8. https://doi.org/10.1177/0022034518759915. Epub 2018 Feb 26.
55. Kotsakis GA, et al. A network meta-analysis of interproximal oral hygiene methods in the reduction of clinical indices of inflammation. J Periodontol. 2018;89(5):558–70.
56. Worthington HV, MacDonald L, Poklepovic Pericic T, Sambunjak D, Johnson TM, Imai P, Clarkson JE. Home use of interdental cleaning devices, in addition to toothbrushing, for

preventing and controlling periodontal diseases and dental caries. Cochrane Database Syst Rev. 2019;4:CD012018.

57. Sälzer S, Graetz C, Dörfer CE, Slot DE, Van der Weijden FA. Contemporary practices for mechanical oral hygiene to prevent periodontal disease. Periodontol. 2000;2020(84):35–44. https://doi.org/10.1111/prd.12332.

58. Sanz M, Del Castillo AM, Jepsen S, Gonzalez-Juanatey JR, D'Aiuto F, Bouchard P, Chapple I, Dietrich T, Gotsman I, Graziani F. Periodontitis and cardiovascular diseases. Consensus report. Glob Heart. 2020;15(1):1. https://onlinelibrary.wiley.com/doi/full/10.1111/jcpe.13189.

59. Sanz M, Kornman K, Working Group 3 of the Joint EFP/AAP Workshop. Periodontitis and adverse pregnancy outcomes: consensus report of the Joint EFP/AAP Workshop on Periodontitis and Systemic Diseases. J Periodontol. 2013;84:S164–9. https://aap.onlinelibrary.wiley.com/doi/epdf/10.1902/jop.2013.1340016?saml_referrer.

60. Sanz M, Ceriello A, Buysschaert M, Chapple I, Demmer RT, Graziani F, Herrera D, Jepsen S, Lione L, Madianos P, Mathur M. Scientific evidence on the links between periodontal diseases and diabetes: consensus report and guidelines of the joint workshop on periodontal diseases and diabetes by the International Diabetes Federation and the European Federation of Periodontology. Diabetes Res Clin Pract. 2018;137:231–41. http://www.cataniamedica.it/wp-content/uploads/2018/03/Articolo-Originale.-Documento-di-consenso-tra-European-Federation-of-Periodontology-e-International-Diabetes-Federation.pdf.

61. Sanz M, Del Castillo AM, Jepsen S, Gonzalez-Juanatey JR, D'Aiuto F, Bouchard P, Chapple I, Dietrich T, Gotsman I, Graziani F. Periodontitis and cardiovascular diseases. Consensus Report Glob Hear. 2020;15(1). https://onlinelibrary.wiley.com/doi/full/10.1111/jcpe.13189.

62. Winning L, Linden GJ. Periodontitis and systemic disease. Bdj Team. 2015;2:15163. https://www.researchgate.net/profile/Lewis-Winning/publication/284812476_Periodontitis_and_systemic_disease/links/565ab86f08ae1ef9297ffb6c/Periodontitis-and-systemic-disease.pdf.

63. Hajishengallis G, Chavakis T. Local and systemic mechanisms linking periodontal disease and inflammatory comorbidities. Nat Rev Immunol. 2021;21:426–40. https://doi.org/10.1038/s41577-020-00488-6.

64. Figuero E, Sanchez-Beltran M, Cuesta-Frechoso S, et al. Detection of periodontal bacteria in atheromatous plaques by nested polymerase chain reaction. J Periodontol. 2011;82:1469–77.

65. World Health Organisation. Non communicable diseases. 2021. https://www.who.int/news-room/fact-sheets/detail/noncommunicable-diseases.

66. World Health Organisation. Health Topics—non communicable diseases. https://www.who.int/health-topics/noncommunicable-diseases#tab=tab_1.

67. Greenberg BL, Kantor ML, Jiang SS, Glick M. Patients' attitudes toward screening for medical conditions in a dental setting. J Public Health Dent. 2012;72(1):28–35. https://pubmed.ncbi.nlm.nih.gov/22316147/.

68. Laurence B. Dentists consider medical screening important and are willing to incorporate screening procedures into dental practice. J Evid Based Dent Pract. 2012;12(3 Suppl):32–3. https://pubmed.ncbi.nlm.nih.gov/23253828/.

69. Leader D, Vujicic M, Harrison B. Could dentists relieve physician shortages, manage chronic disease? Health Policy Institute Research Brief. American Dental Association. 2018. http://www.ada.org/~/media/ADA/Science%20and%20Research/HPI/Files/HPIBrief_1218_1.pdf?fbclid=IwAR01Nvqk8rpqP_HkqXcVllPpmBecq8GHzIbScp03NJl0N0lBbay0gFvXKns. Accessed 4 Aug 2021.

70. Warreth A, Abuhijleh E, Almaghribi MA, Mahwal G, Ashawish A. Tooth surface loss: a review of literature. Saudi Dent J. 2020;32(2):53–60. https://doi.org/10.1016/j.sdentj.2019.09.004. Epub 2019 Sep 24.

71. Adult Dental Health Survey 2009—Tooth Surface Loss. Adult Dental Health Survey 2009—Summary report and thematic series—NHS Digital.

72. Bartlett D, Dattani S, Mills I, et al. Monitoring erosive toothwear: BEWE, a simple tool to protect patients and the profession. Br Dent J. 2019;226:930–2. https://doi.org/10.1038/s41415-019-0411.

73. Bartlett D, Ganss C, Lussi A. Basic Erosive Wear Examination (BEWE): a new scoring system for scientific and clinical needs. Clin Oral Investig. 2008;12(Suppl 1):S65–8. https://doi.org/10.1007/s00784-007-0181-5.

74. Chin S, Keum C, Woo J, et al. Successful weight reduction and maintenance by using a smartphone application in those with overweight and obesity. Sci Rep. 2016;6:34563. https://doi.org/10.1038/srep34563.

75. NHS. Eat well. https://www.nhs.uk/live-well/eat-well/. Accessed 1 Oct 2021.

76. UK Government. Delivering better oral health: an evidence-based toolkit for prevention. Delivering better oral health: an evidence-based toolkit for prevention—GOV.UK. www.gov.uk. Accessed 1 Oct 2021.

77. Cambridge and Peterborough Clinical Commissioning group. https://www.cambridgeshireandpeterboroughccg.nhs.uk/health-professionals/patient-pathways/hypertension-programme/resources-to-improve-management-of-hypertension/strengthening-healthy-lifestyles/very-brief-interventions/. Accessed 1 Oct 2021.

78. NICE. Making Every Contact Count. https://stpsupport.nice.org.uk/mecc/index.html. Accessed 1 Oct 2021.

79. Dental Compliance Limited. https://dentalcompliance.ie/safe-disposal-of-gypsum-plaster-old-models/.

80. Sakshi S. Casting a green future. Casting a green future: recycling the gypsum dental products. https://in.dental-tribune.com/news/casting-a-green-future-recycling-the-gypsum-dental-products-sakshi-sharma/. Accessed 1 Oct 2021.

81. Riley P, et al. Oral splints for patients with temporomandibular disorders or bruxism: a systematic review and economic evaluation. Health Technol Assess. 2020;7:1–224. https://doi.org/10.3310/hta24070.

82. Bosetti C, Carioli G, Santucci C, Bertuccio P, Gallus S, Garavello W, Negri E, La Vecchia C. Global trends in oral and pharyngeal cancer incidence and mortality. Int J Cancer. 2020;147(4):1040–9. https://doi.org/10.1002/ijc.32871.

83. Keeping ST, Tempest MJ, Stephens SJ, Carroll SM, Simcock R, Jones TM, Shaw R. The cost of oropharyngeal cancer in England: a retrospective hospital data analysis. Clin Otolaryngol. 2018;1:223–9. https://doi.org/10.1111/coa.12944.

84. MacNeill AJ, Lillywhite R, Brown CJ. The impact of surgery on global climate: a carbon footprinting study of operating theatres in three health systems. Lancet Planetary Health. 2017;1(9):e381–8. http://wrap.warwick.ac.uk/96255/1/WRAP-impact-surgery-global-climate-carbon-footprinting-Lillywhite-2017.pdf.

85. Rizan C, Steinbach I, Nicholson R, Lillywhite R, Reed M, Bhutta MF. The carbon footprint of surgical operations: a systematic review. Ann Surg. 2020;272(6):986–95. https://journals.lww.com/annalsofsurgery/Abstract/2020/12000/The_Carbon_Footprint_of_Surgical_Operations__A.21.aspx.

86. D'Souza G, Kreimer AR, Viscidi R, Pawlita M, Fakhry C, Koch WM, Westra WH, Gillison ML. Case–control study of human papillomavirus and oropharyngeal cancer. N Engl J Med. 2007;356(19):1944–56. https://doi.org/10.1056/NEJMoa065497.

87. Conway DI, Purkayastha M, Chestnutt IG. The changing epidemiology of oral cancer: definitions, trends, and risk factors. Br Dent J. 2018;225(9):867–73. https://www.nature.com/articles/sj.bdj.2018.922.

88. Aveyard P, Begh R, Parsons A, West R. Brief opportunistic smoking cessation interventions: a systematic review and meta-analysis to compare advice to quit and offer of assistance. Addiction. 2012;107(6):1066–73.

89. Papadakis S, Anastasaki M, Papadakaki M, et al. 'Very brief advice' (VBA) on smoking in family practice: a qualitative evaluation of the tobacco user's perspective. BMC Fam Pract. 2020;21:121. https://doi.org/10.1186/s12875-020-01195-w.

90. World Health Organisation. Global status report on alcohol and health. 2018. https://ncdalliance.org/why-ncds/ncd-prevention/harmful-use-of-alcohol.

91. Stead LF, Buitrago D, Preciado N, Sanchez G, Hartmann-Boyce J, Lancaster T. Physician advice for smoking cessation. Cochrane Database Syst Rev. 2013;2013(5):CD000165. https://doi.org/10.1002/14651858.CD000165.pub4.
92. Bonetti D, Young L, Hempleman L, Deas J, Shepherd S, Clarkson J. Exploring the feasibility of general health promotion in UK dental primary care: ENGAGE in Scotland. Br Dent J. 2018;225(7):645–56. https://www.nature.com/articles/sj.bdj.2018.809.
93. Ntouva A, Porter J, Crawford MJ, Britton A, Gratus C, Newton T, Tsakos G, Heilmann A, Pikhart H, Watt RG. Alcohol screening and brief advice in NHS general dental practices: a cluster randomized controlled feasibility trial. Alcohol Alcohol. 2019;54(3):235–42. https://academic.oup.com/alcalc/article/54/3/235/5382320?login=true.
94. Plessas A, Nasser M. Can we deliver effective alcohol-related brief advice in general dental practice? Evid Based Dent. 2019;20(3):77–8. https://www.nature.com/articles/s41432-019-0036-3.
95. Department of Health. UK chief medical officers' low risk drinking guidelines. https://assets.publishing.service.gov.uk/government/uploads/system/uploads/attachment_data/file/545937/UK_CMOs__report.pdf.
96. de Martel C, Plummer M, Vignat J, Franceschi S. Worldwide burden of cancer attributable to HPV by site, country and HPV type. Int J Cancer. 2017;141(4):664–70. https://www.ncbi.nlm.nih.gov/pmc/articles/PMC5520228/.
97. Centers for Disease Control and Prevention. HPV and Oropharyngeal Cancer. 2020. https://www.cdc.gov/cancer/hpv/basic_info/hpv_oropharyngeal.htm.
98. UK Government. Joint Committee on Vaccination and Immunisation: statement on the delivery of the HPV vaccine. https://assets.publishing.service.gov.uk/government/uploads/system/uploads/attachment_data/file/726319/JCVI_Statement_on_HPV_vaccination_2018.pdf.
99. Arnell TL, York C, Nadeau A, Donnelly ML, Till L, Zargari P, Davis W, Finley C, Delaney T, Carney J. The role of the dental community in oropharyngeal cancer prevention through HPV vaccine advocacy. J Cancer Educ. 2019;14:1–6. https://doi.org/10.1007/s13187-019-01628-w.
100. Gilkey MB, McRee ML. Provider communication about HPV vaccination: a systematic review. Hum Vaccin Immunother. 2016;12(6):1454–68. https://doi.org/10.1080/21645515.2015.1129090.
101. Longevity TL. Putting the mouth back into the (older) body. https://blogs.bmj.com/bmj/2017/01/10/time-to-put-the-mouth-back-in-the-body/.
102. Rakhra D, Walker TW, Hall S, Fleming CA, Thomas SJ, Kerai A, Horwood JP, Waylen AE. Human papillomavirus (HPV) and its vaccine: awareness and opinions of clinical dental students in a UK dental school. Br Dent J. 2018;225(10):976–81. https://www.nature.com/articles/sj.bdj.2018.1024.

A Guide to How to Reduce the Impact of PPE in Your Dental Practice

Chantelle Rizan, Darshini Ramasubbu, Sheryl Wilmott, Alexandra Lyne, and Brett Duane

6.1 PPE in the Dental Setting

Personal protective equipment (PPE) (see Fig. 6.1) is worn by individuals whilst at work to protect them against one or more risks to personal health and safety, which may include biological, chemical, or physical hazards. Whilst use of PPE is part of standard infection control precautions within dental settings, its use has increased since the COVID-19 pandemic. In part, this is due to recommendations such as those from the UK Health Security Agency that all members of the dental team (including reception and administrative staff) should wear fluid-resistant (type IIR) surgical masks and use hand hygiene measures across all dental settings (including the waiting room and reception areas), and also that patients are now required to wear face coverings/masks [1]. It is estimated that, in England, between April 2020 and May 2021, around 444 million items of PPE were ordered by dentists and orthodontists, using either an e-portal through which non-acute settings in England, such

C. Rizan (✉)
Brighton and Sussex Medical School, Brighton, UK
e-mail: c.t.rizan@bsms.ac.uk

D. Ramasubbu · B. Duane
Trinity College Dublin, Dublin, Ireland
e-mail: ramasubd@tcd.ie; brettdu@tcd.ie

S. Wilmott
Leeds Teaching Hospitals NHS Trust, Leeds, UK
e-mail: sheryl.wilmott@nhs.net

A. Lyne
University College London, London, UK
e-mail: alexandra.lyne@nhs.net

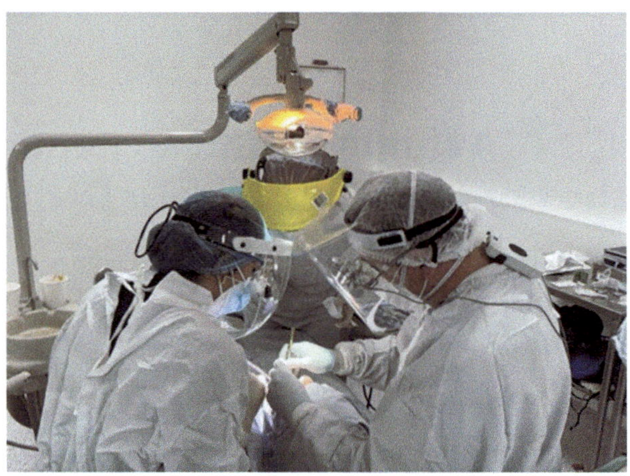

Fig. 6.1 PPE in the dental clinic at Universidad de Javeriana, Bogota

as dental practices, are able to order PPE free of charge (406 million), or by wholesalers serving dentists directly (38 million) [2]. Table 6.1 summarises guidelines (current at the time of writing) for the use of PPE when providing dental treatment. These were issued by the UK government's Department of Health and Social Care (DHSC), in collaboration with Public Health Wales, Public Health Agency Northern Ireland, Health Protection Scotland, Public Health Scotland, Public Health England, and NHS England [3].

In light of the COVID-19 pandemic (current at the time of writing), PPE requirements are dependent upon whether clinical treatment involves an aerosol-generating procedure, defined as procedures likely to be associated with release of airborne particles (<5 μm) from the patient's respiratory tract [3]. Common procedures include use of an ultrasonic scaler (including piezoelectric), high speed air/electric rotor (>60,000 rpm), Piezo surgical handpiece, air polisher, and 3-in-1 syringe (air and water together) [4]. Treatments unlikely to be associated with the generation of such aerosols include examinations (without use of a 3-in-1 syringe), extractions, re-cementation of crowns, hand scaling, impressions, intra-oral radiographs, inhalation sedation, and use of local anaesthetic [4].

For non-aerosol-generating dental procedures, current UK guidelines recommend use of hand hygiene, disposable gloves, disposal plastic apron, fluid-resistant (type IIR) surgical mask, and eye/face protection across all patients [3]. These same pieces of PPE are recommended for aerosol-generating procedures performed on patients with low risk of COVID-19 (Table 6.1).

However, for medium- and high-risk patients undergoing an aerosol-generating procedure PPE guidelines differ and, in this instance, a disposable gown and filtering facepiece 3 mask (FFP3) or hood are required in place of the apron and surgical mask (alongside hand hygiene, disposable gloves, and eye/face protection) [3].

Table 6.1 Personal protective equipment guidelines for PPE use in dental care settings

Clinical setting	Patient risk category	Hand hygiene	Disposable gloves	Fluid-resistant (type IIR) face mask	FFP3 or hood	Eye/face protection	Disposable plastic apron	Disposable gown
Waiting room/reception/ non-clinical treatment	Low/SICP	X		X				
	Medium	X		X				
	High	X		X				
Clinical care not involving generation of aerosols	Low/SICP	X	X	X		X	X	
	Medium	X	X	X		X	X	
	High	X	X	X		X	X	
Aerosol-generating procedure	Low/SICP	X	X	X		X	X	
	Medium	X	X		X	X		X
	High	X	X		X	X		X

PPE to be worn by all individuals undertaking or assisting with the procedure, adapted from UK Department of Health and Social Care guidelines [3]. SICP = standard infection control procedures. FFP3 = filtering facepiece 3

> **Box 6.1 Covid-19 Patient Risk Category**
> **COVID-19 patient risk category.** Adapted from UK Department of Health and Social Care guidelines Department of Health and Social Care (DHSC), Public Health Agency (PHA) Northern Ireland, Health Protection Scotland (HPS), Public Health Scotland, Public Health England, and NHS England. COVID-19: infection prevention and control dental appendix. 2020. Available at: https://www.gov.uk/government/publications/wuhan-novel-coronavirus-infection-prevention-and-control (accessed 16 July 2021).
>
> - High risk
>   - Patients with confirmed SARS-CoV-2
>   - Patients with symptoms of COVID-19 (either awaiting or who have declined a test)
>   - Patients who have had contact with a COVID-19 positive case who are suspected of having COVID-19 based upon clinical assessment and are awaiting test results
>   - Untriaged patients with unknown symptoms
> - Medium risk
>   - Asymptomatic patients but do not have a test result confirming negative SARS-CoV-2 status, for example, because they are
>   - awaiting a test result
>   - have declined a test
>   - testing is not required or is unfeasible
>   - Patients who have been exposed to a COVID-19 positive case but who are clinically determined to be asymptomatic
> - Low risk
>   - Asymptomatic patients who have had a negative SARS-CoV-2 test within 72 h of treatment (and have self-isolated since the test date), have had no known recent exposure to a COVID-19 patient, and have no other known infection transmitted via droplets or aerosols
>   - Patients who have recovered from COVID-19 ($\geq$14 days since onset) and are at least 48 h clear of any fever or respiratory symptoms

6.2 Environmental Impact of PPE

The environmental impact of PPE is considerable since PPE is traditionally single-use and made of predominantly plastics and petroleum-based synthetic rubbers (derived from fossil fuels), with plastics being responsible for around 8% of all global oil production [5]. The carbon footprint (estimate of associated direct and indirect greenhouse gas emissions) of the three billion items of PPE distributed for use by health and social care services (including dental services) in England in the first 6 months of the COVID-19 pandemic has previously been estimated at over

Table 6.2 Estimates of carbon footprint of PPE components

Area of protection	Options		Carbon footprint (g CO_2e/use)
Hands	Non-sterile nitrile glove (one)		26 [6]
	Latex glove (one)		210 [8]
	One pair of nonlatex examination gloves		68 [9]
	One pair of nonlatex sterile gloves		800 [10]
	Hand washing	With liquid soap and water	12 [11]
		With bar soap and water (note this is not recommended in healthcare settings) [12]	6 [13]
	Sanitiser hand gel	Ethanol based	4 [13]
		Isopropanol based	3 [13]
Body	Single-use gown		65 [6]
			905 [6]
			310 [14]
			1000 [11]
			430 [15]
	Reusable gown		295 [6]
			218 [14]
			510 [11]
			210 [15]
Mouth/nose	Single-use	FFP3 (cup fit)	125 [6]
		FFP3 (duckbill)	76 [6]
		FFP2	59 [15]
		Type IIR fluid-resistant surgical mask	20 [6]
			15–32 [16]
		Type II surgical mask	13 [6]
		'Surgical mask' (not otherwise specified)	18 [17]
			19 [15]
	Reusable	Type IR mask	4 [16]
		Cotton mask	3–18 [17]
Eye/face protection	Single-use face shield		231 [6]
			330 [15]
	Reusable visor		63 [15]

Please note in some instances figures have been derived from data within papers. FFP = Filtering facepiece, CO_2e = carbon dioxide equivalents

106,000 tonnes CO_2e (carbon dioxide equivalents) [6]. We can therefore estimate that of the approximately 400 million items distributed within dental settings over a 1-year period during the pandemic (assuming similar composition of PPE types) [2], this would equate to a carbon footprint of over 14,000 tonnes CO_2e. This would constitute approximately 2% of the annual total carbon footprint of dental services (675,000 tonnes CO_2e), as estimated before the pandemic [7].

Table 6.2 summarises estimated carbon footprints for different PPE components. Whilst this is not intended to be a comprehensive review, it provides a general sense of the carbon footprint associated with different types of PPE, with highest impacts for heaviest items (such as gowns), and lower impacts for reusable items when compared to single-use equivalents. Comparing values between different sources should be performed with caution due to the differences in products evaluated, assumptions in processes along the whole product life cycle, and system boundaries. Carbon footprints provide an estimate of direct and indirect emissions associated with a given product or processes, and where other greenhouse gases are included, these are equated to carbon dioxide equivalents (CO_2e). It is also acknowledged that there are many ways in which the use of PPE impact on the environment beyond greenhouse gas emissions (carbon footprint) which can be considered using a life cycle approach, and these are evaluated in detail within some of the studies referenced. For simplicity, in this chapter, we have focused on carbon footprint due to the number of products evaluated. Individuals seeking to make alternative product comparisons should draw upon full life cycle assessments which take into account a range of environmental impacts, thus ensuring a holistic approach is taken.

6.3 Opportunities to Mitigate Environmental Impact of PPE

6.3.1 Reduce

When considering ways to mitigate environmental impact we must consider opportunities to reduce consumption as a top priority. In the context of PPE, we must ensure that reduction strategies are aligned with maintaining safe levels of protection—both for dental staff and patients. For example, it is of course necessary for healthcare workers to wear gloves where they are likely to come in contact with blood, bodily fluids, or hazardous chemicals. Gloves may also play a role also in reducing cross-transmission of microorganisms. However, there is an opportunity to rationalise glove use where this is no clear indication for their use, given that hand hygiene (either using soap and water or hand sanitiser) has been recommended by the World Health Organization [18] and Centers for Disease Control and Prevention [19] as methods for preventing spread of microorganisms including SARS-CoV-2. It is recommended that when hand sanitiser is used it should contain at least 60% alcohol and the efficacy of ethanol or isopropyl alcohol-based hand sanitiser against SARS-CoV-2 have been demonstrated [20]. It is worth noting that research points towards the environmental benefits of using hand gel over washing hands with soap, (with isopropanol-based sanitisers marginally more advantageous over ethanol-based solutions, and the use of bar soap having lower environmental impact compared with liquid soap) [13]. Most decontamination documents, for example, HTM0105 do not however recommend bar soap [21].

In dentistry, most procedures involve contact with mucous membranes or bodily fluids so, at a minimum, will require the use of non-sterile gloves. However, glove use can be rationalised by adequate planning for each appointment and ensuring that all necessary equipment for each patient procedure is easily accessible before gloves are donned. Collaborative working between the dental nurse and dentist will also reduce the number of times gloves have to be changed during each single appointment.

Focusing on gloves is especially important given that these are thought to be responsible for just under half of the total carbon footprint of PPE used during the first 6 months of the pandemic [6]. This is also aligned with the Gloves Off

Campaign, initiated by Great Ormand Street Hospital to reduce over-use of gloves, and rationalising glove use has been supported by UK government policy [22]. These initiatives draw on evidence that the prolonged or inappropriate use of gloves results in cross-contamination of microorganisms to staff and patients and is also associated with contact dermatitis amongst healthcare staff [23]. Whilst evidence points towards the environmental benefits of use of hand hygiene over glove use, it should be noted that hand hygiene is recommended in addition to glove use and should be considered as part of a risk assessment in both regards.

There may be other opportunities to explore relating to rationalising PPE use, including other high impact items such as aprons—especially where members of the dental team do not have direct contact with the patient and for procedures with low risk of aerosol generation. There are also opportunities for sessional use of certain PPE items (continued use across a session of work across multiple patients in a given clinical setting). Sessional use of face masks (including type IIR, FFP3/FFP2/N95 respirators) and eye protection is supported by guidelines from the NHS Chief Dental Officer for England [24].

With the considerable costs associated with PPE reduction strategies would also hold economic benefits (the UK Government budgeted £15 billion for PPE in England during 2020–2021) [25]. We are also aware of risk of labour rights abuses within commonly used PPE items, including gloves, surgical masks, and gowns [26]. It is likely that reducing consumption of PPE will have associated benefits to the triple bottom line (environmental, financial, and social elements of sustainability).

6.3.2   Reusables

Reusable options are currently available for several items of PPE, and comparative carbon footprinting studies support the environmental benefits of these over their single-use equivalents [6, 11, 14–17]. For example, reusable gowns are commonplace in operating theatres, and a systematic review indicates that opting for reusable gowns would be beneficial to our carbon footprint, water footprint, and reductions in waste generation [27]. There are opportunities for further reductions in the use of reusable gowns within dental settings. For example, by opting for non-sterile gowns which are processed using standard healthcare laundering and with minimal bulk packaging (in a similar manner to medical scrubs), and reserving sterile gowns (requiring additional decontamination processing and additional packaging) for where these are clinically required. There are a number of reusable face masks currently being used in healthcare settings, including type IIR masks, with four- to eightfold carbon benefits over their single-use equivalents, supported by life cycle assessment [16]. Use of reusable visors, with use of disinfectant wipes in-between uses, has also been associated with carbon benefits [15].

We are aware of the development of reusable aprons, and it may be that reusable gloves (likely thicker and more durable) would be appropriate for certain tasks (although we are unaware of their current use in clinical settings). Given that most evidence indicates significant environmental benefits associated with reusables, their development and use should be encouraged. In the transition to reusables, we should encourage active maintenance and repair as part of circular economy principles thus extending the products' lifespan and maximising its material use.

6.3.3   Recycling and Alternative Waste Processing

It is important to choose the lowest carbon safe waste management option when disposing of PPE. Guidelines from NHS England indicate that PPE used for treating suspected or confirmed COVID-19 patients in dental settings (likely equating to high-risk patients—Table 6.1) must be disposed of as infectious waste, which involves disposing of PPE in the orange bag infectious waste stream (except where the PPE is contaminated with chemicals, in which case, it must be disposed of as clinical waste in the yellow bag) [28]. Clinical waste must be treated via high temperature incineration [29] which has the highest carbon footprint (1074 kg Co_2e/tonne waste) of typical healthcare waste streams [30]. Infectious waste can be managed in this manner, but can also be treated via alternative processes before being disposed of in a non-hazardous waste stream, which may include recycling, landfill, or low temperature incineration (i.e. using autoclave, chemical disinfection, dry heat, microwaves—using electromagnetic waves at a frequency between radio waves and infrared, macrowaves—using low-frequency radio waves, or dry heat) [29]. Since the carbon footprint of using an autoclave followed by low temperature incineration with energy from waste equates to around half that of high temperature incineration (569 kg CO_2e/tonne waste) [30], it is important for dental practices to commission/hire infectious waste management services using such alternative treatments for the disposal of their infectious waste.

For non-covid PPE (likely equating to that used to manage low-risk patients—Table 6.1), this can be disposed of as offensive waste (in yellow and black tiger striped bags) [28]. Options here include low temperature incineration with energy from waste, landfill, or recycling [29]. The carbon footprint of low temperature incineration with energy from waste gives rise to significant reductions compared with the waste streams previously discussed due to the use of lower temperatures, generation of energy, and also the recovery of some materials (such as scrap metal and bottom ash which can be used in road construction), estimated at 172 kg CO_2e/tonne [30]. It is worth noting that there is conflicting evidence on the relative impact of landfill compared with incineration (likely dependent on temperature of incineration, recovery of energy, and technologies used). This has been estimated at 1185 kg CO_2e/tonne for landfill of PPE specifically in an Indian setting [31], and at 1190 kg CO_2e/tonne for landfill of general hospital waste in China [32].

Adoption of recycling (following alternative treatment for infectious waste PPE, and as the primary mode for offensive waste PPE) likely holds the greatest environmental benefits. We are aware of initiatives that recycle polypropylene masks and gowns converting them into polypropylene blocks which can then be used to manufacture bottles, bins, and toolboxes [33]. However, this constitutes downcycling (the production of an item of lower grade and specification), and the positive benefit of recycling resulting from reduced need to extract virgin raw materials is also assigned to the product made out of recycled materials (e.g. the toolbox). The open loop 'recycled content' method of allocation allocates the environmental impact of transport and processing of recycled waste to the recycled product (e.g. toolbox), rather than the original material (e.g. surgical masks). The environmental benefits (i.e. reduction in need to extract new virgin raw materials) is also assigned to the recycled product using this allocation method. We will therefore only realise the full potential of recycling within the healthcare sector when we increase the proportion of recycled materials (i.e. recycled content) of healthcare products. PPE items, including plastic aprons, may be good starting candidates for this as these are non-critical items which would not typically come into contact with nonintact skin or mucous membranes.

It is unclear how best to manage PPE waste generated in treating patients at medium risk of COVID-19 (Box 6.1). However, NHS guidelines indicate that for PPE waste generated in community pharmacy, primary care optical settings or where clinical staff are working in people's homes, PPE may be double bagged and stored for at least 72 h, after which it can be disposed of as domestic waste. It would, therefore, seem practical/sensible to isolate waste for 72 h before disposing as per standard operating procedures.

6.3.4   Low Carbon Manufacture and Distribution

There are opportunities for manufacturers to reduce the environmental impact of a given item of PPE through choices made in the manufacturing and distribution process, and opportunities for procurers to purchase from suppliers aligned with these principles.

Modelling of alternative transportation methods/systems for PPE distribution indicates that use of air freight for overseas transport (from typical countries of origin for PPE to the UK) increases the carbon footprint by 50%, compared with shipping [6]. Furthermore, where domestic manufacture is adopted, this has the potential to reduce the carbon footprint by over 10% (due in part to the removal of overseas transportation) and from the use of lower carbon electricity sources found in the UK, compared with countries traditionally manufacturing PPE (including Malaysia and China) [6].

Using low carbon energy sources in the manufacture of PPE (and any reprocessing involved in reusables) has potential to have a large impact on the carbon footprint of a given product, and this is predominantly determined by country of manufacture. For example, countries with a high proportion of coal-based electricity, such as Australia, have a carbon footprint per unit of energy usage of over twice that of the European average, which in turn is eight times higher than Icelandic electricity which is powered predominantly by geothermal and hydropower energy [34].

It is also important to eliminate unnecessary packaging wherever possible, which can be aligned with opting for non-sterile options where clinically appropriate. For example, whilst sterile gloves are recommended for procedures involving incision of mucosa or drilling into bone (most commonly during surgical extractions), it is important not to use sterile gloves unless clinically necessary as these are associated with additional packaging, and are typically heavier than non-sterile equivalents, and also go through additional processes which themselves hold a carbon burden (including sterilisation and additional quality checks for any holes and imperfections). This all translates to a higher carbon footprint, and sterile gloves have been associated with over a tenfold higher carbon footprint compared with nitrile non-sterile gloves [35]. Further research is required to determine whether changing from non-sterile nitrile to sterile gloves is beneficial for unplanned surgical extractions, with preliminary evidence indicating that whilst non-sterile gloves have a higher bacterial load pre-operatively, this did not reach the threshold load required for an infection and can be considered clinically irrelevant [36]. However, since this consideration was taken from a conference abstract, further research would be necessary to inform policy here.

6.4 Challenges and Opportunities for Sustainable PPE

Potential challenges for transitioning towards sustainable PPE which may be addressed at a national level include funding schemes currently used in England, whereby single-use PPE is centrally funded via an e-portal, whereas dental practices would typically need to fund reusable alternatives themselves. This financial disincentive needs to be rebalanced, taking into account the true cost of use of reusables vs single-use PPE [2]. Furthermore, national guidelines need to be updated in support of reusable alternatives where their safety and efficacy have been demonstrated. Moving towards sustainable use of PPE will also require engagement and education of dental staff on the ground, including opportunities to rationalise use where possible, and on the use of lowest carbon waste streams.

Whilst the COVID-19 pandemic has presented an immediate threat to human health globally, climate change has been posed as the greatest threat to population health in the twenty-first century [37], and we must do all we can to mitigate the harm to planetary health (and therefore human health) through use of PPE. In this chapter, we have outlined various mechanisms by which this can be achieved, such as

- reduction strategies (e.g. rationalising glove and apron use, and sessional use of PPE where appropriate)
- adopting reusable alternatives, and encouraging innovation where these are not available
- using low carbon waste management
- optimising manufacture and distribution (including domestic manufacture, low carbon energy sources, and reducing packaging)

This has the potential to have a large impact on the carbon footprint of PPE, especially when put together. A study by Rizan et al. found that through a combination of a) rationalising glove use, b) use of reusable gowns and face shields, c) recycling, and d) domestic manufacture, it was possible to reduce the carbon footprint of PPE by 75% [6].

Take Home Points for the Dental Team

- Reduce the use of PPE when possible, through rationalising or sessional use
- Use reusable alternatives where possible
- Improve funding for reusable PPE products
- Select products with minimal packaging
- Choose manufacturers with sustainable processes (especially avoiding air freight) where possible
- In the future, choose recycled PPE products where available

References

1. Department of Health and Social Care (DHSC) PHWP, Public Health Agency (PHA) Northern Ireland, Health Protection Scotland (HPS), Public Health Scotland, Public Health England and NHS England. Covid-19: infection prevention and control dental appendix. https://www.scottishdental.org/covid-19-infection-prevention-and-control-dental-appendix-2/.
2. Department of Health and Social Care. Experimental statistics—personal protective equipment distributed for use by health and social care services in England: 10 May to 30 May 2021. 2021. https://www.gov.uk/government/statistics/ppe-distri.
3. Department of Health and Social Care (DHSC) PHWP, Public Health Agency (PHA) Northern Ireland, Health Protection Scotland (HPS), Public Health Scotland, Public Health England and NHS England. COVID-19: infection prevention and control dental appendix.
4. NHS Scotland Dental Clinical Effectiveness Programme. Mitigation of aerosol generating procedures in dentistry. Version 1.2. 2021. https://www.sdcep.org.uk/wp-content/uploads/2021/04/SDCEP-Mitigation-of-AGPs-in-Dentistry-Rapid-Review-v1.2-April-2021.pdf. Accessed 16 July 2021.
5. Thompson RC, Moore CJ, vom Saal FS, Swan SH. Plastics, the environment and human health: current consensus and future trends. Philos Trans R Soc Lond Ser B Biol Sci. 2009;364(1526):2153–66.
6. Rizan C, Reed M, Bhutta MF. Environmental impact of personal protective equipment distributed for use by health and social care services in England in the first six months of the COVID-19 pandemic. J R Soc Med. 2021;114(5):250–63.
7. Duane B, Lee MB, White S, Stancliffe R, Steinbach I. An estimated carbon footprint of NHS primary dental care within England. How can dentistry be more environmentally sustainable? Br Dent J. 2017;223(8):589–93.
8. Usubharatana P, Phungrassami H. Carbon footprints of rubber products supply chains (fresh latex to rubber glove). Appl Ecol Environ Res. 2018;16(2):1639–57.
9. Hasan J, Lyne A, Ashley P, Duane B. Non-sterile examination gloves and surgical sterile gloves: which are more sustainable? Journal of Hospital Infection 2021. Volume 118, Page 87–89. https://doi.org/10.1016/j.jhin.2021.10.001.
10. Hasan J, Lyne A, Ashley P, Duane B. Non-sterile examination gloves and surgical sterile gloves: which are more sustainable? J Hosp Infect. 2021;118:87–9. https://doi.org/10.1016/j.jhin.2021.10.001.
11. Duane B, Pilling J, Saget S, Ashley P, Pinhas A, Lyne A. Hand hygiene with hand sanitizer versus handwashing. What are the planetary health consequences? Environ Sci Pollut Res Int. 2022;29(32):48736–47.

12. Department of Health, UK. Decontamination in primary care dental practice (HTM 01–05). 2013.
13. Duane B, Pilling J, Saget S, Ashley P, Pinhas A, Lyne A. Hand hygiene with hand sanitiser versus handwashing. What are the planetary health consequences? Environ Sci Pollut Res Int. 2022;29(32):48736–47.
14. Vozzola E, Overcash M, Griffing E. Environmental considerations in the selection of isolation gowns: a life cycle assessment of reusable and disposable alternatives. Am J Infect Control. 2018;46(8):881–6.
15. Almutairi W, Saget S, Mc Donnell J, Tarnowski A, Johnstone M, Duane B. The planetary health effects of COVID-19 in dental care: a life cycle assessment approach. Br Dent J. 2022;233(4):309–16. https://doi.org/10.1038/s41415-022-4906-2. Epub 2022 Aug 26.
16. UCL Plastic Waste Innovation Hub for NHS. A LCA comparison between single-use and Revolution-ZERO reusable face masks. 2021. https://cdn.website-editor.net/2db15d5a7bc74 4a6b8edc8c9c5ad27cd/files/uploaded/08%2520March%25202021%2520Revolution-Z.
17. Schmutz M, Hischier R, Batt T, Wick P, Nowack B, Wäger P, et al. Cotton and surgical masks—what ecological factors are relevant for their sustainability? Sustainability. 2020;12(24):10245.
18. World Health Organisation. Coronavirus disease (COVID-19) advice for the public. 2021. https://www.who.int/emergencies/diseases/novel-coronavirus-2019/advice-for-public. Accessed 16 July 2021.
19. Centers for Disease Control and Prevention. Hand Hygiene FAQs. 2020. https://www.cdc.gov/handwashing/faqs.html. Accessed 16 July 2021.
20. Kratzel A, Todt D, V'kovski P, Steiner S, Gultom M, Thao TTN, et al. Inactivation of severe acute respiratory syndrome coronavirus 2 by WHO-recommended hand rub formulations and alcohols. Emerg Infect Dis. 2020;26(7):1592–5.
21. NHS England. Decontamination in primary care dental practices. https://www.england.nhs.uk/publication/decontamination-in-primary-care-dental-practices-htm-01-05/.
22. UK Department of Health and Social Care. Personal protective equipment (PPE) strategy: stabilise and build resilience. 2020. https://www.gov.uk/government/publications/personal-protective-equipment-ppe-strategy-stabilise-and-build-resilience.
23. Loveday HP, Wilson JA, Pratt RJ, Golsorkhi M, Tingle A, Bak A, et al. epic3: national evidence-based guidelines for preventing healthcare-associated infections in NHS hospitals in England. J Hosp Infect. 2014;86(Suppl 1):S1–70.
24. NHS Office of Chief Dental Officer England. Standard operating procedure, transition to recovery. A phased transition for dental practices towards the resumption of the full range of dental provision. Version 3. 2020. https://www.england.nhs.uk/coronavirus/wp-content/uploads/sites/52/2020/06/C0575-dental-transition-to-recovery-SOP-4June.pdf. Accessed 16 July 2021.
25. National Audit Office. The supply of personal protective equipment (PPE) during the COVID-19 pandemic. 2020. The supply of personal protective equipment (PPE) during the COVID-19 pandemic UK Government Department of Health and Social Care. Accessed 16 July 2021.
26. British Medical Association. Labour rights abuse in global supply chains for PPE through COVID-19—issues and solutions. 2021. https://www.bma.org.uk/media/4288/ppe-labour-rights-abuse-in-global-chains-for-ppe-through-covid-july-2021.pdf. Accessed 16 July 2021.
27. Overcash M. A comparison of reusable and disposable perioperative textiles: sustainability state-of-the-art 2012. Anesth Analg. 2012;114(5):1055–66.
28. NHS England. COVID-19 waste management standard operating procedure. Version 4. 2021. https://www.england.nhs.uk/coronavirus/wp-content/uploads/sites/52/2021/01/C0995-covid-19-waste-management-guidance-sop-v4.pdf. Accessed 16 July 2021.

29. Department of Health. Environmental and sustainability Health Technical Memorandum 07–01: safe management of healthcare waste. 2013. https://assets.publishing.service.gov.uk/government/uploads/system/uploads/attachment_data/file/167976/HTM_07-01_Final.pdf. Accessed 16 July 2021.
30. Rizan C, Bhutta MF, Reed M, Lillywhite R. The carbon footprint of waste streams in a UK hospital. J Clean Prod. 2021;286:125446.
31. Kumar H, Azad A, Gupta A, Sharma J, Bherwani H, Labhsetwar NK, et al. COVID-19 Creating another problem? Sustainable solution for PPE disposal through LCA approach. Environ Dev Sustain. 2021;23(6):9418–32.
32. Zhao W, van der Voet E, Huppes G, Zhang Y. Comparative life cycle assessments of incineration and non-incineration treatments for medical waste. Int J Life Cycle Assess. 2009;14:114–21.
33. Royal Cornwall Hospitals NHS Trust. Recycling unit answers the covid mask mountain problem. 2021. https://www.royalcornwall.nhs.uk/recycling-unit-answers-the-covid-mask-mountain-problem/. Accessed 16 July 2021.
34. Database: SimaPro Version 9.10 (PRé Sustainability, Amersfort, Netherlands), Ecoinvent database (version 3.6).
35. Jamal H, Lyne A, Ashley P, Duane B. Non-sterile examination gloves and sterile surgical gloves: which are more sustainable? J Hosp Infect. 2021;118:87–95. https://doi.org/10.1016/j.jhin.2021.10.001. Epub ahead of print.
36. Creamer J, Davis K, Rice W. Sterile gloves: do they make a difference? Am J Surg. 2012;204(6):976–80.
37. Watts N, Adger WN, Agnolucci P, Blackstock J, Byass P, Cai W, et al. Health and climate change: policy responses to protect public health. Lancet. 2015;386(10006):1861–914.

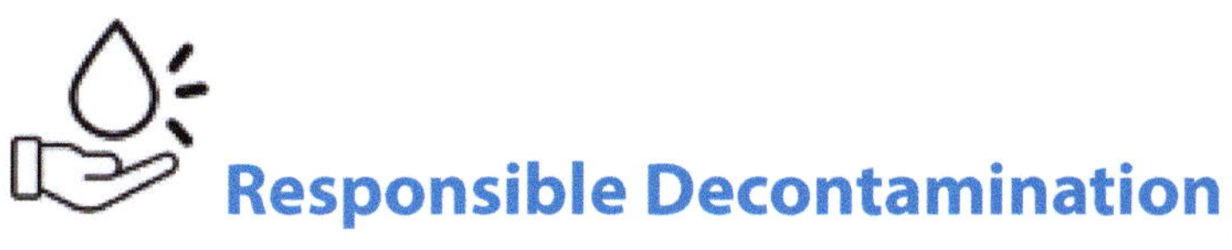

7

Responsible Decontamination

Brett Duane, Nick Armstrong, Sara Harford, Viviana,
Allan Pinhas, Hira Ahmed, and Darshini Ramasubbu

7.1   Introduction

Before describing the links between decontamination and sustainability, we will briefly define a few terms. Decontamination experts please move to Sect. 7.3.

This chapter focusses on cleaning (using washer disinfectors), disinfection (using surface wipes, suction disinfection, and waterline disinfection), and sterilisation (using autoclaves). This chapter is written by a collection of dentists and people with interests in sustainability. It is not meant to be a guide to effective decontamination, more for people to consider the planet as we continue to make use of the decontamination process.

Decontamination describes a combination of processes used to render reusable items safe for further use and handling, for patients and staff. It is essential to reduce the risk of infection transmission between both patients and staff and staff and patients. The stages involved in the decontamination or 'reprocessing' of instruments are cleaning, disinfection, inspection, and sterilisation include:

B. Duane (✉) · H. Ahmed · D. Ramasubbu
Trinity College Dublin, Dublin, Ireland
e-mail: brettdu@tcd.ie; hira.ahmed@dental.tcd.ie; ramasubd@tcd.ie

N. Armstrong
Irish Dental Association Quality and Patient Safety Committee, Dublin, Ireland

S. Harford
Centre for Sustainable Healthcare, Oxford, UK

Viviana
Javeriana University, Bogota, Colombia
e-mail: aldanac@javeriana.edu.co

A. Pinhas
University of Cincinnati, Cincinnati, OH, USA
e-mail: pinhasa@ucmail.uc.edu

- Cleaning is the process that physically removes soiling including large numbers of microorganisms and the organic material on which they thrive [1].
- Disinfection describes a process that eliminates many or all pathogenic microorganisms on inanimate objects, except for bacterial spores [1].
- Inspection refers to the process of inspecting the equipment before sterilising.
- Sterilisation refers to a physical or chemical process that completely kills or destroys all forms of viable microorganisms from an object, including spores. Sterility is an absolute condition—an item is either sterile or not sterile [2].

7.2 Recommendations for Instrument Decontamination and Autoclaving

7.2.1 Washer Disinfector

The emphasis on infection prevention and control has resulted in the emergence of the automated washer disinfector into the dental decontamination procedure. Washer disinfectors are medical appliances, equipped to clean and disinfect reusable instruments and supplies before sterilisation. The rationale behind the use of this device is to minimise the risk of transmission of infectious pathogens and percutaneous injuries to dental staff; prior to the introduction of the washer disinfectors, instruments were rinsed by hand. The typical cycle consists of five steps as follows:

Flush: Gross debris, such as blood, bone, bodily fluids, and other solid waste is removed by water heated to less than 45 °C.

Wash: Any remaining contaminants (e.g. proteins, microorganisms) are removed using chemical (detergents) and mechanically using appropriate equipment.

Rinse: Any remaining detergent from the wash stage is eliminated by rinsing with water.

Thermal disinfection: The load is held in the chamber at a pre-set temperature and time for disinfection—for example, 90 °C for 1 min.

Dry: The contents of the washer disinfector are introduced to heated air to eliminate moisture.

The washer disinfector consumes 15 mL of water per instrument and around 0.011 KWh (around 0.22 Euro Cent per hour).

7.2.2 Autoclave

To kill microorganisms, the instruments need to be exposed to steam at 134–137 °C at 2.1–2.25 bar gauge pressure for at least 3 min see Fig. 7.1 [1] instruments may also be sterilised at 121–124 °C for 15 min at 1.15 Bar or 126–129 °C for 10 min at 1.50 Bar.

Although the water and electricity use varies between autoclaves, our own research shows that an autoclave uses 7 mL of water per instrument, and 0.024 KWh (costing within Ireland around €0.5 per h).

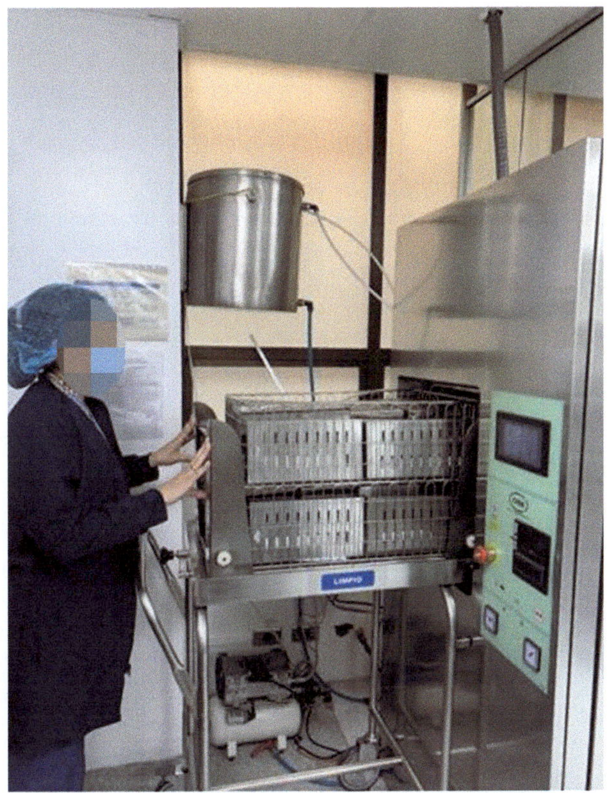

Fig. 7.1 Person using an autoclave, Universidad de Javeriana, Bogota

7.2.3 Recommendations for Cleaning Waterlines

The biofilm needs to be continually reduced (and monitored) within waterlines. Each practice should have a protocol for cleaning waterlines. There are two elements to this:

1. Dentists should use high quality water such as that produced by reverse osmosis, or sterile water, distilled water. In Ireland, the potable bottled water standard as set by the EU is 100 cfu/mL (colony forming unit) of bacteria [3]. In the USA, the standard is somewhat higher (500 cfu/mL) [4].
2. *Cleaning the waterlines regularly*. There are many systems on the market for this purpose. It is crucial that the manufacturers' instructions are followed.

7.2.4 Recommendations for Suction System Cleaning

It is important to disinfect the suction system tubing and that any adaptors used are decontaminated. There are several suction cleaning solutions on the market and the cleaning solution should be non-foaming [5]. Suction tip holders should preferably be autoclavable.

7.2.5 Recommendations for Surface Disinfection

Surfaces in a dental surgery may become contaminated with infective material, and there is evidence that contaminated surfaces can result in the transmission of pathogens in healthcare facilities [6, 7].

Zoning simplifies the decontamination process. Zoning defines particular areas which may be contaminated during the treatment of patients; only these surfaces need disinfection between patients. This will save time and result in less cleaning chemicals being used. There are many surface cleaning products on the market including a number of environmentally friendly ones. Difficult-to-clean areas can be covered by plastic barriers.

7.2.6 Recommendations for Cleaning Prosthesis

Prior to dental practices forwarding prosthesis and other similar work on to laboratories, all items must be disinfected. There are several products on the market for cleaning prosthesis—and sodium hypochlorite is frequently used. Stone working models should be covered with a barrier to prevent contamination. Laboratory work returned from the laboratory should disinfected before fitting.

7.3 An LCA of Hypothetical Products

There is little evidence to suggest what is the most sustainable decontamination process in healthcare settings, there has been, however, some research looking at reusable instruments versus disposable instruments. In a recent paper by Rizan (author of our PPE chapter), the environmental impact of reusable instruments is considerably lower than single-use instruments, and this has been evaluated in a number of studies [8]. A recent paper also looked at the efficacy of wipes, comparing reusable cotton wipes with microfibre wipes, and also looking at disposable wipes [9]. We will discuss this paper alongside our findings in this chapter.

To try and understand the sustainability of various products used within the decontamination and sterilisation process, we 'mocked up' the different items within a selected number of decontamination/sterilisation products.

The astute reader may be able to guess the type of products shown below however, for commercial sensitivity, we have anonymised all these products. In addition, the LCA database we use, ecoinvent, (one of the most comprehensive databases of products), does not always contain the exact chemical we use. Therefore, the list below excludes some products and substitutes others (see Table 7.1).

A life cycle analysis (LCA—see Chap. 1) was performed to understand the relationship between each of the following products. The reference was one procedure performed per patient. The ecoinvent database v3.6.1 was used, with Open LCA software 1.10.3 to calculate the environmental impact factors. The results can be seen in Table 7.2.

The most significant resource use from decontamination processes of dentistry with respect to human health (carcinogenic/non-carcinogenic effects) comes from the surface wipes, followed by the act of disinfecting a prosthesis.

The impact from a climate change perspective for these surface wipes is approximately 124 g of carbon equivalent emissions (almost the same as the carbon equivalent emissions of a new car travelling for 1 km [11]. Disinfecting a prothesis is approximately 30 g.

Table 7.1 Hypothetical decontamination products

Product name	Product components	Product use
Water disinfectant tablets twice a day	Ammonium chloride, 5.44 mg, benzoic acid, 9.6 mg, citric acid, 128 mg, EDTA 32 mg, and soda ash 22.24 mg Packaging: individual Al foil wrap 0.054 g per tablet, and 50 wrapped tablets packaged in cardboard box weighing 18.3 g	Use 2 tablets for 15 patients every day dissolved in 700 mL water
Liquid shock treatment every 3 months (750 patients)	Sodium hydrogen sulphate 20 g, citric acid 20 g, hydrogen peroxide without added water in 50% state, 40 g, tap water one litre. Container is a plastic bottle weighing 102.2 g	For 750 patients, use 336 mL dissolved in 1 L of water
Suction disinfectant (UK)	Ammonium chloride 115 g, EDTA 4.5 g, potassium hydroxide 5 g, sodium pyrophosphate 44 g, water 834 g. Container is a plastic bottle weighing 85.2 g	Use 20 mL daily in 980 mL water, divided by 15 patients per day
Suction disinfectant Colombia	Sodium hydroxide 50%, 40 g, sodium hypochlorite 15%, 35 g, water 985 g. Container is a plastic bottle weighing 85.2 g	Use 48 mL daily in 452 mL water, divided by 15 patients per day
Surface wipe 1	Surface wipe contains 11.28 g each of ammonium chloride, phenol, benzoic compound and ethylene glycol and 15.42 g water. Wipe is a non-woven polypropylene wipe 5.11 g. Plastic container is a 100 g plastic polyethylene bag containing 200 wipes	Use 4 wipes per patient. Dispose of wipes in hazardous waste. Recycle plastic bottle
Surface wipe 2	Surface wipe contains 0.0776 g ammonium chloride and 3.8 g of water. Wipe is a non-woven polypropylene wipe 1.63 g. Plastic container is a 100 g PET tub containing 200 wipes which is refilled and reused three times before disposal	Use 4 wipes per patient. Dispose of wipes in hazardous waste. Recycle plastic bottle
Surface wipe 3 spray with tissues	Spray contains 20 g of sodium hydroxide in 1 litre of water. Container is a plastic PET bottle weighing 94.2 g. Wipes are tissues weighing 3.6 g for 4 tissues *Note a spray can cause issues with people with respiratory problems. This product should only be used as a 'dip' as a spray creates an aerosol [10]	Use 1.08 mL per patient × 4 tissues per patient. Dispose of wipes in hazardous waste. Recycle plastic bottle

(continued)

Table 7.1 (continued)

Product name	Product components	Product use
Prosthesis disinfectant (UK)	To make up solution, use 13.33 g sodium hypochlorite (15%) and 165 g sodium chloride in one litre water. Container is a plastic bottle weighing 102.2 g	Soak prosthesis in 50 mL of disinfectant and 450 mL of water. Use once only
Prothesis disinfectant (Colombia)	Sodium hydroxide 50%, 40 g, sodium hypochlorite 15%, 35 g, water 985 g. Container is a PET bottle weighing 85.2 g	Soak prosthesis in 50 mL of disinfectant and 450 mL of water. Use once only
Autoclave process	No chemicals required	We assumed 7 instruments per patient, and 60 instruments per cycle, we used 2.33 KWh per patient and 700 mL per water
Washer disinfectant Methyl pentane	2-methylpentane 0.75 g, benzothiadiazole-compound 75 g, 724 g water. Container is a plastic bottle weighing 55 g	We assumed 7 instruments per patient, and 53 instruments per cycle, assuming always fill, and not over fill. We used 2.63 KWh per patient, and 5.35 L of water mixed with 1.32 mL of washer disinfectant
Washer disinfectant part A	Citric acid 241 g, tap water 929 g. Container is a plastic bottle weighing 70.4 g	We assumed 7 instruments per patient, and 53 instruments per cycle, assuming always fill, and not over fill. We used 2.63 KWh per patient, and 5.35 litres of water mixed with 1.19 mL of washer disinfectant A and B
Washer disinfectant part B	EDTA 50 g, ethanol 100 g, alcohol 10 g, potassium hydroxide 20 g, sodium cumenesulphonate 100 g in 1 litre water. Container is a PET bottle weighing 70.4 g	

The use of solutions to disinfectant prosthesis per patient is approximately the same as the environmental impact of wiping down clinical surfaces after each patient.

To gauge the effect decontamination might have on average environmental impact levels, normalised scores were calculated. The normalised results are displayed in Fig. 7.2.

Readers may remember that a normalised result is calculated based on one person's/'average Joe's' share of all emission and resource use in the world for 1 year (see Fig. 7.2) [12].

The y axis shows the normalised results. To clarify, a score of '1' would mean that the decontamination process represents one years' worth of the environmental impact. As depicted, the use of surface wipes therefore creates close to what an average person would impact in one day on this planet with respect to carcinogenic and non-carcinogenic effects.

The normalised results for our decontamination products again demonstrate that 'surface wipe 1' has the most environmental impact, followed by the disinfection of prosthesis, and surface wipe 2 and 3. The reader should however accept these results with caution as the LCA process comes with a wide range of assumptions. However, the analysis does give the reader some useful points to consider.

Table 7.2 Environmental impact factors for different decontamination and sterilisation processes

	Surface wipe 1	Surface wipe 2	Surface wipe 3 spray with tissues	Water disinfectant twice a day	Liquid shock treatment every 3 months (750 patients)	Suction disinfectant UK	Suction disinfectant Colombia	Prosthesis Disinfectant (UK)	Prothesis Disinfectant (Colombia)	Autoclave process	Washer disinfectant Methyl pentane	Washer disinfectant part A	
ecosystem quality - freshwater ecotoxicity	1.02091	0.03604	0.03008	0.00056	0.0007	0.00211	0.00331	0.06051	0.05135	0.00333	0.00973	0.01739	CTU
climate change - climate change land use and land use change	7.41E-05	2.17E-05	0.00028	2.50E-06	3.69E-07	1.06E-06	1.48E-06	2.01E-05	2.31E-05	8.36E-06	2.40E-06	1.78E-05	kg CO2-Eq
ecosystem quality - freshwater eutrophication	3.2573E-05	6.4923E-06	8.092E-06	8.9103E-08	9.2773E-08	4.318E-07	6.0628E-07	9.1753E-06	9.4559E-06	2.0145E-06	7.0744E-06	8.1931E-06	kg P-Eq
ecosystem quality - terrestrial eutrophication	0.00081	0.00023	0.00017	3.4079E-06	2.8198E-06	1.2248E-05	1.4733E-05	0.00023	0.00023	7.6316E-05	0.00015	0.0002	mol N-Eq
resources - dissipated water	0.03597	0.00999	0.00815	0.00061	0.00024	0.00116	0.00118	0.01582	0.01839	0.004	0.02448	0.02765	m3 water-Eq
human health - respiratory effects, inorganics	3.1382E-09	8.2626E-10	9.6961E-10	1.8994E-11	1.1918E-11	4.8745E-11	5.5483E-11	8.5477E-10	8.6226E-10	1.1904E-10	3.6639E-10	5.8747E-10	disease incidence
resources - land use	0.32146	0.09319	0.71942	0.00435	0.0026	0.01091	0.00985	0.16813	0.15358	0.0534	0.05158	0.1021	points
climate change - climate change biogenic	0.00019	5.7333E-05	0.00021	3.5251E-05	1.2112E-06	2.4931E-06	3.9338E-06	5.9661E-05	6.142E-05	1.949E-05	5.3236E-06	1.0849E-05	kg CO2-Eq
human health - photochemical ozone creation	0.00028	8.0635E-05	4.4817E-05	8.3906E-07	8.1296E-07	3.3638E-06	4.7124E-06	7.5555E-05	7.3381E-05	2.0264E-05	4.2314E-05	5.3402E-05	kg NMVOC-Eq
human health - ozone layer depletion	4.0065E-08	1.5093E-08	3.2946E-09	2.3831E-11	7.0198E-10	1.7839E-09	4.3697E-09	7.8165E-08	6.8273E-08	5.4159E-10	2.5464E-10	3.0652E-09	kg CFC-11-Eq
human health - non-carcinogenic effects	9.5506E-09	1.7637E-09	7.7381E-09	4.4864E-11	3.2793E-11	1.5997E-10	1.7281E-10	2.7717E-09	2.6471E-09	8.6061E-10	2.1561E-09	2.6193E-09	CTUh
human health - ionising radiation	0.0062	0.00179	0.0011	2.0629E-05	2.8601E-05	0.0001	0.00019	0.00293	0.00293	0.00079	0.00022	0.00042	kg U235-Eq
resources - fossils	2.24684	0.67587	0.20095	0.00333	0.00555	0.02164	0.03316	0.54754	0.5175	0.18916	0.21118	0.26866	MJ
human health - carcinogenic effects	3.2626E-09	4.3889E-10	5.9457E-10	1.8684E-11	1.0141E-11	5.5611E-11	4.508E-11	7.9022E-10	6.6572E-10	1.6778E-10	4.5549E-10	5.4614E-10	CTUh
climate change - climate change fossil	0.12333	0.03629	0.01991	0.00023	0.00033	0.00132	0.00193	0.03147	0.03016	0.01127	0.01394	0.01746	kg CO2-Eq
climate change - climate change total	0.1236	0.03637	0.0204	0.00027	0.00033	0.00132	0.00194	0.03155	0.03024	0.01129	0.01395	0.01749	kg CO2-Eq
ecosystem quality - marine eutrophication	8.1005E-05	2.4663E-05	2.0803E-05	4.4723E-07	3.295E-07	2.4209E-06	1.7044E-06	2.7626E-05	2.6565E-05	7.1336E-06	1.5077E-05	2.0741E-05	kg N-Eq
ecosystem quality - freshwater and terrestrial acidification	0.00038	0.0001	9.3088E-05	1.5263E-06	1.4377E-06	6.3503E-06	7.3004E-06	0.00011	0.00011	4.0942E-05	0.0001	0.00012	mol H+-Eq
resources - minerals and metals	5.8812E-07	4.9347E-07	9.1274E-08	2.3738E-09	1.8685E-08	5.5651E-08	1.1098E-07	2.0813E-06	1.7339E-06	2.6546E-08	4.1872E-08	1.3806E-07	kg Sb-Eq

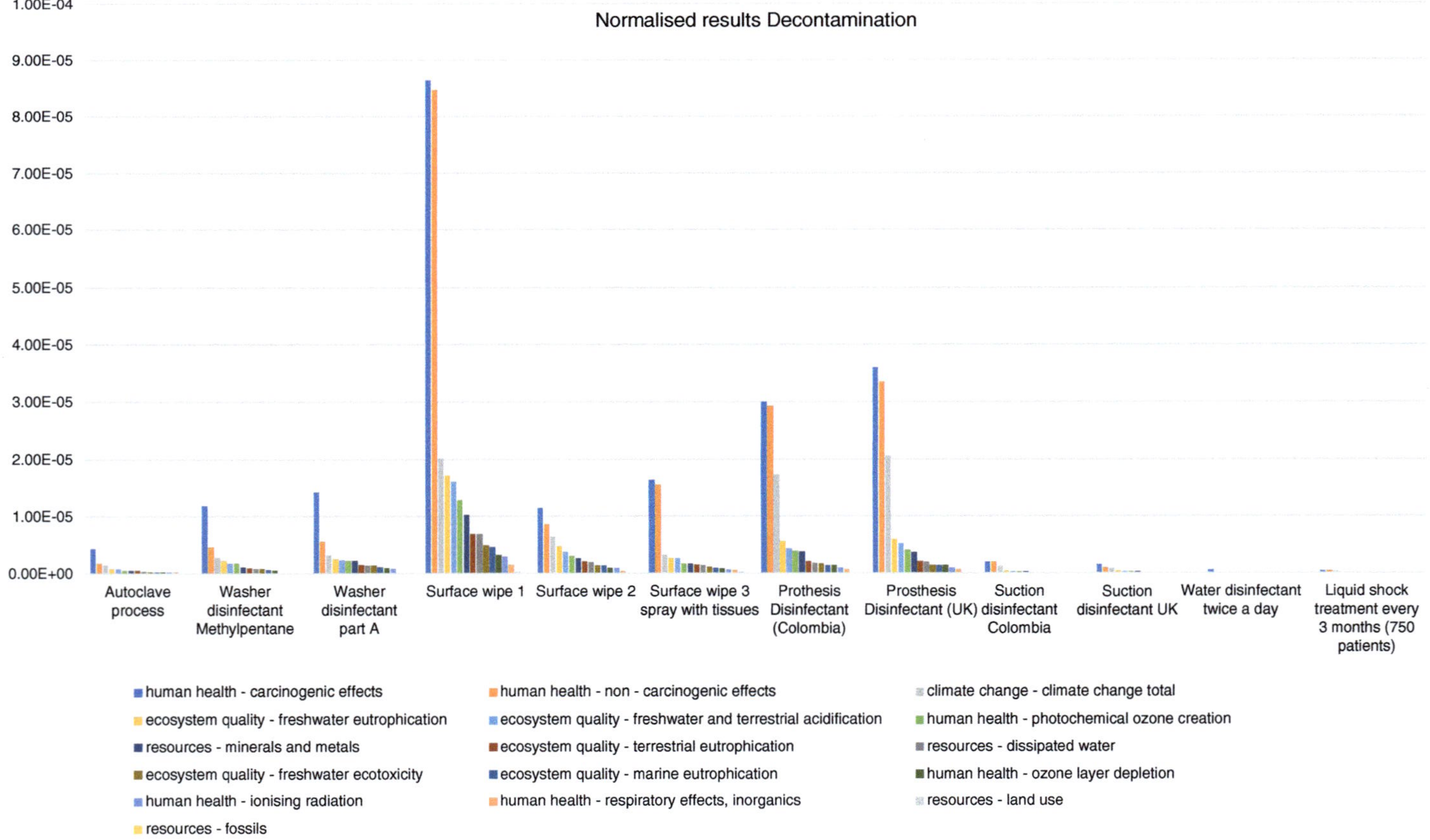

Fig. 7.2 Normalised results: decontamination

To reduce space, for each process, we will now show the contributing factors of four environmental scores: the highest three normalised scores, and the contributing factors to carbon equivalent emissions.

As there are many recurring themes, we will exclude the results for water disinfectant and suction disinfectant as these have less of an environmental impact from an LCA perspective than the other decontamination products.

7.3.1 Surface Wipe 1

In this chapter, we analysed three surface wipes to understand the differences between the wipes. For surface wipe 1, the wipe is heavy (I would say lush), for surface wipe 2 the wipe is lighter, and for surface wipe 3 the operator provides their own tissues.

There are four main reasons surface wipe 1 is less environmentally sustainable. The first is the actual wipe (producing it and disposing of it), the second is the container that the wipe comes in. Thirdly, from an ozone layer depletion perspective, the benzoic compound has some contribution (see Fig. 7.3).

7.3.2 Surface Wipe 2

In surface wipe 2 (see Fig. 7.4) the wipe weighed less than surface wipe one; and therefore has comparatively less contribution from a climate change perspective. The plastic container and the wipe are significant contributors to ozone layer

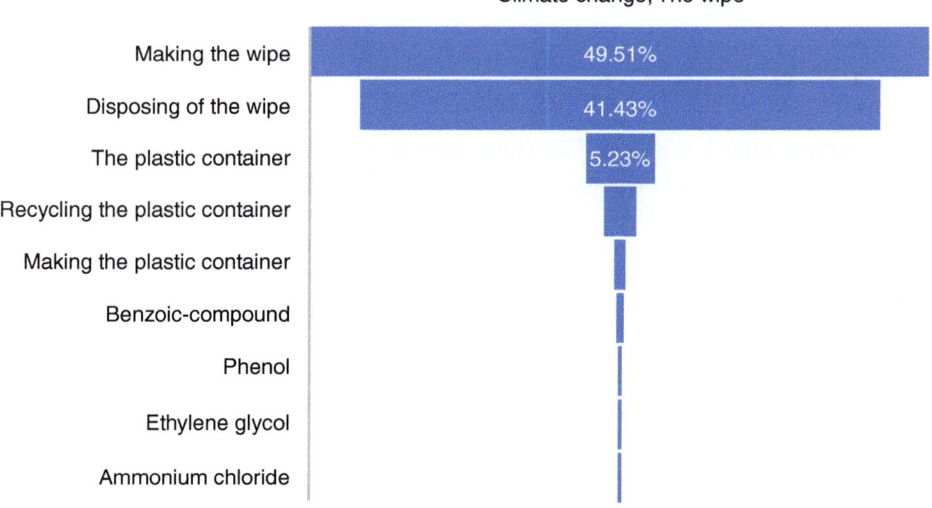

Fig. 7.3 Impact factors from surface wipe 1

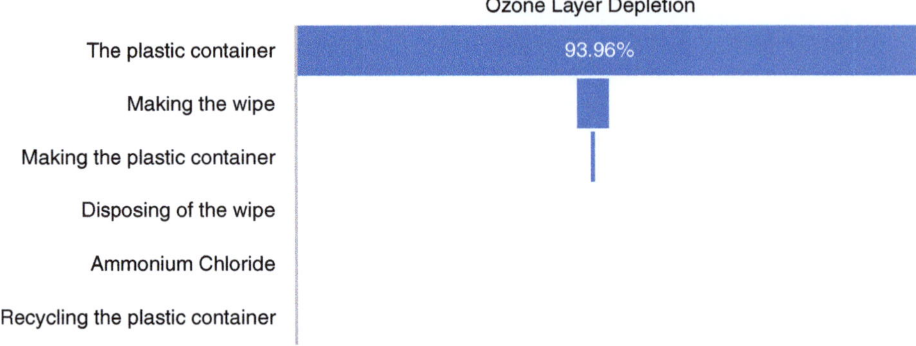

Fig. 7.4 Impact factors from surface wipe 2

depletion, minerals and metals, cancer effects and climate change, with ammonium chloride having much less of an impact. In this case, the relatively small human health cancer effects from ammonium chloride were related to the building of the chemical factory producing the ammonium chloride, and the production of sodium chloride.

The other significant concern with wipes is the packaging they come in. If manufacturers could reduce the amount and weight of the packaging, (or provide refills), significant environmental savings could be made.

To reduce the weight of packaging manufacturers might consider making the decontamination chemicals water soluble, (e.g. in tablet form/or in a condensed formula). Such a product would allow the solution to be made up in-house on a daily basis (instead of in its current ready-to-use formula). This would reduce the size, weight, and amount of packaging required.

7.3.3   Surface Wipe 3

In surface wipe 3, see (Fig. 7.5) where spray is used with tissues, the main concern is the production and disposal of the tissue paper rather than the spray itself. In this example/scenario, however, the plastic container's environmental contribution (i.e. the container the spray comes in) is greatly reduced because the volume of the spray alone is much smaller than the combined volume of the spray and wipes.

From this analysis the actual chemical used does not seem to impact on the highest environmental scores.

The advantage of using dry tissues (rather than wet wipes) is that they need less robust packaging (as they are less likely to be damaged in transit, are less heavy, and there is no risk of liquid evaporation).

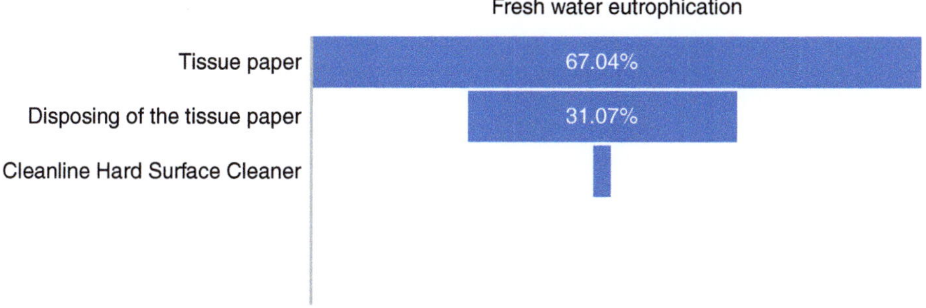

Fig. 7.5 Impact factors from surface wipe 3 with tissues

7.3.4 Sustainable Wipes

Some people have questioned whether cloth towels can be used. From a reduction in plastic and packaging perspective, they would be ideal. However, they would require laundering at high temperatures and would have a limited lifespan before they too would need to be replaced (perhaps—based on similar studies looking at gown replacement—after approximately 100 uses) [13]. Life cycle analysis in similar areas (comparing disposable gowns with reusable gowns) have demonstrated environmental superiority for the reusable product [13].

Disposable wipes generally have a consistent wipe-to-cleaning solution ratio provided the lid is closed securely after each use [14].

In contrast, cotton and microfibre cloths may not be compatible with some disinfectants; it's difficult to standardise the amount of liquid required on a dry wipe, and washed cloth/microfibre wipes could remain contaminated with bacteria even after washing [9, 15–18]. There is a potential for more research into this area, possibly using an adenosine triphosphate monitor to check the effectiveness of the various surface cleaning approaches [19].

To conclude, there are several ways to reduce the amount of waste generated when cleaning surfaces:

1. Use refill packs of wipes rather than replenishing supplies with a new drum every time.
2. Make up your own cleaning solution and use tissue.
3. Consider the use of reusable cloths and disinfectant solution especially in area less exposed to spatter.

There are a number of recommendations relating to the use of surface wipes (see Table 7.3).

Table 7.3 Recommendations for surface wipes

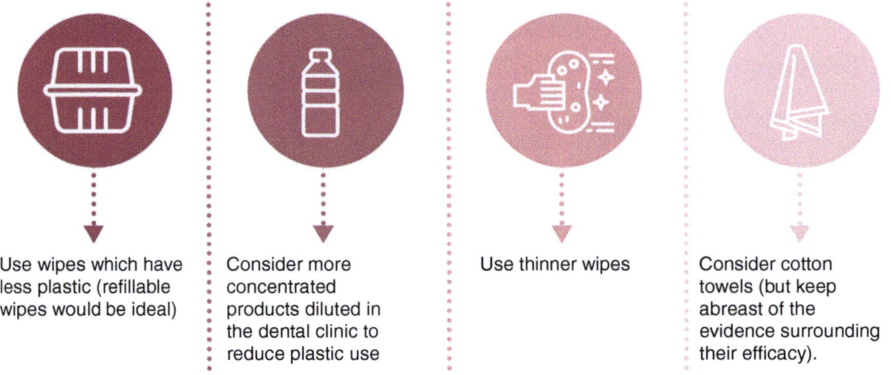

7.3.5 Cleaning Prosthesis

Here we demonstrate the impact factors relating to processes involving disinfecting prosthesis (see Fig. 7.6).

Within these processes most of the environmental impacts originate from the products needed to make a plastic bottle (see Fig. 7.7), the energy (making) the plastic bottle and disposing of it. In this case, the chemicals (sodium chloride and sodium hypochlorite) do contribute to climate change, human health cancer effects, and to a less degree contribute to minerals and metals.

The main reason for the environmental contribution of these products is the environmental impact of building the chemical factory which is, in turn, used to produce the chemicals. From a climate change perspective, the use of electricity and transport is also a big component in the production of sodium chloride and sodium hypochlorite.

In order to reduce the impact of disinfecting prosthesis, companies should consider the use of renewable energy, and either using locally sourced products or sustainable transport systems.

7.3.6 Washer Disinfectant Using Chemicals Part A and B

For the washer disinfector, around 19% of climate change contribution, 17% of non-carcinogenic effects, 16% of human health effects, and 13% of the contribution to freshwater eutrophication comes from the cleaner used within the washer disinfectant. This impact is mostly related to the production of citric acid, sodium cumenesulphonate, the plastic bottle, and the EDTA (ethylenediaminetetraacetic acid). The remainder of the environmental emissions comes from treating the wastewater and the comparatively large amount of electricity consumed by the washer disinfector (see Fig. 7.8).

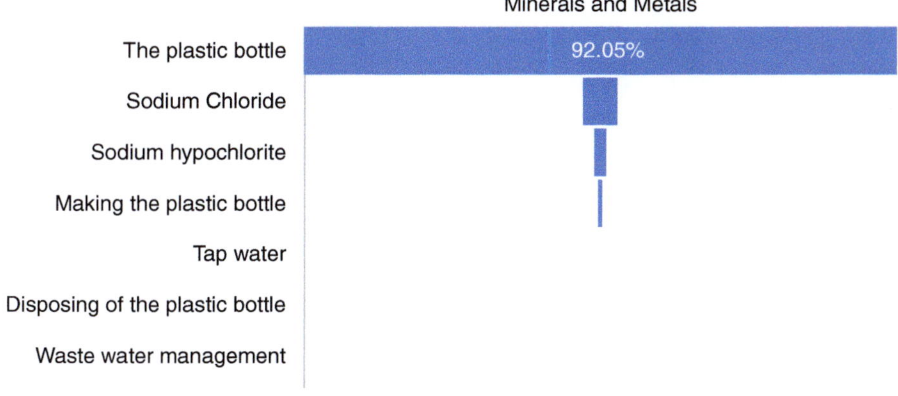

Fig. 7.6 Impact factors from Prosthesis Disinfectant (UK)

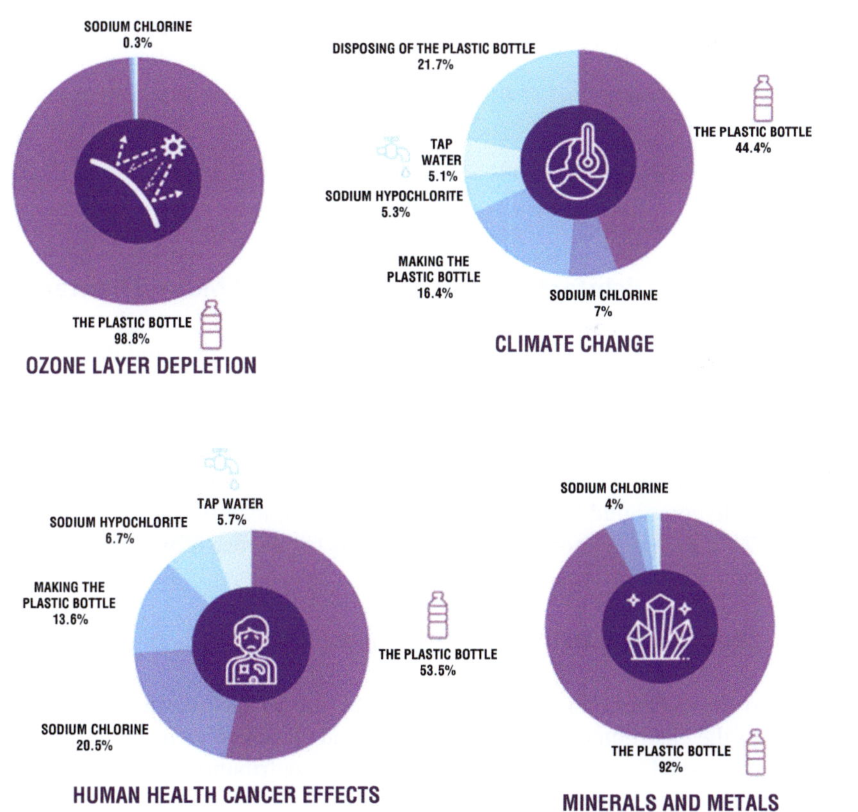

Fig. 7.7 Impact factors from Prothesis Disinfectant (Colombia)

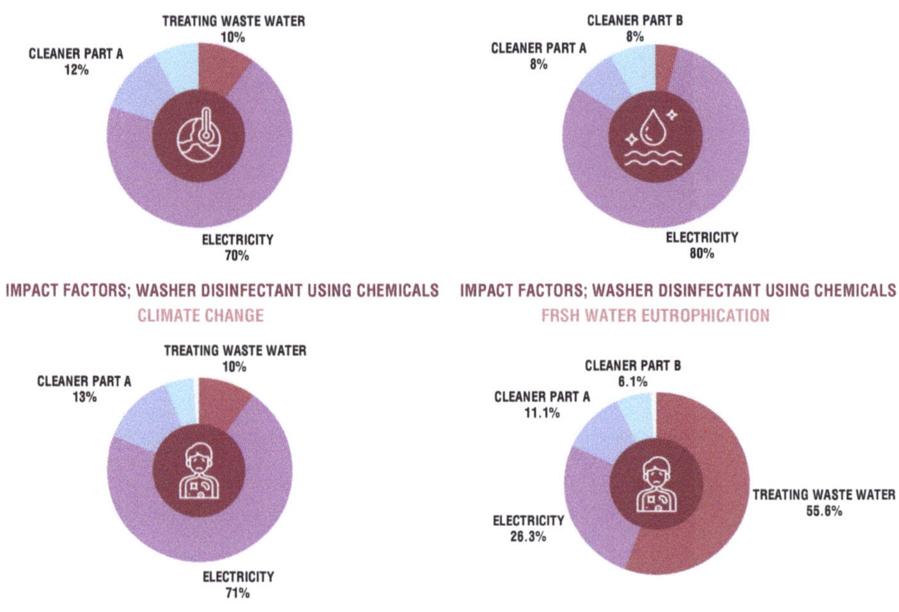

Fig. 7.8 Impact factors: washer disinfectant using chemicals part A and B

7.3.7 Washer Disinfectant Using the Chemical Methyl Pentane

Looking at carbon dioxide equivalent emissions (see Fig. 7.9), and the three worst outcomes from a normalised perspective (human health: carcinogenic effects, ecosytem quality freshwater eutrophication, and freshwater acidification); the majority of environmental emissions do not come from the type of cleaning agent used, but instead comes from the amount of energy used. The 2-methylpentane 0.75 g, benzothiadiazole compound 75 g did not contribute significantly to the footprints.

Table 7.4 summarises some recommendations for the use of washer disinfectors.

7.3.8 Sterilisation Using an Autoclave

Similar to the washer disinfector (but with less of an environmental impact), the majority of the environmental impact from the autoclave comes from the use of coal-based energy (see Fig. 7.10). One exception is the contribution wastewater makes to human health (cancer effects).

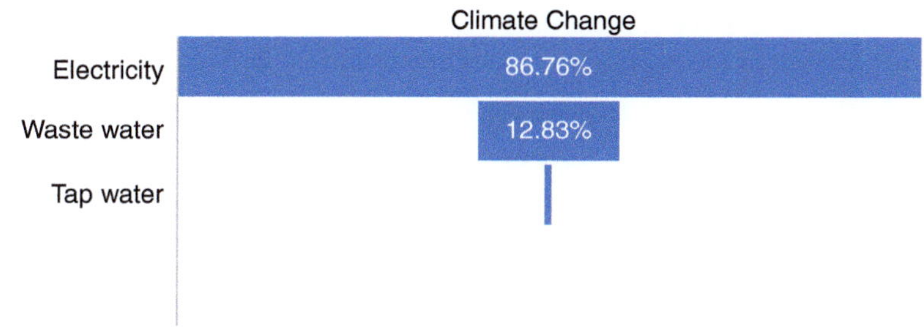

Fig. 7.9 Washer disinfectant using the chemical methyl pentane

Table 7.4 Recommendations for washer disinfectors

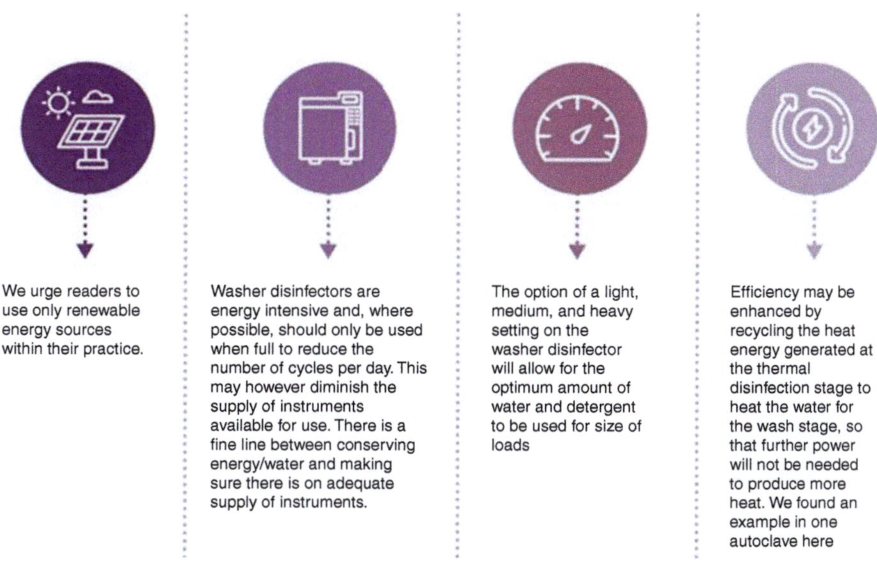

We urge readers to use only renewable energy sources within their practice.

Washer disinfectors are energy intensive and, where possible, should only be used when full to reduce the number of cycles per day. This may however diminish the supply of instruments available for use. There is a fine line between conserving energy/water and making sure there is on adequate supply of instruments.

The option of a light, medium, and heavy setting on the washer disinfector will allow for the optimum amount of water and detergent to be used for size of loads

Efficiency may be enhanced by recycling the heat energy generated at the thermal disinfection stage to heat the water for the wash stage, so that further power will not be needed to produce more heat. We found an example in one autoclave here

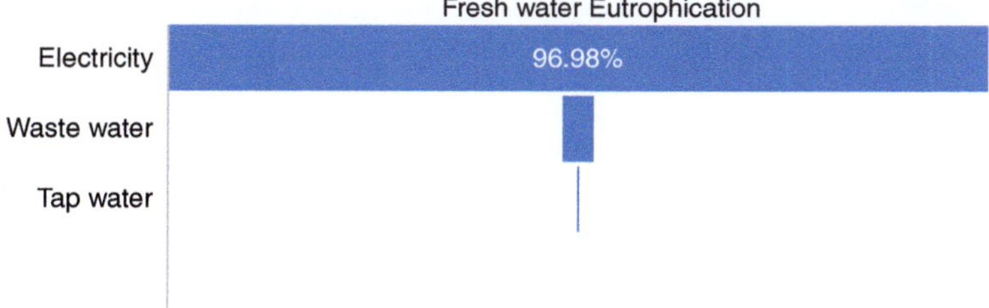

Fig. 7.10 Impact factors from autoclave use

Recommendations for autoclaves.

There are several recommendations for the use of autoclaves. See below:

Autoclaves are high energy users. The main environmental harm comes from the electricity consumed. As the figures from Ecoinvent draw on an electricity source high in coal, substantial environmental savings could be made by changing to green energy, for example, wind energy, installing solar panels, or simply choosing a green energy provider.

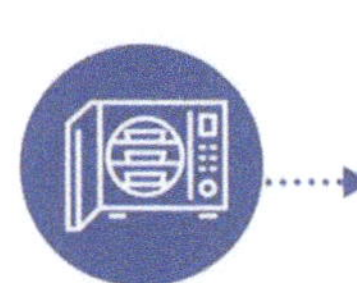

When considering the energy use of an autoclave, smaller is not necessarily better. For example, it takes roughly twice the energy to boil two litres of water / liquid compared to one litre! Thinking about this principle it takes the same energy for all sterilisers to get from temperature A to temperature B and a lesser powered autoclave would just take longer to reach the required temperature. If you increase the time the process takes, you risk heat escaping, with the resulting decrease in efficiency. The purchaser of an autoclave should consider energy efficient autoclaves, e.g. ones that have been manufactured to use less water, and ones that offer economy mode settings (which only use 50% of its heating capacity as and when needed for many of its cycles.

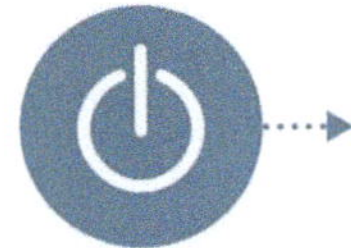

McGain* undertook a year's audit of autoclave use and demonstrated that 40% of the electricity used occurred during standby times. This provides incentives for practices, especially larger practices, to ensure autoclaves are not continuously on standby mode.

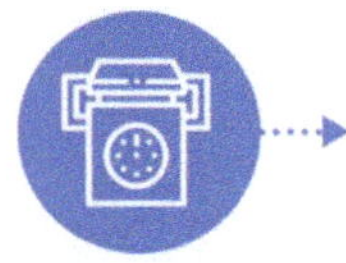

Where product design supports this, consider using a heating and cooling jacket around the autoclave. A jacket can be filled with hot or cold water to provide better temperature control and reduce fluctuations below the sterilisation temperature. There is much better heat transfer to water or any liquid than to air or any gas. A heated jacket would help keep the temperature inside the autoclave more consistent and there would be less heat lost during the sterilisation process.

Secondly, ensure the equipment is regularly serviced, calibrated, and validated to ensure optimal efficiency.

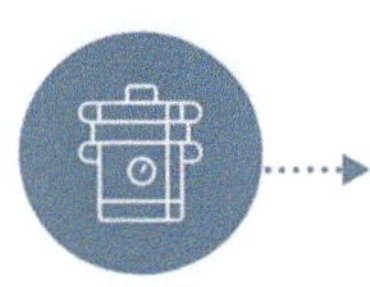

Thirdly, ensure the autoclave is filled to capacity (but, not overfull!). It might also be possible for practices to have a timetable for sterilising instruments so as to avoid having autoclaves set unnecessarily on standby. In a large practice the staff member working in the unit could ensure that the decontamination equipment is used as efficiently as possible with an optimal load for each cycle. It may be possible to recirculate hot water from the autoclave and the final rinse water from the washer disinfectors instead of simply disposing of it. In practices that do not have a dedicated LDU operative, other staff members can agree to process the instruments at designated times throughout the day, thus avoiding unnecessary cycles, and increasing efficiency.

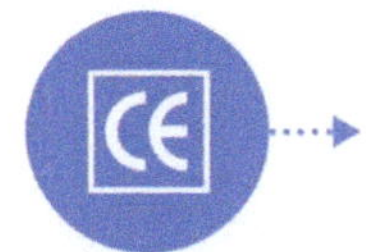

For all dental specific devices, practices should ensure they purchase an EU rated product that is certification marked (CE) or relevant country's current standards?) Practitioners need to ensure that they purchase the appropriate model for the purpose intended; too small a product will result in additional machine cycles, too big a machine will result in low-capacity machine utilisation.

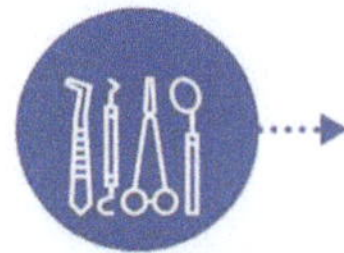

Ensure the dental setting does not use out-dated clinical trays with too many instruments. Ensure operative trays are laid out fit for purpose.

* McGain F, Moore G, Black J. Hospital steam sterilizer usage: could we switch off to save electricity and water? J Health Serv Res Policy. 2016 Jul;21(3):166-71. doi: 10.1177/1355819615625698. Epub 2016 Jan 13. PMID: 26769573.

7.4   Considerations About Chemicals

As a part of sustainability in dentistry, we need to consider the chemicals we use carefully. Safety data sheets (SDS) are available for most chemical products and chemicals should not be purchased if there is no SDS readily available [20]. Ideally, we should only use products which are readily biodegradable to non-toxic and low environmental footprint. However, in reality, environmental sustainability is difficult to understand. The fact is there isn't enough evidence relating to the environmental impact of the chemicals we use. We have therefore written a summary of chemicals commonly used in dental practice (see Table 7.5).

Table 7.5 Comments on commonly used chemicals in decontamination

Chemical	Comment	Avoid/use
2-methylpentane	Toxic to aquatic life and can potentially have a long-term impact on the marine environment. 2-methylpentane consists of volatile organic compounds that disperse within the air. Some constituents are harmful to the environment and cannot be broken down by water treatment plants [21]	Avoid if possible
Benzothiadiazole compound	2,1,3-benzothiadiazole-4-acrylic acid is a biocide. Its release into the environment should be avoided. This chemical is soluble in water and, as a result, is likely to be mobile within soil. Currently, information on its bioaccumulation is unavailable [22]	Avoid if possible
Ammonium chloride	Not classified as harmful to the environment	Use
Benzoic compound	Benzoic compounds (such as benzoic acid and sodium benzoate) are primarily eliminated via biotic mineralisation and are not volatile. For this reason, these compounds are not directly contributory to global warming or deterioration of the ozone layer. However, benzoic acid is derived from chloroform (trichloromethane) and chloroform emissions contribute to ozone depletion. Chloroform contributes to the depletion of the stratospheric ozone layer. However, due to its short lifespan, and predominantly natural sources, it is not included in the Montreal Protocol that regulates the production and uses of ozone-depleting substances [23, 24]	Use

(continued)

Table 7.5 (continued)

Chemical	Comment	Avoid/use
Chlorine	The release of large amounts of chlorine disinfecting agents into the environment can be harmful to aquatic organisms. Chlorine can also damage the cell walls and proteins of living organisms and combine with organic material (such as biofilms) in surface water to produce toxic trihalomethane or haloacetic acid by-products. Additionally, chlorine can react with nitrogen to form carcinogens such as chloramine or N-nitrosodimethylamine. Oxidising disinfecting agents, especially those containing chlorine, can enhance the mobilisation of mercury from amalgam which, if not disposed of correctly, can facilitate the entry of mercury ions into the environment. Furthermore, mercury released into the environment can bioaccumulate in organisms such as fish and disseminate throughout the food chain [25]	Avoid if possible
Citric acid	Biodegradable with low ecological footprint [26]	Use
Dimethyl dioctadecyl ammonium chloride	Associated with low risk of bioaccumulation and toxic to aquatic organisms. Adsorbs into sediment in water [27]	Use
EDTA (ethylenediaminetetraacetic acid)	EDTA, a chelating agent, may facilitate the mobilisation and bioavailability of heavy metals (such as lead) by forming ligand-metal complexes. However, when introduced into the natural environment, EDTA is poorly biodegradable. Its impact on different living organisms is unpredictable and varies depending on the associated metal(s) and the concentration of EDTA. In addition, it has an inhibitory effect on chlorophyll production and cellular division in photosynthetic organisms, unless it is chelated with micronutrients [28]	Avoid if possible
Ethanol 10 g	Ethanol is a water soluble, volatile, biodegradable compound. Ethanol vapour produces air pollutants such as ozone and peroxyacetyl nitrate by reacting with other gases such as nitrogen oxides. At high concentrations, it may be toxic to aquatic life but is associated with low risk of bioaccumulation [29]	Use
Ethylene glycol	In general, ethylene glycol has low toxicity to aquatic organisms and is spontaneously broken down in the natural environment over a period of a few days/weeks [30]	Use

(continued)

Table 7.5 (continued)

Chemical	Comment	Avoid/use
Hydrogen peroxide	When used as intended, hydrogen peroxide is not classed as a persistent substance due to its spontaneous decomposition to oxygen and water. The rate of the reaction can depend on the presence of catalysts in the environment, such as heat. The use of hydrogen peroxide does not pose additional risk of toxicity to aquatic life as the compound is already ubiquitous within natural waters [31]	Use
Phenol	Bacteria assist in the degradation of phenol in aerobic environments (such as fresh and saltwater, sewage, and soil), whereas photochemical reactions and rainfall facilitate decomposition of phenol in the atmosphere. Higher concentrations of phenol may allow for bacteria to acclimate, potentially resulting in diminished decomposition. Although toxic to aquatic organisms, growth and metabolism of specific species of algae, fish, and crustaceans may be sensitive to lower concentrations of phenol [32]	Use with caution
Phenylalanine	An essential amino acid found in foods and medication. Phenylalanine enters the environment via waste streams. It is water soluble and mobile within soil, and it should not be emptied into drains. Information of its effect on wildlife is unavailable [33]	Use
Potassium hydroxide	Generally toxic to aquatic life, with low risk of bioaccumulation. Soluble in water and, as a result, can be highly mobile within soil. In water, potassium hydroxide dissociates into its ionic components which, depending on the system buffering capacity, can raise the pH of the system. Additionally, pH monitoring allows for disruptions in pH to be rapidly detected and corrected and, if potassium hydroxide is used as intended, no significant increase in pH or harm to aquatic life is expected [34]	Use
Sodium chloride	Sodium chloride (table salt) is a naturally occurring inorganic complex. It is not of substantial toxicological concern, nor is it considered particularly harmful to environmental receptors	Use
Sodium cumenesulphonate	Primary method of elimination is via biodegradation in aerobic environments—thus not a persistent compound. No evidence of bioaccumulation or terrestrial and sediment toxicity. Low risk of acute toxicity towards aquatic organisms. Chronic toxicity was seen in invertebrates and algae. Out of all marine life tested, green algae is considered most sensitive to the compound [35]	Use
Sodium hydrogen sulphate	No evidence of either short- or long-term toxicity to terrestrial or aquatic life. Readily biodegradable in aqueous environment [36]	Use

(continued)

Table 7.5 (continued)

Chemical	Comment	Avoid/use
Sodium hydroxide	Dissociates into sodium and hydroxyl ions in aqueous environment and, if not well-buffered, can lead to an increase in pH. Elevated pH beyond the tolerance range (1–2 pH units) of certain species of fish can be lethal and reduce their fertility. Generally, released liquid waste no longer contains sodium hydroxide due to neutralisation by other substances in water; therefore, its effect on aquatic organisms is negligible if used as intended [37]	Use
Sodium hypochlorite	Toxic to aquatic organisms. An unstable compound that usually reacts with organic material in water and is eliminated before reaching the natural environment. Water soluble, releasing chlorine and oxygen gas—neither of which persist in the atmosphere	Use with caution
Sodium pyrophosphate	Hydrolyses into sodium and orthophosphate ions which are nutritious for plants and promotes the growth of aquatic plants. It has no evidence of bioaccumulation or toxic effects on the environment [38]	Use

7.5 Conclusion

It is important that the decontamination of dental premises is carried out to the standard advised by the national authorities. However, there is growing importance to also ensure that dentistry's ecological footprint is kept to a minimum. This chapter made a number of recommendations the clinical team might consider to reduce their decontamination environmental footprint. The main messages in the chapter relate to the need to find less damaging alternatives to the disinfectant wipe; to consider the energy we use and, with the support of our manufacturing colleagues, reduce, reuse, and recycle the plastic within our products.

Take Home Points for the Dental Team

- Reduce packaging.
- Reduce the thickness of wipes.
- Wherever possible, prioritise the use of reusable rather than disposable products.

References

1. Scottish Dental Clinical Effectiveness Programme. Decontamination into practice. Scottish Dental Clinical Effectiveness Programme. 2016.
2. Rutala WA, Weber DJ. Guideline for disinfection and sterilization in healthcare facilities. 2008. https://scholar.google.com/scholar_url?url=http://hica.jp/cdcguideline/dsguide.pdf&hl=es&sa=X&ei=7ZhYYfrqFILemgHVs5GYDg&scisig=AAGBfm2bmGIJqrksMfJVr0xKf3OrnTRbww&oi=scholarr. Accessed Sept 2021.
3. European Council Directive 98/83/EC. 1998. https://eur-lex.europa.eu/legal-content/EN/TXT/?uri=celex%3A31998L0083.
4. Centers for Disease Control and Prevention. Dental Unit Water Quality Dental Unit Water Quality. https://www.cdc.gov/oralhealth/infectioncontrol/summary-infection-prevention-practices/dental-unit-water-quality.html. Accessed Sept 2021.
5. HSE: National Guidelines for IPC in HSE Dental and Orthodontic Services. 2019.
6. Weber DJ, Anderson D, Rutala WA. The role of the surface environment in healthcare-associated infections. Curr Opin Infect Dis. 2013;26(4):338–44.
7. Otter JA, Yezli S, Salkeld JA, JA and French GL. Evidence that contaminated surfaces contribute to the transmission of hospital pathogens and an overview of strategies to address contaminated surfaces in hospital settings. Am J Infect Control. 2013;41(5):S6–S11.
8. Rizan C, Bhutta MF. Environmental impact and life cycle financial cost of hybrid (reusable/single-use) instruments versus single-use equivalents in laparoscopic cholecystectomy. Surg Endosc. 2021;36(6):4067–78. https://doi.org/10.1007/s00464-021-08728-z. Epub ahead of print.
9. Boyce JM. A review of wipes used to disinfect hard surfaces in health care facilities. Am J Infect Control. 2021;49(1):104–14. https://doi.org/10.1016/j.ajic.2020.06.183. Epub 2020 Jun 19.
10. Clausen PA, Frederiksen M, Sejbæk CS, Sørli JB, Hougaard KS, Frydendall KB, Carøe TK, Flachs EM, Meyer HW, Schlünssen V, Wolkoff P. Chemicals inhaled from spray cleaning and disinfection products and their respiratory effects. A comprehensive review. Int J Hyg Environ Health. 2020;229:113592. https://doi.org/10.1016/j.ijheh.2020.113592. Epub 2020 Aug 15.
11. European Environment Agency. Average CO2 emissions from new cars and new vans increased in 2018; European Environment Agency; 2019. https://www.eea.europa.eu/highlights/average-co2-emissions-from-new. Accessed Sept 2021.
12. Tommie Ponsioen. Normalization: new developments in normalization sets, 2014. https://pre-sustainability.com/articles/the-normalisation-step-in-lcia. Accessed Sept 2021.
13. Vozzola E, Overcash M, Griffing E. Environmental considerations in the selection of isolation gowns: a life cycle assessment of reusable and disposable alternatives. Am J Infect Control. 2018;46(8):881–6. https://doi.org/10.1016/j.ajic.2018.02.002. Epub 2018 Apr 11.
14. Sattar SA, Maillard JY. The crucial role of wiping in decontamination of high-touch environmental surfaces: review of current status and directions for the future. Am J Infect Control. 2013;41(5):S97–S104.
15. MacDougall KD, Morris C. Optimizing disinfectant application in healthcare facilities. Infect Control Today. 2006;10:62–7, 589–591. https://www.infectioncontroltoday.com/environmental-hygiene/optimizing-disinfectant-application-healthcare-facilities. Accessed Sept 2021.
16. Boyce JM, Sullivan L, Booker A, Baker J. Quaternary ammonium disinfectant issues encountered in an environmental services department. Infect Control Hosp Epidemiol. 2016;37(3):340–2.

17. Sifuentes LY, Gerba CP, Weart I, Engelbrecht K, Koenig DW. Microbial contamination of hospital reusable cleaning towels. Am J Infect Control. 2013;41(10):912–5.
18. Bergen LK, Meyer M, Høg M, Rubenhagen B, Andersen LP. Spread of bacteria on surfaces when cleaning with microfibre cloths. J Hosp Infect. 2009;71(2):132–7.
19. ATP Monitoring. https://www.aiconline.co.uk/what-is-atp-monitoring/. Accessed Sept 2021.
20. Commission Regulation (EU) 2020/878 of 18 June 2020 amending Annex II to Regulation (EC) No 1907/2006 of the European Parliament and of the Council concerning the Registration, Evaluation, Authorisation and Restriction of Chemicals (REACH).
21. Fisher Scientific 2020 2-Methylpentane Safety Data Sheet. https://www.fishersci.se/store/msds?partNumber=10222652&productDescription=1LT+2-Methylpentane%2C+99%2B%25%2C+pure&countryCode=SE&language=en. Accessed Sept 2021.
22. Fisher Scientific 2019, 2,1,3-Benzothiadiazole-4-carboxylic acid Safety Data Sheet. https://www.fishersci.com/store/msds?partNumber=CC09101DE&productDescription=2%2C1%2C3-BENZOTHIADIAZOLE-4+5GR&vendorId=VN00092202&countryCode=US&language=en.
23. Fang X, Park S, Saito T, Tunnicliffe R, Ganesan AL, Rigby M, Li S, Yokouchi Y, Fraser PJ, Harth CM, Krummel PB. Rapid increase in ozone-depleting chloroform emissions from China. Nat Geosci. 2019;12(2):89–93.
24. Wibbertmann A, Kielhorn J, Koennecker G, Mangelsdorf I, Melber C. Concise International Chemical Assessment Document 26. Benzoic acid and sodium benzoate. International Programme on Chemical Safety. 2000. Accessed 13 Mar 2010.
25. Roberts HW, Marek M, Kuehne JC, Ragain JC. Disinfectants' effect on mercury release from amalgam. J Am Dent Assoc. 2005;136(7):915–9.
26. HERA. Risk assessments-executive summary: substance group: citric acids/salts. https://www.heraproject.com/ExecutiveSummary.cfm?ID=219. Accessed Sept 2021.
27. National Library of Medicine COMPOUND SUMMARY Dimethyldioctadecylammonium chloride. https://pubchem.ncbi.nlm.nih.gov/compound/Dimethyldioctadecylammonium-chloride#section=Non-Human-Toxicity-Values. Accessed Sept 2021.
28. Fisher Scientific Ethylenediamine Tetraacetic Acid Safety Data Sheet. https://www.lewisu.edu/academics/biology/pdf/Ethylenediamine_Tetraacetic_Acid(EDTA).pdf.
29. Willey JD, Avery GB, Felix JD, Kieber RJ, Mead RN, Shimizu MS. Rapidly increasing ethanol concentrations in rainwater and air. NPJ Climate and Atmospheric Science. 2019;2(1):1–5.
30. ATSDR Toxicological Report for Ethylene Glycol. https://www.atsdr.cdc.gov/toxprofiles/tp96-c1.pdf. Accessed Sept 2021.
31. Regulation (EU) No 528/2012 concerning the making available on the market and use of biocidal products Evaluation of active substances assessment report: hydrogen peroxide product-types 1–6. https://echa.europa.eu/documents/10162/cad256b7-8716-80f4-d091-c7bce0305d89. Accessed Sept 2021.
32. Directive WF. Proposed EQS for Water Framework Directive Annex VIII substances: 2,4-dichlorophenol. 2012. https://www.wfduk.org/sites/default/files/Media/2,4-dichlorophenol.pdf. Accessed Sept 2021.
33. National Library of Medicine COMPOUND SUMMARY Phenylalanine. https://pubchem.ncbi.nlm.nih.gov/compound/Phenylalanine#section=Environmental-Fate. https://www.fishersci.se/chemicalProductData_uk/wercs?itemCode=10793541&lang=EN. Accessed Sept 2021.
34. Fisher Scientific Potassium Hydroxide Safety Data Sheet. https://www.fishersci.pt/store/msds?partNumber=10448990&productDescription=1KG+Potassium+hydroxide%2C+Certified+AR+for+analysis%2C+pellets%2C+meets+Ph.Eur.%2C+BP&countryCode=PT&language=en. https://hpvchemicals.oecd.org/UI/handler.axd?id=0cd7a76e-c7bc-4545-b26e-b2c4dbfb9ef9. Accessed Sept 2021.
35. Human & Environmental Risk Assessment on ingredients of household cleaning products Hydrotropes. 2005. https://cdn3.evostore.io/documents/vow/px56969_coshh.pdf. https://www.heraproject.com/files/24-F-HERA%20Hydrotropes%20Sept%202005.pdf. Accessed Sept 2021.

36. European Chemicals Agency Sodium hydrogen sulphate. https://echa.europa.eu/es/registration-dossier/-/registered-dossier/14458/5/4/1. Accessed Sept 2021.
37. Evonik Industry AG GPS Safety Summary Sodium Hydroxide; https://corporate.evonik.com/downloads/corporate/gps-summaries/gps-summary-sodium-hydroxide-(naoh).pdf. https://echa.europa.eu/documents/10162/917becd0-b0a4-4b68-8e5e-c2e466d8641a. Accessed Sept 2021.
38. National Library of Medicine Compound Summary Sodium Hypochlorite. https://pubchem.ncbi.nlm.nih.gov/compound/Sodium-hypochlorite#section=EPA-Ecotoxicity. Accessed Sept 2021.

Supporting People and Their Behaviour in the Dental Setting as Sustainably as Reasonably Achievable

Caoimhin Mac Giola Phadraig, Amarantha Fennell-Wells, Andrew Geddis-Regan, and Katherine Wilson

8.1 Introduction

8.1.1 Dental Behaviour Support

Dental behaviour support (DBS) is a term used to describe the group of strategies that the wider dental care team practice to help patients receive appropriate dental care [1]. Readers may be more familiar with the term *behaviour management techniques*; a term no longer congruent with current concepts of health, function, and participation. DBS is delivered through a range of environmental, communication-mediated, pharmacological and physical interventions, which are sometimes classified as "pharmacological or non-pharmacological", "accepted or controversial", and "basic or advanced" techniques [2–4].

8.1.2 Populations Covered

Dental behaviour support is most pertinent for the population who need or prefer support due to anxiety, age-related issues, certain impairments related to

C. Mac Giola Phadraig (✉)
Trinity College Dublin, Dublin, Ireland

Department of Child and Public Dental Health, Dublin Dental University Hospital, Dublin, Ireland
e-mail: macgiolla@dental.tcd.ie

A. Fennell-Wells
Centre for Sustainable Healthcare, Oxford, UK
e-mail: amarantha@sustainablehealthcare.org.uk

A. Geddis-Regan · K. Wilson
Newcastle University, Newcastle upon Tyne, UK
e-mail: Andrew.Geddis-Regan@newcastle.ac.uk; katherine.wilson@newcastle.ac.uk

© The Author(s), under exclusive license to Springer Nature Switzerland AG 2022
B. Duane (ed.), *Sustainable Dentistry*, BDJ Clinician's Guides,
https://doi.org/10.1007/978-3-031-07999-3_8

disabilities, and those receiving dental procedures that are inherently unpleasant. For many patients in these groups, the type of support defines care delivery and resource usage—think dental general anaesthesia, for example. For most people though, to a greater or lesser degree, DBS is applied inherent in their dental care. For many, this support can be imperceivable—seen by the patient as the dentist simply giving information or building rapport.

The vast majority of care is delivered in a primary care setting, typically local to patients in countries where services are developed. When patients require further support/specialist services, these change the process of care delivery which, subsequently, may then limit access, involve greater travel and involve differential use of resources.

8.2 Choices for Behaviour Support in Dentistry

There are probably as many techniques to support patients to receive dental treatment as there are patient visits. While there is considerable variation internationally, in this chapter we consider four commonly used modalities in western Europe: communication-mediated techniques, inhalation sedation (IS), single drug

Table 8.1 Comparison of behaviour support modalities

	Indications (relative and absolute)	Contraindications (relative and absolute)	Advantages	Disadvantages
Communication-mediated	Mild to severe anxiety. Low to high levels of support need	Need for additional support.	Range of techniques. Non-invasive. Limited potential physiological side effects. Promotes skill building and internalised coping strategies	Often poorly defined. Many techniques lack evidence base
Inhalation sedation	Mild to moderate anxiety. Gag reflex. Specific fear of needles. Low to medium levels of support need	Claustrophobia. Pregnancy. Nasal obstruction. Chronic obstructive airways disease (COAD)	Non-invasive. No biotransformation. Rapid onset. Rapid recovery. Few drug–drug interactions. Easily titratable. Minimal cardiovascular and respiratory effects	Nasal hood may impede access. Patient acceptance of nasal hood. Reliance on correct respiration. Specialised equipment and training needed. Potential for staff health risks. Release of unconverted gas into atmosphere

Table 8.1 (continued)

	Indications (relative and absolute)	Contraindications (relative and absolute)	Advantages	Disadvantages
Intravenous sedation (in primary care)	Moderate to severe anxiety. Gag reflex. Traumatic surgical procedure. Mild medical conditions which may be aggravated by stress. Moderate to high levels of support need	Unstable medical conditions. Hepatic or renal impairment. COAD. Where venous access is not possible. Severe mental health conditions. BMI >40 kg/m^2 Allergy to sedative agents. Pregnancy	Titratable. Reversible. Rapid onset and recovery within one hour. Wide margin of safety	Care support required post-procedurally. Unpredictable in some instances. May cause respiratory depression. Potential for disinhibition
General anaesthesia	Severe anxiety or phobia. Extensive treatment needs or complex procedures. Sedation unsuitable. Where a secure airway is essential to facilitate safe care. Co-delivery with other specialties. High levels of support need.	Simple procedures in patients who do not need GA. Where anaesthetic risks outweigh dental procedural benefits	Facilitated by a dedicated anaesthetist (UK and Ireland). Near guarantee of treatment completion. Behavioural challenges mitigated once anaesthetised	Extensive cost. Highly resource intensive. Limited access to appropriate hospital facilities. Intimidating environment

intravenous sedation (IVS), and general anaesthesia (GA). Table 8.1 gives a basic summary of their features. In doing so, we accept loss of detail and descriptive accuracy to benefit from meaningful comparison. Each of these four techniques dictates its own training requirements, staffing levels, equipment, infrastructure, governance, and environmental impact. In practice, the features of these modalities differ so much that they often hold separate points in the patients' continuum of care. While these techniques are often applied in combination, for example, the use of a sedative to enable induction or the use of hypnotic suggestion for efficacious IS; in this chapter, we will consider them individually. Often, the selection of one approach can be seen as the decision not to adopt an alternative. We do not consider local anaesthesia as a separate modality since it is crucial to appropriate use across all modalities, even GA. We introduce the indications, contraindications, advantages, and disadvantages for behaviour support techniques in Table 8.1.

8.2.1 Communication-Mediated Dental Behaviour Support Techniques

The term *communication-mediated DBS* covers a wide array of DBS techniques that are practised through communication with the patient in the dental setting and is synonymous with the term non-pharmacological behaviour management. Techniques included in this category vary greatly. Some relate to basic universal approaches like distraction or purposive communication through our words, expression, behaviour, and environment, or like establishing a relationship based on mutual trust and even by applying alternative communication methods like picture stories. This category also includes specific theory-driven interventions such as applied behaviour analysis, where principles of behaviourism are applied to support behaviour and exposure-oriented therapies such as systematic desensitisation or Cognitive Behaviour Therapy (CBT), which normally involve elements of repeated exposure to dental stimuli. A broad range of techniques lie in between.

8.2.2 Inhalation Sedation

Inhalation sedation (IS) is a form of conscious sedation where the administration of a variable mixture of nitrous oxide and oxygen is used to induce a state of psycho-pharmacological sedation. It is widely accepted as a safe and effective technique due mainly to the favourable pharmacological properties of nitrous oxide. Its most common application is in paediatric dentistry, where it has a very high success rate. Inhalation sedation is increasingly used among adult patients, particularly those with comorbidities that contraindicate the use of intravenous techniques. Since it undergoes no biotransformation when circulating around the body, once exhaled its analgesic and sedative effects cease to affect patients directly [5]. However, this form of sedation does affect patients and populations indirectly due to the release of nitrous oxide into the environment, as discussed later. See Sect. 8.3.3.

8.2.3 Intravenous Sedation

Intravenous sedation (IVS) is a form of conscious sedation where sedative agents are administered intravenously. While there is significant variation internationally, in the UK intravenous sedation with the single drug midazolam is considered a standard conscious sedation technique in primary care for adults and young people over the age of 12 years [6, 7]. Midazolam is a short acting benzodiazepine, stored in vials and administered IV through cannulae. IV sedation is often delivered by a single operator sedationist, with a trained team, in general dental practice. In addition to the use of midazolam, a combination of drugs such as fentanyl and midazolam is used in hospital settings, typically administered by an anaesthetist. Other combinations of drugs are routinely used in other parts of the world.

8.2.4 General Anaesthesia

For some patients, general anaesthesia (GA) is the only approach by which comprehensive dental care can be facilitated. For other patients, GA is a preference (or an approach perceived to be preferable) to the use of local anaesthesia or conscious sedation alone. GA leads to a of loss of consciousness and insensibility to painful stimuli [8]. In a hospital setting, it is generally administered by an anaesthetist. The use of a managed airway and the full remit of drugs available mean anaesthetists have a significant degree of control over physiological systems. Once a patient is anaesthetised, treatment is generally easily facilitated. For some patients, however, communication-mediated DBS, sedation or clinical holding is required to prepare them for entering the theatre environment. Pre-, intra-, and postoperatively, GA can be associated with significant risk, especially when systemic health is poor or a patient has a compromised airway. The use of GA, therefore, is carefully considered and often reserved for those with the greatest potential to benefit from such an approach [9].

8.3 Factors Influencing Selection and Application of Behaviour Supports

The clinical judgement involved in selecting an appropriate behaviour support technique is determined by the clinician and patient balancing the risks and benefits of alternative options; occasionally, other people are also consulted, for example, a family member or anaesthetist. This process is underpinned by the ethical principles of least restriction, duty of care, reasonableness and proportionality in efforts to select the 'correct' approach. Patient assessment is the foundation of appropriate behaviour support selection, and it should be framed within the patients' expressed need and preference. The patients' physical health also needs to be considered because knowledge of such conditions will inform the choices available. For example, severe liver disease may contraindicate IV sedation with midazolam, whereas some cyanotic congenital heart defects will contraindicate the use of general anaesthesia. While an in-depth discussion on adjunct selection is outside the scope of this publication, factors usually considered when selecting behaviour supports are listed in Table 8.2. Traditionally, environmental factors have not been central in this decision-making process. We elaborate further on this aspect in the next section.

8.3.1 Sustainability of Different Techniques

So far, in this chapter, we have introduced the topic of behaviour support in dentistry. As demonstrated therein, there are various established criteria to consider before selecting the most appropriate technique(s). In the next section, we will explore the sustainability of these alternatives and introduce a novel factor to consider when selecting adjuncts: environmental sustainability.

Table 8.2 Factors considered in selecting behaviour supports

Ethical	• Duty of care
	• Right to health
	• Right to access of healthcare
	• Right to autonomy
	• Right to minimal restriction
Patient	• Preference
	• Physical health
	• Psychological health
	• Dental anxiety
	• Social circumstance
	• Age
	• Behaviour
	• Communication preference
Operator	• Skills
	• Training
	• Preference
	• Cognitive bias
Procedure	• Urgency
	• Extent
	• Complexity
	• Suitability
	• Cost
	• Logistics
Service	• Availability of pharmacological and psychological services
	• Care pathways
	• Supports
	• Acceptability
	• Appropriateness
Sustainability	1. Environmental resources (consumed by each behavioural support method)
	• Travel fuel (patients and staff)
	• Procurement: (1) plastics, (2) paper, (3) pharmaceuticals, (4) other resources
	• Human resources and associated environmental impact (including administration)
	• Water, electricity, gas
	2. Environmental waste (produced by each behavioural support method)
	• Traditional materials and equipment waste as listed above, which links with procurement
	• Emissions to air and water
	• Travel-associated particulate matter
	• Pharmaceutical waste

8.3.2 Communication-Mediated DBS

Given that each visit on average involves 24 km of return travel and the emission of 3 kg CO_2e, at scale, the need for repeat attendance increases the environmental impact of dental care. Where support need is minimal, it is reasonable to assume that communication-mediated DBS does not drive additional environmental impact. However, as the need for support increases, it is likely the dental team will need to lengthen the procedure time to some degree which, in turn, will increase the length of appointment. Relative to alternative options, communication-mediated behaviour support does not allow for multiple treatments per session. The length of a single session in general practice is limited by a patient's psychological and physical fatigue. Put simply, it is hard to accept a long session of dental care, so treatment plans tend to be divided into manageable sessions of repeated attendance. The environmental impact is exacerbated when communication-mediated behaviour support is delivered as a separate, additional appointment to the actual operative appointment or where care is fragmented to accommodate support need. Examples include graded exposure, CBT, acclimatisation, and systematic desensitisation. All of these techniques traditionally involve repeated exposure to dental stimuli meaning that they work through repeated visits. All involve a patient engaging with an explicit or implicit hierarchy of fear-evoking stimuli, practice or rehearsal, to greater or lesser degrees. CBT and systematic desensitisation, for example, may take up to 10 additional visits, whereas acclimatisation and desensitisation visits typically involve only a couple. Whenever possible, environmentally more sustainable approaches should be considered in this area. One session therapy (OST—an exposure therapy based on a single, therapist-guided, visit), online CBT, virtual reality based exposure, or introductions to clinics and team members via tele-dentistry could all be options. Prevention and early intervention of dental disease, dental anxiety, and behavioural problems offer obvious environmental returns.

In summary, the environmental impact of communication-mediated behaviour support can be mitigated through prevention, early intervention, and maximising the treatments provided per session, limiting physical attendance for exposure-related approaches, and considering reasonable alternative approaches when multiple visits are needed and this is suitable to the patients' needs and preferences.

8.3.3 Inhalation Sedation

The use of nitrous oxide for inhalation sedation (IS) introduces a unique set of environmental challenges regarding clinical attendance, infrastructure, and pharmaceutical disposal.

To carry out treatment using inhalation sedation, a minimum of two staff with accredited training will be required. Both will need to wear appropriate PPE for each individual case. Children will need to have an adult present and travel to and from the clinic can be in a variety of ways: e.g. on foot, public transport, car, or taxi. Adults can attend on their own, or with an escort who can travel as above. The number of visits the patient will require depends on the plan, patient preference and coping capacity.

Children can generally tolerate treatment with IS for 30–40 min. If attending for extractions, treatment can usually be completed in one to two visits. However, where complex restorative treatment is required, the amount of work that can be completed may be more limited, necessitating repeat visits, and therefore increasing travel-associated emissions. The response to IS among children can be unpredictable, and this may result in mouth breathing and increased exhalation into the dental environment rather than through the active scavenging system, which is present as part of double-layered mask. Careful assessment of nitrous oxide products must be taken because nitrous oxide is a powerful climate pollutant, and one of the major long-lived greenhouse gases targeted by the first UNFCCC climate change accord or Kyoto Protocol [10]. It is estimated that nitrous oxide is 298 times more potent than carbon dioxide and can remain in the atmosphere for up to 150 years. Some scientists also describe the gas as the dominant ozone-depleting substance of the twenty-first century. It is estimated that an equivalent of 6% of global carbon dioxide emissions result from nitrous oxide, out of this, 1% originates from medical use in the healthcare sector [11]. This estimation demonstrates that healthcare nitrous oxide emissions have a global impact.

The first step in reducing the environmental impact of nitrous oxide relates to the nature of the delivery system. Dedicated IS units are used to administer a variable mixture of nitrous oxide and oxygen. These units may be stand alone, using portable gas cylinders, or piped systems. Recent investigations of acute hospital sites have shown that vast quantities of piped nitrous oxide products are wasted as a result of antiquated infrastructure, poor product management, and departmental disconnect; this loss is before the nitrous oxide even reaches patients [12]. This evidence has led to quality improvement projects successfully decommissioning obsolete piped systems and has also encouraged further consideration around the use of nitrous oxide products.

Efforts are being made to limit the uncontrolled release of nitrous oxide within clinical settings due to its acute and physiological effects as regulated in working environments by COSHH. Risk reduction is obtained through: selective administration, reducing the length and frequency of use, using minimal flow rate of gases, minimising the concentration of nitrous oxide, appropriate titration, and compulsory scavenging equipment. All active dental breathing systems are designed to a) generate enough flow to scavenge at the recommended 40–45 L/min for the duration of the procedure, and b) carry away the waste gases exhaled by the patient during the procedure to the outside of the surgery and building [13, 14].

However, concern regarding nitrous oxide release should not stop at the surgery door. Typically, nitrous oxide scavenging prevents accumulation in the clinical setting, but anything collected is vented directly into the local environment as there is no provision for its collection and molecular reconfiguration, known as gas capture technology. Nitrous oxide is not metabolised in the body, and its constant molecular state means that all release counts towards Scope 1 emissions.

To mitigate nitrous oxide emissions and use scavenging effectively, services in Sweden have progressed beyond double-layer masks, i.e. nasal hoods currently used in dental settings. Gas capture technology, known as capture and cracking, has been developed: a suction system evacuates exhaled nitrous oxide gas through a full coverage facemask, transporting it through to a nitrous oxide destructor. The destructor purifies the nitrous oxide by breaking it down into oxygen and nitrogen, forming a closed circuit. This is already being used in the equivalent of three large Swedish health boards, with one region installing nitrous oxide destruction systems in all of their emergency hospitals [11].

Measures such as these in areas where nitrous oxide is used often (e.g. maternity wards) can significantly reduce the emissions of nitrous oxide from the health sector. In dentistry, it is not so easy to control nitrous oxide due to the nature of treating the oral cavity—a full facemask covering both the nose and mouth would prevent dental treatment. Therefore, environmental scavenging, capture, and cracking of nitrous oxide is imperative for the dental setting at the present moment in time; we must also be open to novel efficacious inhalation sedation options with a much smaller planetary impact. There is a lot of potential for reducing the climate impact from hospitals and other healthcare facilities by targeting the emissions of nitrous oxide.

8.3.4 Intravenous Sedation

The use of intravenous (IV) sedation introduces a unique set of environmental challenges mainly incorporating dental attendance and equipment. IV sedation has many nuances that increase travel and its associated environmental considerations. Firstly, robust patient assessment is an essential pre-requisite for safe and effective treatment under intravenous sedation and must take place on a separate day to the actual treatment visit. Secondly, access to intravenous sedation may be limited to specific general dental practices, community clinics, and secondary care units. In some areas, the structure of service provision means local facilities may be limited with reliance on patient referral to distant centres thus having an additional environmental impact. Thirdly, patients are advised, where possible, to travel home post-treatment in private transport. They should not use low carbon travel options, such as walking or cycling, owing to the postoperative effects of the sedative agent. Finally, chaperones are necessary for IV sedation, with the resulting need for transport to accompany the patient to the clinic and/or to the patient's residence if they live alone.

The main issues relating to sustainability at the treatment visit relate to equipment and drugs, together with their associated packaging and sterilisation where appropriate. All of these require energy to develop, produce, and transport. Unlike other pharmacological approaches, there are no gaseous emissions, apart from oxygen in some instances. Figure 8.1 illustrates a typical set up for single drug IV sedation.

Fig. 8.1 IV sedation setup

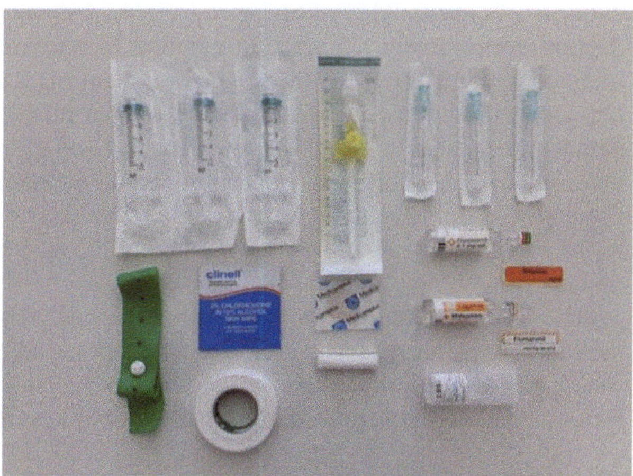

Typical setup for IV sedation with midazolam without oxygen supplementation.

Each episode of intravenous sedation typically requires the following single use items, all of which will be presented in their own disposable packaging:

- Cannulation: disposable tourniquet, cannula, surgical wipe, tape.
- Drugs: midazolam, saline, flumazenil.
- Drug administration: 3 5 mL syringes, 3 drawing up needles, 3 labels, plasters, cotton wool swabs.

8.3.5   General Anaesthesia

Once a patient is anaesthetised, operating conditions are typically favourable and the opportunity arises to complete all the necessary dental treatment required as per applicable guidance [9]. There are few instances where it is necessary to use repeated episodes of GA to deliver a single course of dental treatment, meaning that only one episode of GA is typically required. While this may seem to minimise the environmental impact of care by reducing a) the need for patient transport, b) repeated visits, and c) multi-stage procedures, the need to complete all treatment in a single episode of GA means extensive and cautious planning is required.

In the UK and Ireland, GA is limited to hospital settings [15] meaning primary care services typically refer a patient to a specific service when GA is being considered. Typically, a patient will receive one initial primary care dental visit, one visit to a specialist service, the general anaesthesia itself and, a follow up appointment. UK guidelines detail the requirements for pre-operative assessment [16]. For patients with no significant comorbidities, these assessments may be minimal, however, pre-assessment might identify further investigations needed, e.g. ECG or blood tests, at separate appointments. If local anaesthesia alone is possible, many (but not all) of these investigations might not be indicated.

Once a GA is planned, a new set of resources are required to facilitate treatment. Patients are admitted to a hospital setting and discharged from theatre to a ward for a period of postoperative monitoring. Day-case procedures are suitable for the majority of patients [17] meaning overnight stays and the associated resources for this are not routinely required. In addition to ward staff who admit a patient and monitor their recovery, the theatre environment may, at least, include an anaesthetist, an anaesthetic assistant or operating department practitioner, a scrub nurse, a dental nurse, and a minimum of one dentist. Each of these staff members will have an essential and unique role in promoting patient safety, and each one will require protective equipment at all or some parts of the care process. This PPE is in addition to the vast amount of single-use equipment that is specifically used for the patient themselves.

The process of delivering anaesthesia is itself resource intensive. A far more substantial volume of anaesthetic drugs and gases are required than with any other treatment modality. Anaesthesia can be induced either by intravenous or gaseous routes, but either route precedes intubation. A wide variety of drugs may be required to deliver general anaesthesia. These include, but are not limited to, drugs for anxiolysis, induction of anaesthesia, neuromuscular blockage, analgesia, and antisickness drugs. Anaesthesia is often maintained by a range of gases that have substantial environment impacts [18]. An alternative is the use of TIVA (total intravenous anaesthesia) where a drug (such a remifentanil) is continuously delivered to maintain anaesthesia instead of using a gas. This mitigates the use of anaesthetic gases but is not routinely used or viewed as suitable by all anaesthetists and such an approach is not appropriate in every situation [19]. Discussing anaesthetists' choices and simply starting dialogue over GA practices can change professional behaviour without creating conflict. Considering how routine IV sedation uses a single agent, even one episode of GA is clearly less sustainable in terms of drug usage, even if multiple sedation episodes are required.

An additional environmental cost arises in a theatre setting from the routine use of drapes, gowns and sterile covers. It is typical to see multiple full clinical waste bags after each patient in theatre which, as per infection control protocols, are then replaced in readiness for the next patient.

Following a GA and discharge from hospital a patient is expected to be supported for 24 h. Also, from a safety perspective, travel home by public transport is far from ideal—taxi or private car is preferable. Though, ideally, a person should be dentally fit by the end of a single GA, this does not mean that the environmental impact of such an approach is minimal. The preparation required may mean more visits to a clinical environment are needed than would be required with even a multivisit treatment plan using conscious sedation or local anaesthesia. In addition to the anaesthetic risks and cost of GA, its environmental impact should also induce a sense of caution and ensure this approach is not used routinely. Figure 8.2 illustrates a typical anaesthetic gases. Figure 8.3 illustrates a typical setup for anaesthetic equipment used for induction or maintenance of anaesthesia.

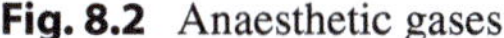

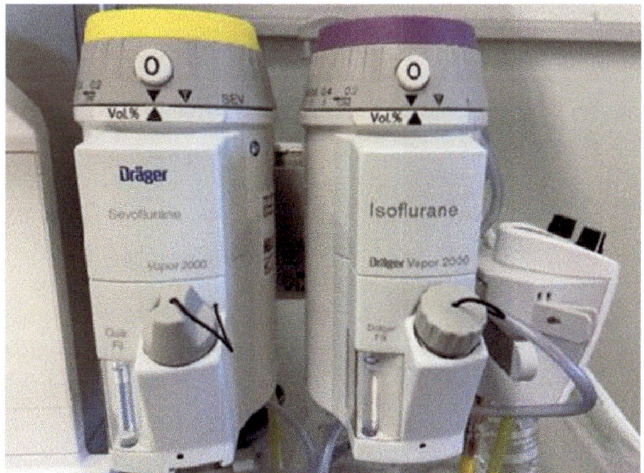

Fig. 8.2 Anaesthetic gases

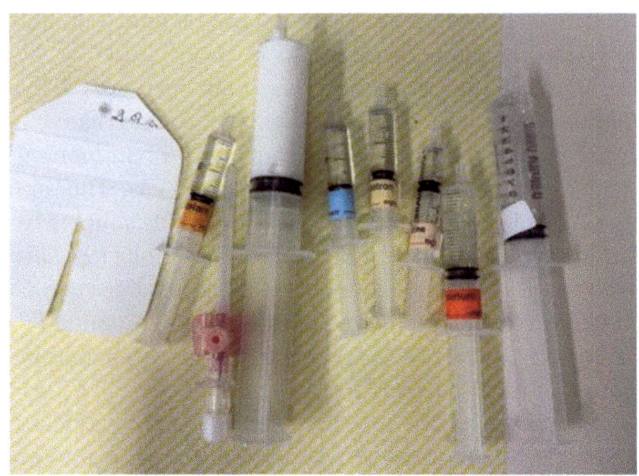

Fig. 8.3 Anaesthetist set up for IV drug delivery

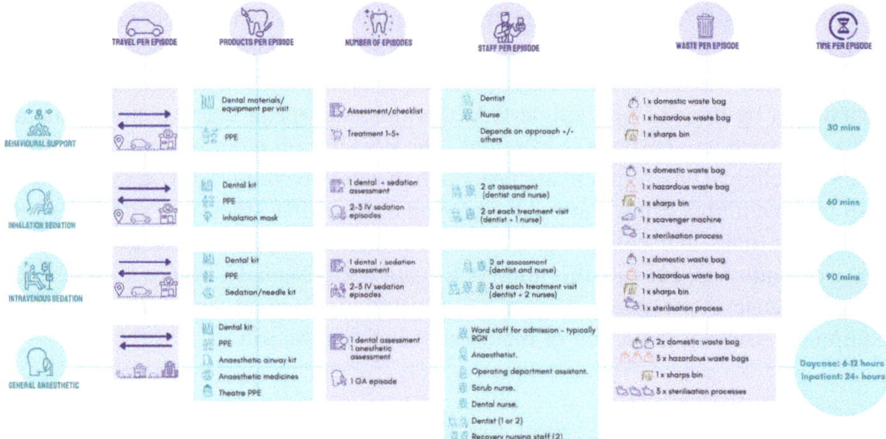

Fig. 8.4 Differential impact of behaviour support techniques on environment

8.4 Comparing Sustainability of Alternative Modalities

For many patients, there is a choice to be made regarding behaviour support techniques, each with their own advantages and disadvantages. Where this choice presents, we argue that clinicians and patients must consider the differential environmental impact of each technique so the behaviour support is as sustainable as reasonably achievable. Variables, such as travel, resources, number of episodes, staff numbers, waste produced, and time required must also be considered. The differential impact of alternatives is further illustrated in Fig. 8.4.

8.5 Sustainability of Dental Behaviour Support (DBS): As Sustainable as Reasonably Acceptable (ASARA)

The above illustrates the need to consider sustainability when selecting and practising all DBS techniques. In this section, we summarise a range of practical steps to mitigate environmental impact of DBS. We do not discuss the benefits of prevention of both oral disease and triggering events that increase the need for behaviour support. Adapting the radiation safety principles of ALARA (as low as reasonably achievable—see Sect. 1.1), we suggest that clinicians operate according to the principles of ASARA (as sustainable as reasonably acceptable). That is, to select and apply DBS techniques in a way that is patient-centred and minimises environmental impact.

8.6 Policy

Policies should be written and based on balanced consideration of all factors relevant to providing DBS; environmental analysis, and planetary impact should be recognised as relevant factors [20]. 'Sustainability' is not simply about offering the least 'carbon intense' option; 'sustainability' means factors pertinent to the individual patient, the population (i.e. as a minimum carbon emission calculation), and overall planetary impact have been considered.

Policy-makers should:

- Ensure person centred DBS is provided as sustainably as reasonably acceptable.
- Develop care pathways that enable sustainable DBS choices for patients and dental teams.
- Ensure a range of local DBS supports, considering travel optimisation in locations with good public transport that minimises both patient and staff travel as well as local contracts, procurements, and supply chains.
- Encourage tele-dentistry as a medium for DBS.
- Incorporate service requirements for the presence and use of environmental technology to capture, neutralise, and/or reuse waste gases.
- Develop low intensity preventive services and health promotion activities, minimising the need for intervention in the first place.

8.7 Leadership

Leadership is required within DBS and the wider dental community to address, support, and establish the changes necessary to reduce the environmental impact of DBS. DBS providers and commissioners need to be guided and informed about how best to decarbonise the delivery of DBS and mitigate its carbon footprint. Leaders in DBS should encourage the profession to:

- Consider patients as partners in their treatment pathways extending understanding of DBS options to include the planetary impact.
- Become carbon literate by embedding planetary health into the context of DBS.

- Innovate in sustainable alternatives to traditional modes of delivering DBS.
- Develop effective methods of preventing and minimising the use of environmentally impactful DBS techniques in dentistry.
- Measure and monitor the environmental sustainability of DBS options using contemporary metrics [21].
- Mediate on behalf of sustainable processes in the recycling and manufacture of equipment and packaging.

8.8 Research and Education

There is a need to educate patients and professionals regarding the environmental impact of DBS options. Many colleges, associations, and postgraduate faculties for medical specialties have declared climate emergencies and formulated subsequent strategies to address and manage individual healthcare groups—similar action is needed specifically relating to dentistry.

Researchers should:

- Develop evidence regarding sustainable DBS using environmental analyses.
- Create and champion specific planet-friendly products and processes for DBS dental professionals and consumers.
- Identify carbon emission "hotspots" within DBS services and clearly illustrate the planetary impact of alternatives.
- Investigate the complex internal drivers and external forces that influence sustainability within DBS.

8.8.1 Dental Education Should

- Embed the concept of sustainability in DBS into undergraduate and postgraduate education.
- Develop the decision-making skills of dental professionals to select and apply DBS adjuncts adopting the principles of ASARA.

8.9 Clinical Practice

Clinically, sustainability within DBS implies selecting care and applying principles prudently to help minimise transport-related emissions, the number of clinical attendances and attendees, as well as emissions and waste [22] to prevent oral disease and conditions requiring resource-intense DBS. Where reasonable, DBS should be practised as follows:

- Plan courses of treatment using sustainable principles, frameworks, and pathways to achieve correct resource use.
- Minimise transport-related emissions.
- Avoid non-essential travel (e.g. by running joint dental/anaesthetic pre-GA assessment clinics).

- Use teledentistry and e-health options where appropriate (e.g. for information gathering and review appointments and, remote communication-mediated techniques such as e-CBT or tele-desensitisation).
- Where reasonable, reduce the number of staff in attendance.
- Where reasonable, maximise treatments undertaken per session.
- Select effective agents.
- Administer medical gases selectively.
- Seek out alternative modalities or alternative drugs.
- Use minimal effective flow rate of gases.
- Minimise the concentration of medical gases.
- Apply appropriate titration where possible with suitable scavenging equipment.
- Ensure there is appropriate infrastructure to minimise emissions and capture gases where possible.

8.10 Conclusion

Patients can be supported in many ways to receive effective and acceptable dental care. The choice of adjunct and the way that adjunct is applied has a modifiable environmental impact. While we cannot disregard the personal responsibilities that we all bear to minimise our need for environmentally costly interventions, the dental team must bear responsibility for the impact that our practices and decisions regarding behaviour support do have. Dental teams should adopt the principles of ASARA when selecting and applying behaviour supports, which implies finding a balance between what is safe, effective, acceptable, and also environmentally sustainable.

Take Home Points for the Dental Team
- Dental behaviour support (DBS) is an essential and valuable aspect of dental care for all patients.
- Different modes of delivery for DBS present different environmental challenges and impacts.
- DBS practitioners should select and apply techniques in a way that is person-centred, safe, effective, and acceptable to the patient.
- DBS should be selected and applied in a way that is as sustainable as reasonably acceptable.
- There are many policy, leadership, educational, research, and clinical opportunities to enhance the sustainability of how dental care is provided to patients.

References

1. Mac Giolla Phadraig C, Newton T, Daly B, et al. BeSiDe time to move behavior support in dentistry from an art to a science: a position paper from the BeSiDe (Behaviour Support in Dentistry) Group. Spec Care Dentist. 2021:1–4. https://doi.org/10.1111/scd.12634.
2. British Society of Paediatric Dentistry. Non-pharmacological behaviour management guideline. (revised 2011). https://www.bspd.co.uk/Portals/0/Public/Files/Guidelines/Non-pharmacological%20behaviour%20management%20.pdf. Accessed 25 June 2021.

3. Clinical Affairs Committee, American Academy of Pediatric Dentistry. Guideline on behavior guidance for the pediatric dental patient. Pediatr Dent. 2015;37:57–5.

4. Roberts JF, Curzon ME, Koch G, Martens LC. Behaviour management techniques in paediatric dentistry. Eur Arch Paediatr Dent. 2010;11(4):166–74.

5. Becker D, M. Rosenberg M. Nitrous oxide and the inhalation anesthetics. Anesth Prog. 2008;55(4):124–30.

6. Standards for Conscious Sedation in the Provision of Dental Care: Report of the Intercollegiate Advisory Committee for Sedation in Dentistry (IACSD). 2020. www.rcseng.ac.uk/dental-faculties/fds/publications-guidelines/standards-for-conscious-sedation-inthe-provision-of-dental-care-and-accreditation/. Accessed 6 July 2021.

7. Conscious Sedation in Dentistry Dental Clinical Guidance. 2017. www.sdcep.org.uk/wp-content/upload/2018/07/SDCEP-conscious-sedation-guidance.pdf. Accessed 6 July 2021.

8. Urban BW, Bleckwenn M. Concepts and correlations relevant to general anaesthesia. Br J Anaesth. 2002;89(1):3–16.

9. Geddis-Regan A, Gray D, Buckingham S, Misra U, Boyle C. The use of general anaesthesia in special care dentistry: clinical guidelines from the British Society for Disability and Oral Health. Spec Care Dentist. 2021;42(S1):3–32. https://doi.org/10.1111/scd.12652.

10. Sulbaek Andersen MP, Sander SP, Nielsen OJ, Wagner DS, Sanford TJ Jr, Wallington TJ. Inhalation anaesthetics and climate change. Br J Anaesth. 2010;105(6):760–6. https://doi.org/10.1093/bja/aeq259. Epub 2010 Oct 8.

11. Dahling S and Wennerhed F. Nordic Know-How 2020: #1 Nitrous Oxide. 2020. https://nordic-shc.org/images/Nordic_know-how_2020_Nitrous_Oxide_2.pdf.

12. Chakera A, Fennell-Wells A, Allen C. Piped nitrous oxide waste reduction strategy. Association of Anaesthetists. 2021. https://anaesthetists.org/Portals/0/PDFs/Environment/Nitrous%20waste%20methodology.pdf?ver=2021-04-26-115439-240. Accessed May 2021.

13. RA Medical Services Ltd. Explanatory overview of dental nitrous oxide scavenger breathing systems. 2017. https://ramedical.com/explanatory-overview-dental-nitrous-oxide-scavenger-breathing-systems/. Accessed Dec 2020.

14. DH Estates and Facilities Directorate. Medical Gases Health Technical Memorandum 02–01: medical gas pipeline systems. Part A: Design, installation, validation and verification. 2006. http://www.bcga.co.uk/assets/HTM_02-01_Part_A.pdf. Accessed Dec 2020.

15. Department of Health. A conscious decision—a review of the use of general anaesthesia and conscious sedation in primary dental care. London: Department of Health; 2000.

16. Key W, Swart M. Chapter 2: Guidelines for the provision of anaesthesia services for preoperative assessment and preparation 2019. London: Royal College of Anaesthetists; 2019.

17. Bailey CR, Ahuja M, Bartholomew K, Bew S, Forbes L, Lipp A, et al. Guidelines for day-case surgery 2019. Anaesthesia. 2019;74:778–92.

18. Royal College of Anaesthetists. Your anaesthetic and the environment. https://rcoa.ac.uk/patient-information/about-anaesthesia-perioperative-care/your-anaesthetic-environment.

19. Nimmo AF, Absalom AR, Bagshaw O, Biswas A, Cook TM, Costello A, Grimes S, Mulvey D, Shinde S, Whitehouse T, Wiles MD, et al. Guidelines for the safe practice of total intravenous anaesthesia (TIVA) Joint Guidelines from the Association of Anaesthetists and the Society for Intravenous Anaesthesia. Anaesthesia. 2019;74(2):211–24.

20. Duane B, Stancliffe R, Miller FA, Sherman J, Pasdeki-Clewer E. Sustainability in dentistry: a multifaceted approach needed. J Dent Res. 2020;99(9):998–1003. https://doi.org/10.1177/0022034520919391.

21. Duane B, Ashley P, Saget S, Richards D, Pasdeki-Clewer E, Lyne A. Incorporating sustainability into assessment of oral health interventions. Br Dent J. 2020;229(5):310–4. https://doi.org/10.1038/s41415-020-1993-9.

22. Duane B, Lee M, White S, Stancliffe R, Steinbach I. An estimated carbon footprint of NHS primary dental care within England. How can dentistry be more environmentally sustainable? Br Dent J. 2017;223:589–93. https://doi.org/10.1038/sj.bdj.2017.839.

Buying Sustainably and Ethically for the Dental Practice (Procurement)

Eleni Pasdeki-Clewer, Sheryl Wilmott, and Brett Duane

9.1 Sustainable Procurement

Improving oral health requires resources and products that may have significant environmental impacts. The way in which dental practices source these (resources and products), and the types of materials and products that they choose (where choice is possible), can help reduce the environmental impacts of dentistry.

9.2 Type of Product

When one looks across Europe, the healthcare sector currently has 2.8 million beds in approximately 13,000 hospitals. In providing this care, the different healthcare sectors purchase, use and dispose of a considerable number of single-use products, building materials, pharmaceuticals, and medical devices. Many of these products have components and/or by-products that can be toxic to staff and patients and can also have serious environmental impacts (e.g., drugs, chemicals, radiation, infectious hazards, air and water pollution). Dentistry forms part of the greater healthcare sector and, as such, has a responsibility to manage and reduce its share of these impacts.

To get a scale of the challenge, within the English NHS Dentistry system, the purchasing of dental goods and services accounts for 19% of the overall carbon

E. Pasdeki-Clewer (✉)
Amersham, England, UK

S. Wilmott
Leeds Teaching Hospitals NHS Trust, Leeds, UK
e-mail: sheryl.wilmott@nhs.net

B. Duane
Trinity College Dublin, Dublin, Ireland
e-mail: brettdu@tcd.ie

impacts of dentistry [1]. Whilst carbon is not the only environmental impact, it is by far the most pressing one and, as such, serves as a good proxy for sustainability.

The English NHS dentistry system calculation was based on analysis carried out using a spend-based model with data from the financial year 2014/15. Whilst the spend-based carbon accounting methodology is imperfect and sensitive to price changes, it offers the authors an acceptable estimation of where the biggest impacts lie which helps us move on from identifying problems to solving them.

There are, of course, alternative ways to estimate the contribution of purchased dental goods and services towards the overall carbon footprint. A life cycle assessment (LCA) (see Chap. 1) provides more accurate results; however, it is resource intensive and costly to undertake.

Analysing and reducing the impacts of our procurement decisions (what we buy) is an integral part of any environmental strategy. When embarking on carbon foot printing, it is advisable to bear in mind that the ultimate goal is to identify ways of reducing emissions and focus action on where it is most likely to bring about the biggest benefits. Striving for analytical accuracy can become a distraction. Deciding on the most effective carbon accounting methodology should be informed by the balance between accuracy and cost.

Dentists and oral healthcare professionals may influence, and ultimately reduce, these impacts through the following interventions:

1. Buy less (buy smarter, be more efficient, improve stock control, review expiry dates) (see Sect. 9.3).
2. Buy better (products with improved impacts, from sustainable suppliers, with minimal or least impactful packaging) (see Sect. 9.4).
3. Educate patients (on effective use of products, preventative care) (see Chap. 5).
4. Collaborate to accelerate the pace of change (work with suppliers, industry groups, and health systems to make this happen) (see Sect. 9.5).

These four interventions will form the basis of this chapter.

9.3 Buy Less

It is often said that the most sustainable purchasing decision is the product you didn't buy. One of the easiest ways to rethink your need and buy less is to opt for reusable devices over disposable, or single-use ones.

Many healthcare practitioners now choose, or are compelled to use, single-use devices. Some of these are mandatory, for example, endodontic files, others are chosen for convenience, for example, disposable gowns. Whilst the former are medically necessary to reduce infection risks, the latter are potentially not.

On the face of it, single-use instruments, and the need to produce, package, transport, and then dispose of them, appears to be less ecologically sound. This may often be true; however, such decisions should be based on analysis of the pros and cons of each approach using an LCA or equivalent (i.e. how much energy, carbon and resources each product uses). Until environmental guidance in this area is available, dentists need to consider the appropriate cross-infection and de-contamination guidance (e.g. HTMO5—Health Technical Memoranda) when choosing instruments [2].

In Byrne's paper [3], we looked at the environmental impact of a disposable dental kit compared with a recycled kit. As anticipated, the disposable kits had a significantly higher environmental impact across all categories including minerals and metals, climate change, freshwater use, etc. (see Fig. 9.1).

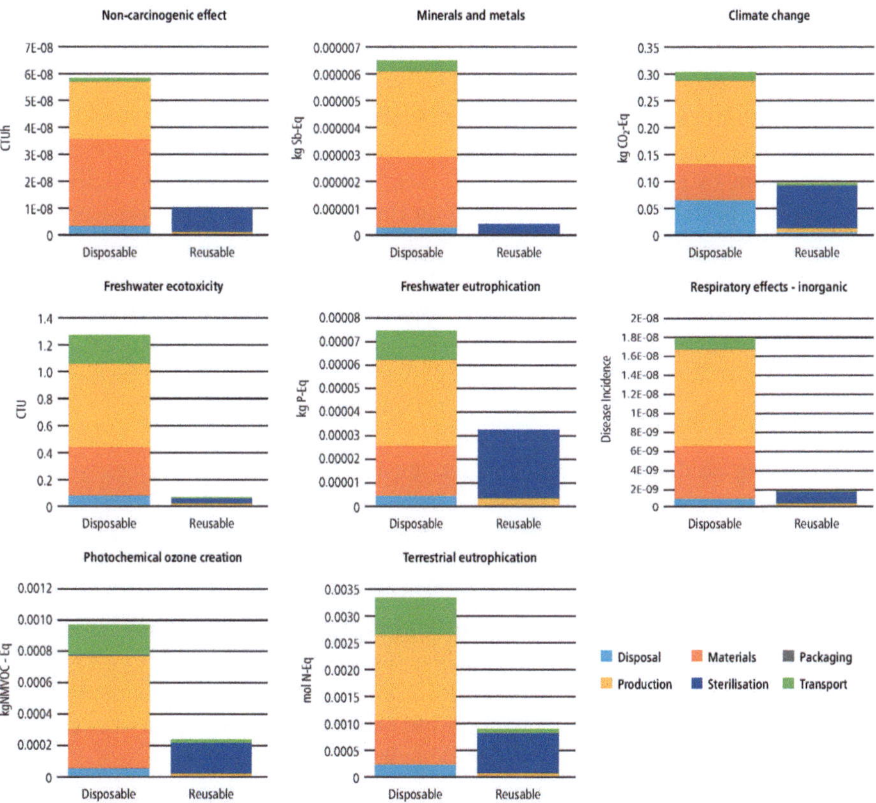

Fig. 9.1 Contribution analysis for reusable versus disposable examination kits

From this analysis, it is clear manufacturing/production is the largest contributor to the environmental impacts of a kit. It contributes between 18 and 69% towards the disposable kit, and less in the reusable kit, Unger and Landis' study of single-use versus reusable dental burs aligns with Byrne's study, demonstrating a 40% larger CO_2 emission-total associated with disposable burs [4].

On the other hand, from a decontamination perspective, we understand that the evidence behind using reusable versus disposable wipes is less robust [5]. Single-use disposable wipes offer a more consistent approach to decontamination, but they do have a significant life cycle impact (see Chap. 7). We suspect reusable wipes have a lower environmental footprint, but the quality of the wipe and the ability for decontamination (with a potential for cross-contamination) may be less. Currently, there is no definitive evidence that one is better than the other.

9.3.1 Stock Control

Appropriate stock management should be considered a requirement by the dental team. One hospital in Australia, for example, implemented a stock management system to provide staff with efficient access to products to deliver safe patient care in the right place, at the right time. For financial and environmental reasons, the dental team needs to ensure supplies are used in date order and not available for use beyond their expiry date and, to that end, only order the number of supplies needed. Consideration should also be given to the environmental consequences of transporting the goods to the practice together with the packaging they come in.

There are several ways to reduce the need to buy, including:

- Focussing on the most used items the most expensive items, or ones with short shelf lives.
- Having a system or a designated person to oversee stock management.
- Minimising orders.
- Checking items routinely and having a well-organised stock room.
- Auditing what you use yearly; this may make you consider your most frequently purchased products, and to analyse their sustainability.
- Establishing supplier partnerships with companies who support your sustainability ideals—ask questions about shelf-life extension, for example, what could go wrong if shelf life is exceeded (see Table 9.1).

Table 9.1 Suggested questionnaire for manufacturers

Nos	Sustainability question	Score = 0	Score = 1	Score = 2
1a	Does the supplier have an approach to manage their environmental impact?	No	In progress	Yes*
1b	If no, are they willing to put one in place?	No	Unsure	Yes
2a	Can the supplier trace the product back to the original country of origin?	No		Yes
2b	If yes, please state the country of origin			
3	Are substantial amounts of activity in the supply chain undertaken where no effective labour standards legislation (or enforcement of these standards) exists?	Yes or no, and the product is produced in a country which ranks poorly on the ITUS list (see notes)	No. The product is produced in the following country__________, a country which ranks moderately on the ITUC list (see notes).	No. The product is produced in the following country__________, a country which ranks highly on the ITUC list (see notes below)
4a	Is the product content: (please tick all that apply)	None of this content		Biodegradable Recyclable Contains recycled content Reusable Remanufactured
4b	If no, is the supplier/manufacturer willing to change their product content?	No		Yes
5	Is the delivery of the product undertaken in an efficient manner to reduce emissions to the local environment?	No	Sometimes	Yes
6a	Is the product's packaging: (please tick all that apply) content/reusable/remanufactured?	No, this does not apply to this product's packaging		Biodegradable Recyclable Contains recycled content Reusable Remanufactured
6b	If no, is the supplier/manufacturer willing to change their packaging?	No		Yes
7	Would the supplier be prepared to collect all packaging from their products?	No		Yes

1 Generally, it is useful for a supplier to have a policy with a robust implementation plan supported by a measurement and public reporting structure. A dental practice should consider whether it has its own policy and plan first in order that it can 'practice what it preaches' (see Duane for advice.)

2 This question can be useful for dental practices to help them understand the environmental and social requirements within the country. There are a number of ways dental practices can consider different countries. The Environmental Performance Index ranks a country's performance in sustainability related matters. [48] Within this index Switzerland ranks highest, with the UK having a score of 6 and China a score of 120. Although this index is a broad-brush approach to determining the sustainability of products, countries who score highly exhibit excellent commitment to public health protection, the preservation of natural resources and reductions in greenhouse gases.

3 Similar to other areas of healthcare, information relating to ethical manufacturers of dental products is hard to find. [49] There is, however, a useful index of countries produced by the International Trade Union Confederation (2018) which ranks countries for worker's rights. This may assist dental practices when considering where they purchase products from.

4 The terms reduce, reuse and recycle all help to cut down on the amount of waste that is produced. The ideal product/packaging would conserve as much as possible natural resources, landfill, space and energy. [50] The manufacturing/packaging sector can be innovative and materials, such as biological based materials, may partially replace crude oil as an input material for plastics in the future.

5 The SDU's (Sustainable Development Unit) Health Outcomes of Travel Tool (HOTT) will assist organisations to measure the impact their travel has on environmental indices, including air and noise pollutions. [51] This can assist suppliers in helping reduce the NHS impact on the environment from travel associated emissions.

6 See 4

7 In some French supermarkets recycling bins are placed at exits with a view to encouraging consumers to remove packaging from items purchased before they leave the supermarket. [52] Increasingly some companies are taking back their own products to recycle or repurpose and this can include their packaging. [53]

9.4   Buy Better

In this section, we explore the concept of the *ideal product*; its characteristics, physical performance, and/or attributes (see Box 9.1).

> **Box 9.1 The Ideal Product**
> The ideal product will be optimally balanced across the following considerations:
>
> 1. Safe for the patient
> 2. Fit for purpose
> 3. Not fossil fuel based
> 4. Grown—but able to be reused repeatedly, or able to be reused with local processing
> 5. Supplied in sustainable or minimal packaging
> 6. Biodegradable into harmless natural environmental elements
> 7. Easy to clean and reuse, where possible
> 8. Simple, i.e. not a complex product difficult to recycle
> 9. Transported with clean vehicles or 'made' at the point of care
> 10. Produced with renewable energy
> 11. Manufactured in ways that do not involve abuse of labour
> 12. Involving suppliers and supply chains that espouse good environmental management and protection
> 13. Inexpensive

Let's consider some of the principles mentioned above in more detail.

9.4.1 Safe for the Patient and the Dental Team

The product must be safe for the patient. In reality, insufficient research has been undertaken to know the exact safety of each product we use. From a restorative perspective, we are aware that there is potential health harm when mercury is released from amalgams [6].

A review of the literature comparing the use of amalgam versus composite restorations showed only some differences between amalgam and composite resin in terms of renal, neuropsychological, and psychosocial function; however, no consistent or clinically important harms were found [7].

Concerns have been raised regarding the materials in composites—such as bisphenol A diglycidyl methacrylate (bis-GMA)—however, the amount of bis-GMA released is probably less than that released from plastic food and drink containers [7].

Of course, the safety of a restoration is not the only consideration within dental practices. We also know that the use of chemicals can cause global deaths and additional disability-adjusted life years (DALYs). A review of cleaners showed a deterioration in lung function in people who cleaned domestically and identified a need to prevent exposure of cleaning agents to reduce this deterioration. Significantly more research is needed to help healthcare professionals understand which products are safe and which less so. Until this happens, dental teams should reduce the amount of chemicals being used and consider training staff about the chemicals that are purchased. There are often alternatives to the cleaning products being used in the non-clinical areas of dental practices. 'Healthcare Without Harm' provides a good description of alternatives to many household products online, with government buying standards available for cleaning products [8]. Alternatives include the use of vinegar, baking soda, lemon juice, and ordinary household soap.

9.4.2   Fit for Purpose

Products used within the dental practice need to be fit for purpose. Ideally, any restoration placed lasts a considerable amount of time; however, we know this isn't always the case. Low-certainty evidence suggests that composite resin restorations have almost double the failure rate of amalgam restorations. The risk of restoration fracture does not appear to be higher with composite resin restorations, but there is a much higher risk of developing secondary caries [9]. As a profession, we need to be advocating low frequency sugar diets and optimising the use of fluorides to reduce the need for any restoration, and then do all we can to ensure restorations last.

We need to also ensure that if we opt for more sustainable preventive options. One example is to ensure that any non-nylon bristles in a toothbrush are as effective at removing plaque as nylon bristles. We urgently need more research in this area.

9.4.3   Not Fossil Fuel Based

In recent years, healthcare practices have increasingly gravitated towards single-use or single-patient solutions for patient safety and efficiency purposes. Plastic has served the health sector well in providing inexpensive and customisable products for patients. However, single-use plastics have significant environmental impacts not only because they pollute but also from an embedded carbon perspective, as they are the product of an energy-intensive process [10]. Whilst the evidence in support of a shift away from fossil-based to bio-based plastics is still developing, bio-based solutions are increasingly being considered as viable alternatives [11, 12].

Bio-based polymers are a fast-developing sector [13]. They have great potential for bringing about added benefits when compared to conventional plastics; not only are they decoupled from fossil fuels but also they can have improved properties [13, 14]. Feedstocks for bio-based plastics do not compete with or displace food-crops—but rather act as part of the broader industrial symbiotic relationships that can support our transition to a more circular economy [15–17].

An example of a waste-based bio-plastic is MarinaTex. MarinaTex is a bioplastic of equal strength to low-density polyethylene (LDPE) and is made using waste products from the fishing industry [18].

Our ideal situation is a process where a product can be used, then recycled in-house, or shredded, autoclaved and then reconstituted into a new product. In our toothbrush study [19], we demonstrated that a toothbrush recycling scheme (not currently available) produced only 10.3% of the carbon footprint of a conventional toothbrush which is not recycled [19]. Even though bamboo brushes seem better from a carbon perspective, imagine the amount of land that would be required to grow sufficient bamboo to manufacture enough brushes for the whole planet!

The thinking we would like to encourage with this analysis is that of a conscious consumer; one who considers the impact of the product they are buying on a whole-life basis before making a purchasing decision.

9.4.4   Grown: But Able to Be Reused Repeatedly, or Able to Be Reused with Local Processing

Ultimately, in the manufacturing of dental products, our objective should be to move towards renewable materials and resources. This means, wherever possible, opting for products that are a) made from materials that are grown rather than being fossil-based, b) that require minimal land-use, or c) can be grown on non-arable land (so as not to displace food crops).

In our example of dental products, alternatives to plastic toothbrushes could be sold and/or promoted, for example, bamboo toothbrushes or toothbrushes with replaceable heads.

In order to make a more informed product choice, the reader needs to consider the different definitions of products. According to European Bioplastics, a plastic material is defined as a bioplastic if it is either biobased, biodegradable, or features both properties [20]. The term 'biobased' means that the material or product is (partly) derived from biomass (plants). Biomass used for bioplastics stems from, for example, corn, sugarcane, or cellulose. A product is able to be called biobased even if it only has, for example, 1% of its mass from a grown product.

Care should be taken to avoid unintended consequences, for example, bio-based materials may be mistaken for virgin plastics in waste management processes and therefore compromise segregation and recycling rates.

9.4.5   Supplied in Sustainable Packaging

9.4.5.1 Recycling and Packaging

The dental team should also consider how manufacturers manage both packaging and recycling, i.e. they need to consider the fundamental principles of 'reduce, re-use, and recycle'. This might include, for example, consolidation of delivery, reusing packaging, and the size, type of material and quality of the packaging itself. Packaging should be minimal, recyclable without marketing and promotional impact. There are examples of manufacturers who are beginning to promote their 'greener' products in packaging that 'sells' the greener idea, for example, unbleached paper, no plastic coating, minimal design, and inking [21].

In Duane's paper, we showed the benefits of recycling, in this instance, a toothbrush [22]. The power of recycling can be seen from both a climate change perspective and a disability-adjusted life year perspective. Based on a leading European factory that produces 28 million toothbrushes per year, a potential 374 tonnes of carbon equivalent emissions can be removed by simply replacing plastic blister packaging with a printed, recycled cardboard—as well as reducing the DALY harm by 25 years.

If we could overcome, the decontamination issues with recycling toothbrushes as part of a circular economy, we could reduce the environmental footprint of a plastic toothbrush to just 10% of its current impact [22].

Ideally, manufacturers should provide recycling information for their products in user manuals and/or offer to recycle the equipment they produce. Requesting such information might encourage manufacturers to make products that are easily recyclable, can be upcycled, or re-purposed. Some companies have programmes that take back and recycle their own equipment to ensure the disposal of all electronic products and materials are managed appropriately. Recycling could in turn generate cost savings for dental practices: for more information, see Waste within the dental practice, in this series (Chap. 10).

Box 9.2 Circular Economy

A circular economy is an alternative to a traditional linear economy (make, use, dispose) in which we keep resources in use for as long as possible, extract the maximum value from them whilst in use, then recover and regenerate products and materials at the end of each service life.

As part of the European Union's Circular economy action plan, the EU is introducing measures such as making sustainable products the norm, empowering consumers, and focussing on areas where the potential for circularity is high, such as in dentistry, batteries, packaging, and plastics. The plan would ensure also less waste is produced.

9.4.6 Biodegradable into Harmless Natural Environmental Elements

First, we would like to discuss the difference between *biobased, bioplastic*, and *biodegradable*.

> **Bioplastics** are a whole family of materials with different properties and applications. According to European Bioplastics, a plastic material is defined as a bioplastic if it is either biobased, biodegradable, or both [20].
>
> **Biobased:** The term 'biobased' means that the material or product is (***partly***) derived from biomass (plants). Biomass is used for bioplastics stems from, for example, corn sugarcane or cellulose.
>
> **Biodegradation** is a chemical process during which microorganisms that are available in the environment convert materials into natural substances such as water carbon dioxide and compost (artificial additives are not needed). The process of biodegradation depends on the surrounding environmental conditions (e.g. location or temperature) on the material and on the application [20].

The reader should ensure they are familiar with this definition.

A biobased plastic doesn't necessarily biodegrade. A biodegradable plastic isn't necessarily biobased. In Fig. 9.2, we can see that there are bioplastics that are derived from fossil fuels and bioplastics which are derived from plant material (but doesn't need to be 100% plant, i.e. it could include some fossil fuel plastic). From a biodegradable perspective, bioplastics don't necessarily biodegrade, and even when they do they may not biodegrade into harmless materials.

To summarise the term 'Biobased' does not equal 'biodegradable'.

The property of biodegradation does not depend on the resource basis of a material but is rather linked to its chemical structure. In other words, 100% biobased plastics may be non-biodegradable, and 100% fossil-based plastics can biodegrade (but not necessarily into harmless matter).

With this in mind, we advocate that any product used in dentistry should be 100% biodegradable into harmless natural environmental elements. To do this, it needs to be 100% of plant matter.

9.4.7 Easy to Clean and Reuse, Where Possible Without Causing More Harm Than Good

Single-use plastics are used both in medical settings and everyday life. Convenience, sterility and relatively low purchasing cost make their use widespread. Using the 'reduce, reuse, and recycle', model can help in the reduction of overall plastic use. Opting for products that follow this model will help promote a change in the market

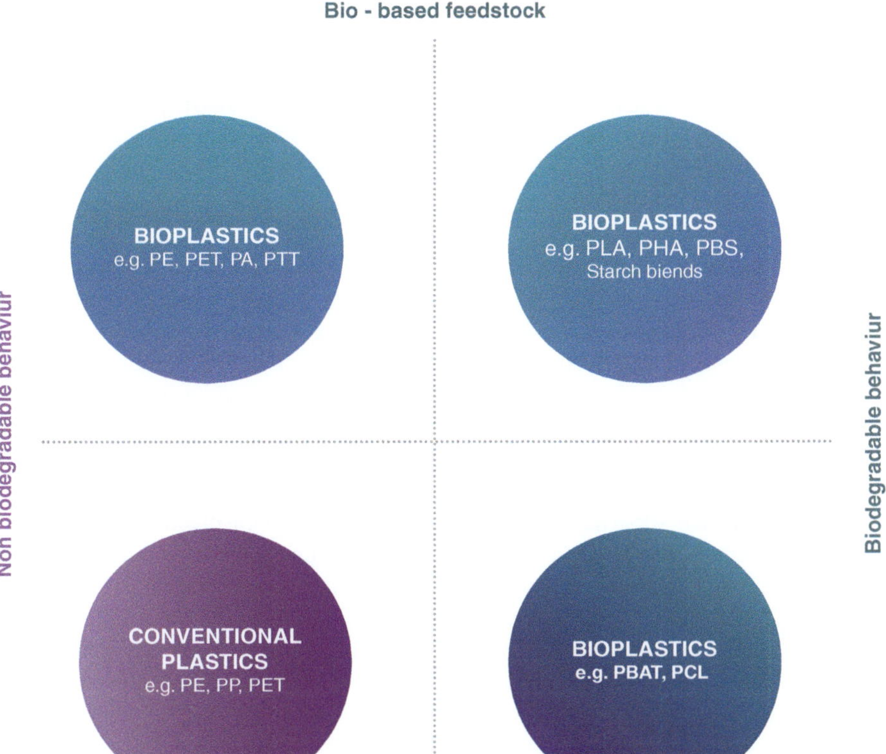

Fig. 9.2 Complexity of the term bioplastics

and drive an increase in the supply and availability of such products. For example, some suppliers offer disposable wipe refills for their plastic containers, thus allowing the containers to be reused time and time again. Opting for such products will not only establish them in the market but also encourage their growth.

9.4.8 Simple, i.e. Not a Complex Product That's Difficult to Recycle

The problem with a number of oral hygiene products is their complexity (see Chap. 11 for more detail). We need to ensure, wherever possible, that products can be easily broken down into recyclable parts.

The amount of plastic being recycled varies from country to country and also relates to the actual type of plastic. In Europe, the amount varies from 4.5% (furniture) to 39.9% (packaging) [23]. This variation stems from issues around contamination and the sheer diversity of the products being disposed of. To assist in the recycling process, oral health products need to be clearly marked with recycling codes to add in this process. Future technology might help with chemical recycling processes, such as pyrolysis which are able to convert plastic waste that is not easily recyclable through mechanical means into monomers that can subsequently be built up into polymers [24, 25].

One example of a difficult-to-recycle product is an electric toothbrush. This is because, for example, it has multiple components, nylon bristles are difficult to remove, and toothbrushes are considered to be contaminated, thus resulting in them presumably being placed in landfill waste. We are aware that the company Terracycle [26] takes a wide variety of spent oral health products and uses chemical and mechanical recycling processes to convert them into a variety of serviceable products, such as outdoor furniture and decking, plastic shipping pallets, watering cans, and storage containers.

In some French supermarkets, recycling bins have been placed at exits with a view to encouraging consumers to remove the packaging from the items they have bought before they leave the supermarket. Increasingly some companies are actively taking back their own spent products to recycle or repurpose, including the packaging. In Lynes' toothbrushing paper, we hypothesised the creation of supermarket recycling bins for toothbrushes and calculated the environmental savings inherent in this process [22].

9.4.9   Transported with Clean Vehicles or Locally

Although not factored directly into our dental carbon footprint [27], dental practices should consider the carbon emissions and the air pollution impact associated with the way they purchase goods. Carbon emissions and air pollution impact will be reduced if the products purchased came from one logistics centre in a single delivery and, ideally, were produced locally. Products that are transported in bulk have surprisingly low travel-associated carbon emissions, for example, bananas [28]. Products that are air freighted, or express transported separately, have much higher footprints [29].

The dental team should ensure that someone is always available to accept deliveries, thus avoiding the need for a repeat journey by the delivery company.

From a dental laboratory perspective, the closest laboratory will have the lowest travel-associated carbon emissions and is therefore assumed to have a lower air pollution impact. Larger practices may be able to influence their dental laboratory to bulk-deliver their products. They might also be able to influence their laboratory to become more sustainable, perhaps utilising similar sustainable initiatives as discussed in the BDJ series [30–36].

It may also be possible for a practice to reduce its overall travel-associated carbon footprint and air pollution impact by combining a staff members' commute with the laboratory drop off and/or pick up.

We know that air pollution is a significant cause of both population and planetary harm [37]. We also know that locally made products can significantly reduce overall environmental emissions. Within the toothbrush study by Lyne [19], transport accounted for more than half of the contribution of nearly all environmental factors.

9.4.10 Produced with Renewable Energy

Products manufactured using renewable energy have a much lower environmental impact than products produced from an energy source which is predominantly high in fossil fuels. The use of renewable energy can be facilitated by supplier engagement and a push towards renewable energy use throughout the manufacturing supply chain. Both buyers/consumers and legislators have a role to play in driving this change.

In our toothpaste study [19], we noted that the electricity used for manufacturing contributed 10% to the overall climate change impact of 1 tube of 1450 ppm sodium fluoride toothpaste. If the manufacturing process was undertaken using renewable energy (see our chapter on renewable energy, Chap. 4), these impacts would be significantly reduced (perhaps almost negligible) across most areas.

Although the origin of a fuel source might be complicated for the dental team to understand, there are two points than can be considered, i.e. the products country of origin and asking the manufacturer whether reusable energy was used in making the product. In 2020, 36.6% of world-wide energy was generated from renewable sources. Some common areas where dental products are manufactured include Europe (renewable energy 49.2%), Germany (renewable energy 56.3%), China (renewable energy 40.6%), the United Kingdom (renewable energy 45.2%), and the United States (renewable energy 25.4%). It is therefore more likely that, for example, if a product is made in Germany, that the manufacturing process would use renewable energy compared with a similar product being produced in the United States [38].

9.4.11 Manufactured in Ways That Do Not Involve Abuse of Labour

Mahmood provides a useful outline of the many concerns associated with the production of healthcare goods and the abuse of labour rights in countries with low wage costs, a high prevalence of unskilled workforce, and poor governance practices [39]. As Mahmood suggests poor labour conditions should concern all those in health care. These labour conditions include inadequate wages, long exhausting working hours, bullying, harassment violence, and even imprisonment.

The BMA has produced a workbook to help identify and protect labour rights in healthcare supply chains [40]. It contains both policy-driven interventions and practical steps that can be taken by procurement teams. Today's globalised, and largely opaque, supply chains add to the challenge of ensuring these rights are observed throughout the supply base. Off-the-shelf, due diligence IT products abound and may be a useful investment for procurement teams to consider. Collaboration is crucial in effecting change; often buyers have limited influence over suppliers when acting independently of each other. Collaboration amongst the procurement profession (supporting and driving industry-specific approaches for high-risk sectors, and engaging with pressure groups and government organisations), will help edge closer to more transparent and cruelty-free supply chains. However, it is important to maintain perspective and be realistic about expectations and anticipated outcomes from such approaches—progress is generally slow and new labour exploitative approaches may emerge in the meantime.

9.4.12 Involving Suppliers and Supply Chains That Espouse Good Environmental Management Protection

The high environmental impact of dental products and services is not solely because of the manufacturing processes that were involved in their making. Ultimately, we should be aiming to buy and use *sustainable products* from *sustainable suppliers*. There are several ways in which a procurer may explore a supplier's environmental credentials, and equally many ways for a supplier to showcase their progressive work in this area. So as to avoid engaging with suppliers that have a lack of commitment or poor governance practices, corporate-level environmental credentials could be an area for consideration during the supplier selection process. This is an effective yet relatively high-risk approach, which is dependent on sector maturity, criticality of the supplier and can also lead to delays in sourcing; setting the environmental bar too high may exclude suppliers whose products are a good solution but who may lack corporate environmental credentials. Environmental credentially also be included within the terms and conditions of thus binding the supplier to certain expectations (note: whether the supplier is adhering to these would need to be explored directly with the supplier) [41]. The most realistic intervention is likely to come in the shape of 'supplier-relationship-management' programmes, involving collaboration with contracted suppliers to create transparency and improvement programmes. The questionnaire (see Table 9.1) includes suggested questions that could be used to frame this requirement to a dental practice's suppliers.

However, because the levels of spend are so high in health care, the medical community also has the capacity to influence and impact global trade, and consequently global health.

9.4.13 Inexpensive

Clearly the issue of practice expenses is pivotal to any well-managed business, and any product needs to be affordable!

> Buying better example: Grocery items when purchasing supermarket-type items, such as tea and coffee, the dental team should consider the purchasing of items with social or environmental accreditation such as Fairtrade or Rainforest Alliance items. As one example, Fairtrade is a governance system designed to deliver sustainable livelihoods and development opportunities to small-scale independent farmers, who often struggle to gain fair access to markets. The Fairtrade system guarantees a fair price to farmers and includes participatory governance, capacity building, and long-term performance goals for buyers.

Box 9.3 Stationery Suggestions
Buying better example: Stationery

- Print in black and white—not colour
- Print using both sides of the paper (double-sided)
- Ensure printer default settings are on environmentally friendly printing
- Print in a smaller font size
- Reuse non-identifiable paperwork a second time, for example, for writing notes/appointments down
- Use recycled paper or, if not appropriate/acceptable, use sustainably produced paper, for example, FSC (Forest Stewardship Council) certified paper
- Don't buy glossy, coloured, or plastic-coated paper
- Prioritise electronic communication, invoicing, etc.
- Send emails with links to appropriate educational videos rather than handing out leaflets/paper information (e.g. YouTube)
- Make use of reusable or refillable products, or products made from post-consumer production (e.g. the household waste we all produce)
- Use stationery with recycle symbols to facilitate appropriate waste management
- Purchase wooden furniture from forestry certification programmes. Examples of these are the Forest Stewardship Council (FSC), DEFRA's timber and procurement policy, and the Programme for the Endorsement of Forest Certification (PEFC).

9.5 Collaborating to Accelerate the Pace of Change

Globally, the dental profession needs to consider how they can influence manufacturers to become more environmentally sustainable. Activism may be a way for the dental team to influence procurement. Activism has been successful in a number of campaigns seeking to improve working conditions; one example being the successful pressure put on Nike to change its employees' working conditions. Other successful campaigns by Greenpeace have encouraged companies such as Nike to stop dumping toxic chemical waste into waterways [42].

The dental team needs to question the industry regarding the sustainability of their products. The Green Impact Tool encourages the dental team to engage directly with manufacturers and to communicate their practices' sustainability, ethical, and labour commitment [43]. In larger NHS healthcare settings, healthcare professionals are bound by procurement regulations; however, most dental teams are free to source items from whichever supplier they choose.

9.5.1 Sustainability and Ethical Procurement Questionnaire

In our BDJ paper, we discussed the use of the sustainability and ethical procurement questionnaire which we developed. This questionnaire is similar to those used within other areas, for example, at Kaiser Permanente [44]. If dental practices consider using only companies who provide sustainable and ethical products, a significant environmental change could result. Practices could also establish buying cooperatives with other practices to increase their influence in the marketplace. The questionnaire we have inserted (see Table 9.1) has been reproduced with permission from our BDJ procurement paper [35].

The questionnaire should be considered a checklist to encourage dental practices to consider various factors when purchasing products. A scoring system is also suggested to rank viable alternatives. Products which score more highly on this table could be prioritised against others (see Table 9.1).

Procurement consists of a series of stages, including planning, supplier sourcing, preparation of documents, invitation to tender, evaluation, and contract management. At each stage, there are a number of opportunities to make the process more sustainable. To avoid 'greenwashing', a procurement tender should include detailed environmental specifications (these can be sourced from Table 9.1). Each specification should use an evaluation criterion.

Take Home Points for the Dental Team

- Around one fifth (19%) of the dental footprint is embedded within the goods and services that the dental team buys.

- The dental team should not consider single-use goods unless mandated through patient safety and/or legislation.
- The dental profession needs to influence suppliers to become more environmentally sustainable in manufacture, packaging, travel, recycling, and reuse.

References

1. Duane B, Berners Lee M, White S, Stancliffe R, Steinbach I. An estimated carbon footprint of NHS primary dental care within England. How can dentistry be more environmentally sustainable? Br Dent J. 2017;223:589–93.
2. NHS England. Decontamination in primary care dental practices. https://www.england.nhs.uk/publication/decontamination-in-primary-care-dental-practices-htm-01-05/.
3. Byrne—Awaiting acceptance. contact BDJ for more information. https://www.nature.com/articles/s41415-022-4912-4.
4. Unger SR, Landis AE. Comparative life cycle assessment of reused versus disposable dental burs. Int J Life Cycle Assess. 2014;19:1623–31.
5. Boyce JM. A review of wipes used to disinfect hard surfaces in health care facilities. Am J Infect Control. 2021;49(1):104–14. https://doi.org/10.1016/j.ajic.2020.06.183. Epub 2020 Jun 19.
6. Mulligan S, Kakonyi G, Moharamzadeh K, Thornton S, Martin N. The environmental impact of dental amalgam and resin-based composite materials. Br Dent J. 2018;224:542–8.
7. Khangura SD, Seal K, Esfandiari S, et al. Composite resin versus amalgam for dental restorations: a health technology assessment. Health Technology Assessment Report No. 147. Ottawa (ON): Canadian Agency for Drugs and Technologies in Health; 2018. https://www.ncbi.nlm.nih.gov/books/NBK531946/.
8. Health Care Without Harm. Cleaners and disinfectants. 2019. https://noharm-uscanada.org/issues/us-canada/cleaners-and-disinfectants.
9. Rasines Alcaraz MG, Veitz-Keenan A, Sahrmann P, Schmidlin PR, Davis D, Iheozor-Ejiofor Z. Direct composite resin fillings versus amalgam fillings for permanent or adult posterior teeth. Cochrane Database Syst Rev. 2014;3:CD005620. https://doi.org/10.1002/14651858.CD005620.pub2.
10. BPF. How is plastic made? A simple step-by-step explanation. https://www.bpf.co.uk/plastipedia/how-is-plastic-made.aspx#:~:text=In%20the%20refining%20process%2C%20crude,a%20large%20amount%20of%20plastic.
11. Walkerab S, Rothmanab R. Life cycle assessment of bio-based and fossil-based plastic: a review. 2020; Journal of Cleaner Production, 261:121158.
12. European Council. All products based on fossil fuels could be made from biomass—Dr. Philippe Mengal. https://ec.europa.eu/research-and-innovation/en/horizon-magazine/all-products-based-fossil-fuels-could-be-made-biomass-dr-philippe-mengal.
13. Cywar RM, Rorrer NA, Hoyt CB, et al. Bio-based polymers with performance-advantaged properties. Nat Rev Mater. 2021;7:83–103. https://doi.org/10.1038/s41578-021-00363-3.
14. Nicholson SR, Rorrer NA, Carpenter AC and Beckham GT. Manufacturing energy and greenhouse gas emissions associated with plastics consumption. Joule. 2021. https://doi.org/10.1016/j.joule.2020.12.027.
15. British Plastics Federation. Bio-based plastics: feedstocks, production and the UK market. https://www.bpf.co.uk/plastipedia/polymers/biobased_plastics_feedstocks_production_and_the_uk_market.aspx.
16. Rameshkumar S, Parameswaran S, O'Connor KE, Babu R. Bio-based and biodegradable polymers—state-of-the-art, challenges and emerging trends. Curr Opin Green Sustain Chem. 2019;21:75–81.

17. Lambert S, Wagner M. Environmental performance of bio-based and biodegradable plastics: the road ahead. Chem Soc Rev. 2017;46(22):6855–71. https://doi.org/10.1039/c7cs00149e.
18. MarinaTex. A home compostable alternative to plastic film. https://www.marinatex.co.uk.
19. Lyne A, Ashley P, Saget S, Porto Costa M, Underwood B, Duane B. Combining evidence-based healthcare with environmental sustainability: using the toothbrush as a model. Br Dent J. 2020;229(5):303–9. https://doi.org/10.1038/s41415-020-1981-0.
20. European Bioplastics. https://www.european-bioplastics.org/bioplastics/.
21. Beardwood. Colgates bamboo toothbrush. https://beardwood.com/updates/sustainable-packaging-design-colgates-bamboo-toothbrush/.
22. Duane B, Ashley P, Saget S, Richards D, Pasdeki-Clewer E, Lyne A. Incorporating sustainability into assessment of oral health interventions. Br Dent J. 2020;229(5):310–4. https://doi.org/10.1038/s41415-020-1993-9.
23. European Parliament News. Plastic waste and recycling in the EU: facts and figures. https://www.europarl.europa.eu/news/en/headlines/society/20181212STO21610/plastic-waste-and-recycling-in-the-eu-facts-and-figures.
24. Chemical and Engineering news. Plastic has a problem; is chemical recycling the solution? https://cen.acs.org/environment/recycling/Plastic-problem-chemical-recycling-solution/97/i39.
25. Armenise S, Syieluing W, Ramírez-Velásquez J, Launay F, Wuebben D, et al. Plastic waste recycling via pyrolysis: a bibliometric survey and literature review. J Anal Appl Pyrolysis. 2021;158:105265. https://doi.org/10.1016/j.jaap.2021.105265.
26. Terracycle. How we recycle. https://www.terracycle.com/en-GB/about-terracycle/how_we_solve.
27. Public Health England. Carbon modelling within dentistry. https://assets.publishing.service.gov.uk/government/uploads/system/uploads/attachment_data/file/724777/Carbon_modelling_within_dentistry.pdf. Accessed 30 June 2021.
28. The Guardian. What's the carbon footprint of…a banana? https://www.theguardian.com/environment/green-living-blog/2010/jul/01/carbon-footprint-banana. Accessed Apr 2018.
29. CO_2 emissions from freight transport: an analysis of UK data. http://www.greenlogistics.org/SiteResources/d82cc048-4b92-4c2a-a014-af1eea7d76d0_CO2%20Emissions%20from%20Freight%20Transport%20-%20An%20Analysis%20of%20UK%20Data.pdf. Accessed Apr 2018.
30. Duane B, Harford S, Ramasubbu D, Stancliffe R, Pasdeki-Clewer E, Lomax R, Steinbach I. Environmentally sustainable dentistry: a brief introduction to sustainable concepts within the dental practice. Br Dent J. 2019;226(4):292–5. https://doi.org/10.1038/s41415-019-0010-7.
31. Duane B, Ramasubbu D, Harford S, Steinbach I, Swan J, Croasdale K, Stancliffe R. Environmental sustainability and waste within the dental practice. Br Dent J. 2019;226(8):611–8. https://doi.org/10.1038/s41415-019-0194-x.
32. Duane B, Harford S, Steinbach I, Stancliffe R, Swan J, Lomax R, Pasdeki-Clewer E, Ramasubbu D. Environmentally sustainable dentistry: energy use within the dental practice. Br Dent J. 2019;226(5):367–73. https://doi.org/10.1038/s41415-019-0044-x.
33. Duane B, Ramasubbu D, Harford S, Steinbach I, Stancliffe R, Ballantyne G. Environmental sustainability and biodiversity within the dental practice. Br Dent J. 2019;226(9):701–5. https://doi.org/10.1038/s41415-019-0208-8.
34. Duane B, Croasdale K, Ramasubbu D, Harford S, Steinbach I, Stancliffe R, Vadher D. Environmental sustainability: measuring and embedding sustainable practice into the dental practice. Br Dent J. 2019;226(11):891–6. https://doi.org/10.1038/s41415-019-0355-y.
35. Duane B, Ramasubbu D, Harford S, Steinbach I, Stancliffe R, Croasdale K, Pasdeki-Clewer E. Environmental sustainability and procurement: purchasing products for the dental setting. Br Dent J. 2019;226(6):453–8. https://doi.org/10.1038/s41415-019-0080-6.
36. Duane B, Steinbach I, Ramasubbu D, Stancliffe R, Croasdale K, Harford S, Lomax R. Environmental sustainability and travel within the dental practice. Br Dent J. 2019;226(7):525–30. https://doi.org/10.1038/s41415-019-0115-z.
37. Environmental protection agency. Carbon Pollution from Transportation. https://www.epa.gov/transportation-air-pollution-and-climate-change/carbon-pollution-transportation.

38. IEA. Renewables. 2019. https://www.iea.org/reports/renewables-2019.
39. Bhutta MF. Fair and ethical trade in health procurement. Lancet. 2008;372(9654):1935–7. https://doi.org/10.1016/S0140-6736(08)61826-7.
40. British Medical Association. Ethical procurement for health: workbook 2.0,1 a guide and workbook for protecting labour rights in medical supply chains. https://www.bma.org.uk/media/2409/ethical_procurement_for_health_workbook_20_final_web.pdf.
41. Chancery Lane Project. The net zero standard for suppliers. https://chancerylaneproject.org/climate-clauses/the-net-zero-standard-for-suppliers/.
42. Nike. Response to greenpeace report. https://news.nike.com/news/nike-inc%E2%80%99s-response-to-greenpeace-report.
43. Green impact for health toolkit. https://www.greenerpractice.co.uk/gifh-audit.
44. Greenbiz. Kaiser applies new green scorecard. https://www.greenbiz.com/article/kaiser-applies-new-green-scorecard-1b-medical-supply-chain.

Responsible Waste Management: Using Resources Efficiently

Sheryl Wilmott, Eleni Pasdeki-Clewer, and Brett Duane

10.1 Introduction

Sustainability is about the sensible and responsible use of natural resources in order to avoid depletion and to maintain an ecological balance [1]. The current linear production model of manufacturing goods from raw materials, selling them, utilising them, and then disposing of them is unsustainable. Goods production also creates pollutants and green house gases that damage the environment and are harmful to human health [2]. Products used in dentistry are no different. Dentistry must move towards a circular economy. This will reduce its dependence on non-renewable natural resources, and reduce waste production through the development of products which become raw materials for other industries at the end of their useful life [3]. Dentistry must also embrace zero-waste, zero carbon, and low environmental impact concepts.

A responsible waste management strategy provides an action plan for the conservation of energy and resources. This could include making changes to the purchasing and procurement of goods, and making the decision to only purchase from manufacturers who produce responsibly, who reuse and recover their products, and whose packaging and materials can be recycled without unnecessary discharge to the land, water, or air. By doing this, we reduce our negative impact both on the planet and human health [4]. It could also include making changes to waste management behaviours within the dental practice; mininising clinical waste through reusing and recycling helps reduce natural resource use and depletion and is

S. Wilmott (✉)
Leeds Teaching Hospitals NHS Trust, Leeds, UK
e-mail: sheryl.wilmott@nhs.net

E. Pasdeki-Clewer
Independent Consultant, Amersham, UK

B. Duane
Trinity College Dublin, Dublin, Ireland
e-mail: brettdu@tcd.ie

generally associated with lower environmental emissions than landfill. Managing food waste in an appropriate food waste management system generates lower environmental emissions and ensures that beneficial nutrients are returned to the soil [5].

10.2   Types of Dental Waste

Dental practices produce significant amounts of waste. Table 10.1 segregates this waste into streams including recycling waste, food waste, landfill waste, hygiene waste, infectious waste, and chemically contaminated infectious waste. These waste streams are categorised as hazardous (e.g. contaminated clinical waste, sharps, and amalgam) and non-hazardous (e.g. office waste such as paper, landfill/landfill waste, and food waste) [6]. The colours of these waste streams were referred to in our previous BDJ papers; however, here the colours have been removed as there is no international consistency in colour coding. We all need to consider our legal, ethical, and professional duties to ensure waste is appropriately segregated, stored, transported, and disposed of in a way that minimises environmental pollution and damage to human health [7–12].

10.3   Costs and Environmental Emissions

As can be seen in Table 10.1, managing waste effectively has both environmental and financial benefits [21, 22]. An audit undertaken by Plymouth University demonstrated that the two most common waste products within a dental practice were paper (tissues and sterile packaging) and nitrile gloves. The audit demonstrated both financial and environmental savings resulted from appropriate waste segregation [23].

Table 10.1 Types of dental waste and the financial cost of their disposal [13]

Waste type		Cost/credit
Recycling	Glass waste	£32 (cost)–£18 (credit) [14]
	Plastic waste	£140–£330 credit [15]
	Paper waste	£0–£35 credit [16]
	Cardboard	£25–£60 credit [16]
Other disposal methods	Food waste/organic waste	£18–£40 per tonne [17]
	Domestic waste	£80–£123 per tonne [18]
	Hygiene waste	£241 per tonne [19]
	Infectious waste contaminated with chemicals	£457 per tonne [19]
	Infectious waste not contaminated with chemicals	£337 per tonne [19]
	Medicines waste for incineration	Cost not available
	Dental amalgam waste	Cost not available
	Plaster waste	Cost not available
	X ray fixer and developer	Cost not available

Euros were converted into British pounds sterling at £1 = €1.13, correct 4th May 2018 [20]

In general, as waste streams become more complex, waste treatment costs increase accordingly. For example, incineration of contaminated waste is more costly than non-contaminated waste, and landfill is more costly than recycled waste. According to Letsrecycle (a website with current waste management costs), the costs associated with recycling depend on the product; glass, for example, can incur a charge or a credit depending on market conditions, good quality plastic bottles, paper, and cardboard generate income for the person managing these waste streams. However, more complex waste (e.g. healthcare waste) and landfill is expensive to manage.

10.4   Environmental Comparison of Different Waste Streams

An LCA has been used to explore the impact of seven waste streams produced in dental practice. The waste streams are defined in Table 10.2. For information regarding LCA terminology, please see Sect. 1.2.

Table 10.3 shows how 1000 kg of waste produced in dental practice contributes to 16 environmental impact categories. A traffic light system identifies the contaminated waste stream as the biggest contributor to all but four of the impact categories. This waste is usually incinerated, resulting in the production of greenhouse gases, particulate matter, and other pollutant materials. The overall impact of the landfill, plastic, and cardboard waste streams are moderate. However, the plastic waste stream is the principal pollutant of the marine environment, has the most respiratory effects on human health, and is the second highest contributor to freshwater ecotoxicity. Food, plaster, and water waste have the lowest environmental impact in most categories; however, food waste is the largest contributor to photochemical ozone creation, and plaster waste contributes to freshwater and terrestrial acidification.

Measuring environmental impact using an LCA can appear abstract. However, the impact factors can be converted into disability-adjusted life years (DALYs) [25]. For more information on DALYs, the reader is referred to Chap. 1. Measuring the impact of dental waste streams using DALYs shows how disposal of this waste affects human health (see Table 10.4). The traffic light system shows that the contaminated waste stream has the largest impact on human health. This means that for every 1000 kg of contaminated dental waste disposed of, the population loses 0.93 h of healthy life. Compare this to the cardboard stream which contributes to just 0.22 h of DALYs.

Table 10.2 Definitions of the seven waste streams produced in dental practice

Contaminated waste stream	Disposal of 1000 kg of 100% hazardous waste—usually incinerated [24]
Plaster waste stream	Disposal of 1000 kg of 100% natural gypsum waste
Plastic waste stream	Disposal of 1000 kg of mixed various plastics
Cardboard waste stream	Disposal of 1000 kg of mixed waste paperboard using country-specific data (the United Kingdom)
Municipal/landfill waste stream	Disposal of 1000 kg of landfill solid waste using country-specific data (the United Kingdom)
Food waste stream	Processing of 1000 kg of biowaste, kitchen, and garden waste in a home composting process

Table 10.3 Environmental impact of seven dental waste streams per 1000 kg of each waste type

Impact category	Food waste stream	Contaminated waste stream	Plaster waste stream	Plastic waste stream	Cardboard waste stream	Municipal / landfill waste stream	Units
Ecosystem quality - freshwater ecotoxicity	4.89	3889.85	23.89	2337.56	111.76	1767.23	CTU
Ecosystem quality - freshwater eutrophication	1.18E-03	0.69	7.50E-04	0.01	0.01	0.03	kg P-Eq
Ecosystem quality - terrestrial eutrophication	0.35	8.78	0.29	2.27	1.27	1.34	mol N-Eq
Resources - dissipated water	25.83	366.28	1.54	52.25	47.46	46.95	m3 water-Eq
Human health - respiratory effects, inorganics	4.43E-07	3.55E-05	8.71E-06	3.53E-05	6.25E-06	6.07E-06	disease incidence
Resources - land use	23.50	3457.10	519.80	637.97	591.16	692.51	points
Human health - photochemical ozone creation	9.85	2.39	0.68	0.63	0.52	0.43	kg NMVOC-Eq
Human health - ozone layer depletion	2.02E-07	2.90E-04	3.17E-06	6.06E-06	5.18E-06	6.02E-06	kg CFC-11-Eq
Human health - non -carcinogenic effects	2.59E-07	1.40E-04	4.33E-06	5.35E-05	2.51E-05	4.25E-05	CTUh
Human health - ionising radiation	0.49	78.21	1.30	1.90	2.11	2.37	kg U235-Eq
Resources - fossils	110.86	12617.60	220.14	486.81	445.00	495.60	MJ
Human health - carcinogenic effects	7.01E-08	1.00E-04	4.91E-07	9.84E-06	3.65E-06	1.05E-05	CTUh
Climate change - climate change total	25.54	2459.46	9.03	1383.43	679.13	614.33	kg CO2-Eq
Ecosystem quality - marine eutrophication	0.01	0.89	0.03	1.18	0.77	0.76	kg N-Eq
Ecosystem quality - freshwater and terrestrial acidification	0.09	3.79	9.70	0.48	0.34	0.32	mol H+-Eq
Resources - minerals and metals	2.01E-05	0.01	2.77E-05	1.20E-04	0.00	1.10E-04	kg Sb-Eq

Table 10.4 Impact of dental waste streams on human health (DALYs per 1000 kg dental waste)

	Food waste stream	Contaminated waste stream	Plaster waste stream	Plastic waste stream	Cardboard waste stream	Municipal / landfill waste stream
Hours	0.45	0.93	0	0.48	0.24	0.22

10.5 Improving Waste Management Using the Waste Hierarchy

The waste hierarchy [26] identifies opportunities for dental practices to manage their waste by preventing the generation of future waste; initially through reducing the need for a product, and then by managing the waste through four steps:
1. Preparing for reuse
2. Recycling
3. Recovering
4. Disposal

In the United Kingdom, the NHS alone generates 1 in every 100 tonnes of landfill waste and if all of that waste goes to landfill or incineration, around 600–2500 kg of carbon dioxide can be released into the atmosphere [27]. The waste hierarchy (see Fig. 10.1) was developed to provide alternatives to waste disposal therefore reducing the raw material extraction and the greenhouse gases produced by these processes.

10.5.1 Preventing the Generation of Waste

10.5.1.1 Influencing Manufacturers and Suppliers to Produce Less Waste

To consider how we can buy smarter, reduce our waste, and lower our environmental impact, the Procurement chapter (Chap. 9) is a useful resource to turn to.

10.5.1.2 Reducing Paper Use

Within the dental setting, the amount of paper being used can be reduced by making optimum use of telephone calls, text messaging, and electronic patient records. This reduction will save money, resource use, and unnecessary environmental emissions [28]. In 2019, when 200 NHS Trusts switched from virgin to recycled copier paper, £256,000 and the CO_2 equivalent of ten around-the-world flights was saved [29]. Practices would need to ensure that when using such technology, that they are compliant with General Data Protection Regulations (GDPR) [30]. Where the use of paper (or 'documentation') is necessary, and where it does not adversely affect patients with visual impairment, consider changing the default printer settings to double-sided printing and reducing font size or spacing within documents. Aim to use only recycled, non-bleached paper. Use of video conferencing for staff meetings has the potential to reduce the need to print documents. As with any system change, practices should audit the amount of paper they use, as well how they are using it. The results of the audit can be linked to an emission calculator to show the impact on the environment [31].

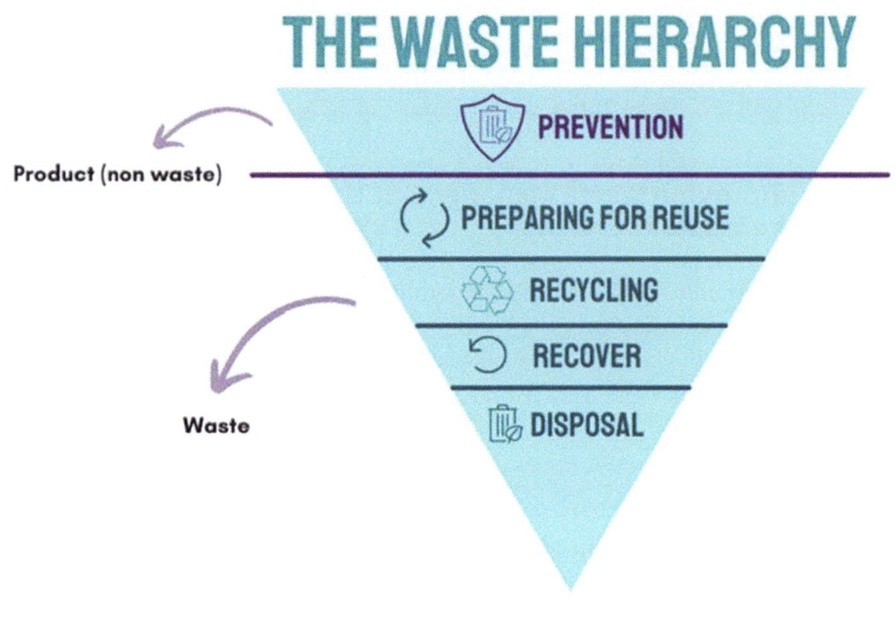

Fig. 10.1 The Waste Hierarchy

10.5.1.3 Reducing Medicines Waste

Dentists in England prescribed 13,235,561 items between 2017 and 2020 [32] and are estimated to be responsible for 10% of antimicrobial prescriptions [33]. There is, therefore, a responsibility to ensure that these medications are disposed of in a way that minimises their environmental impact. Drug metabolites from medications that are disposed of in household waste can leach into ground and surface water from landfill, or enter water systems if they are flushed down the toilet or washed down the drain [34]. These metabolites are not fully removed by water treatment facilities, resulting in contaminated drinking water, genetic changes in aquatic species and bacterial resistance to antibiotics—a significant health impact [35]. Unfortunately, such changes have the biggest impact on low socio-economic status groups, who are more likely to live in areas where medicines waste is disposed of inappropriately [34].

Education is key to the appropriate disposal of medications. Patients who are advised of the correct methods of disposal are more likely to discard medications appropriately [36]. Dentists can reduce the number of medications they prescribe by focusing on preventative care (see Prevention Chap. 6) and prescribing in line with up-to-date guidance. For example, the standard of care for irreversible pulpitis is immediate pulpectomy however, antibiotics continue to be prescribed (in part due to appointment time constraints, procedural challenges such as difficulty achieving anaesthesia, and maintaining a positive clinician–patient relationship) [37, 38].

Take-back schemes (the return of unwanted medications to pharmacies or temporary drop off points), have had some success, although in most countries dentists cannot yet participate in these programmes.

Incineration of medicines waste oxidises the active ingredients and deactivates them. This results in reduced water systems contamination but increases harmful gas emissions [39]. Active ingredients can also be deactivated using non-incineration-based oxidation and hydrolysis processes. For example, activated carbon can deactivate amoxicillin in 7 days. This process, still in development, protects the environment and does not produce harmful emissions [40].

10.5.2 Preparing for Reuse

10.5.2.1 Use of Reusable Instruments

Within dentistry, there is growing evidence of the superiority of reusable instruments compared with disposable instruments with respect to their environmental impact. Bryne et al. [41] carried out an LCA of a reusable examination kit compared with a disposable kit. The environmental impacts identified were mostly from the processing of materials and the type of energy used in their production. The production and use of the disposable kit resulted in around 300 g of CO_2 per use, three times that of the reusable kit. The amount of smog causing atmospheric ozone creation attributed to the disposable kit is around four times that of the reusable kit, with ionising radiation resulting from the disposable kit being 3.5-times larger. Water consumption is four times higher with a disposable examination kit [41].

To truly compare the environmental impact of reusable and disposable instruments, studies need to ensure all environmental costs are taken into consideration including sterilisation, water use, etc. in the life cycle assessment [42].

In essence, dental practices need to consider not just the financial cost, but the overall cost to the planet before purchasing supplies. Eco labels would be very helpful to assist the healthcare team in this regard.

10.5.2.2 Durable Equipment

When dental practices invest in new or replacement equipment, they should research various aspects of the product to ensure that it will have a good lifespan, for example, durability, the length of the warranty, and the cost of replacement parts. Checking product reviews might also help identify common problems other users have had with the item.

All equipment within the practice should be checked regularly and repaired as necessary. Staff should feel comfortable about reporting faults, breakages, or concerns so repairs can be undertaken in a timely manner, and an equipment log and policy document could aid this process.

10.5.2.3 Reuse and Up-Cycle

To help reduce environmental damage created by landfill waste, thought should be given to whether an item (e.g. furniture, computers, printers) could be mended, repurposed, up-cycled, or re-homed. Rather than impulsively disposing of surplus equipment into the various waste streams, practices should devise systems that identify possible avenues for repurposing items. This suggestion would benefit from being written into practice policy [43]. Equipment which no longer meets the practice's needs but is still functional could be donated to local community groups or charities. Alternatively, money could be generated by advertising surplus items for sale on community websites such as Gumtree, Freecycle, or Dentaid (a site for dental-specific items). The NHS uses 'Warp It', a site for functional but unwanted equipment which is also used by schools, universities, charities, and the private sector [44–47].

10.5.3 Recycling

Not only is it a legal requirement in most countries to segregate waste appropriately, it is important for environmental and safety reasons and can also generate financial benefits [48].

10.5.3.1 Recyclable Waste

In the dental surgery, materials such as cardboard, paper, and plastic should be placed in the appropriate recycling bin before operative procedures commence. This avoids cross-contamination of recyclable waste with clinical waste. Positioning recycling bins inside the dental surgery could help facilitate this process. As an example of the possible benefits of well-thought-out waste processes, since Oxford University Hospitals Trust placed recycling bins in one of their operating suites, they now recycle 22% of theatre waste with an annual financial saving of £1300 [49].

10.5.3.2 Food Waste

The Irish Green Healthcare Programme (GHCP) estimates that between 4400 and 5800 tonnes of segregated food waste are produced per annum in Irish healthcare facilities at a cost of 11.6 million euros. In addition, 15–17% of general landfill waste is also comprised of food waste [50]. Disposal of food waste to landfill has a significant environment impact because, as it decomposes, it produces methane gas which is 25 times more potent than CO_2 over a 100-year period [51]. Even when the methane is recaptured, disposal to landfill is the worst available disposal option [52].

To reduce the amount of food waste being sent to landfill, dental practices have three options [53, 54]:

1. Commercial food waste collection—responsible for converting food waste into energy via anaerobic digestion—and use the residual digestate as a soil conditioner.
2. Composting—thus reducing costs associated with food disposal and improving soil quality. Revenue could also be generated by selling the compost produced.
3. Worm farms (vermiculture)—the process of using earthworms to convert organic waste into the world's most nutrient-rich fertiliser.

10.5.4 Recovering Energy from Waste (Waste to Energy)

The term waste to energy describes a waste disposal method of generating energy from incinerated waste, with the end result being that there is no actual waste. The practice is controversial because it is more energy efficient to recycle used materials, than to create new products from extracted virgin material. Furthermore, recycling is cost-effective. There is also evidence that incineration programmes have been prioritised at the expense of investing in recycling [55]. In healthcare environments, the main concern is the public health consequences of burning of solid and regulated waste. Medical waste incinerators release toxic air pollutants and toxic ash, both of which are major contributors of dioxins in the environment [56]. Older incinerator technology and infrequent maintenance schedules have been strongly linked with adverse health effects. Modern incinerators have fewer reported ill effects, perhaps because of inadequate time for adverse effects to emerge. The literature provides conflicting evidence of how problematic this is. A French study (2012) showed all incinerators operating within EU tolerable air quality limits [57], another 2011 paper however showed an increased risk of non-Hodgkin lymphoma and serum organochlorine concentrations in populations living close to solid waste incinerators [58]. As highlighted in the travel chapter in this book, air pollution has become a key public health issue to solve [59].

A cautious approach is required by the dental team when considering waste-to-energy systems, and waste minimisation is essential [60].

10.5.5 Clinical Waste and Landfill

Despite the higher disposal costs for complex waste streams, in many healthcare facilities waste is not managed as well as it could be. In an audit of Irish healthcare settings, researchers found that nappies/incontinence wear was incorrectly identified as landfill waste (29%) rather than their correct waste stream of hygiene waste. In this specific audit, the total landfill waste consisted of 29% nappies/incontinence wear, 18% tissues, 17% food, 16% waste recyclables, and 4% non-risk clinical-type materials. A separate audit of clinical waste identified 66% of waste was disposed of appropriately with the remaining 34% being disposed of incorrectly, i.e. being placed in either the recycled or landfill waste streams [63].

Incorrectly separated waste sent to landfill can be expensive and often contains an assortment of items that should be allocated to recyclable waste, for example, hard plastics and food waste. The correct segregation of food waste items would be more cost-effective and more environmentally sustainable.

Great care must be taken when separating infectious and non-infectious waste; any cross-contamination between the two will necessitate all being classified as infectious. Staff need to be made familiar with the correct disposal route of each instrument used during any procedure, i.e. contaminated and non-contaminated.

Fig. 10.2 Importance of a non-contaminated and contaminated waste zone

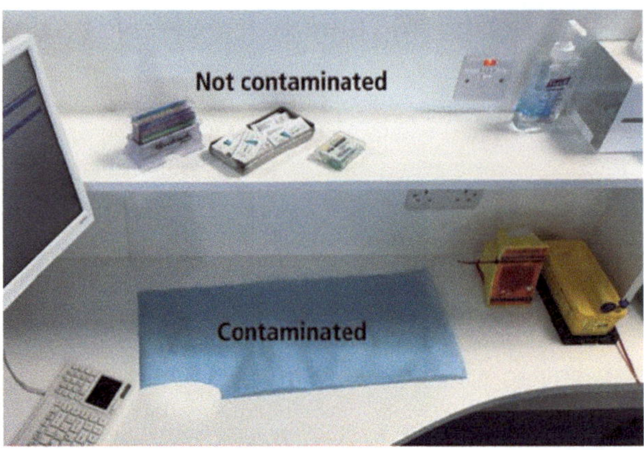

Figure 10.2 depicts the importance of maintaining non-contaminated and con-taminated waste zones.

Staff should be familiar with the waste stream bin colour-coding system in use in their country. Bins should be labelled, giving clear guidance on the specific waste that should be placed in each bin.

The World Health Organization considers waste management training to be 'crit-ical' for healthcare staff and recommends periodic refresher courses [55]. This pro-cess will help ensure correct waste segregation behaviour in practice staff.

10.5.5.1   Location, Availability, and Type of Bins

Within the dental surgery, consideration needs to be given to the availability, type, size, and appropriate location of bins required. Bin location and size is an opportu-nity to use 'nudge theory' to great effect, i.e. by placing appropriate bins in the areas where they are most likely to be used, staff are encouraged to dispose of waste cor-rectly without the need for conscious decision-making. It is, however, important to ensure that unconscious actions do not lead to incorrect items contaminating the recycling waste. For example, in an office/reception setting—where there is likely to be a higher volume of wastepaper—a recycling bin should be placed closer to the source of the waste than a landfill waste bin.

The need for waste bins in sterilisation and decontamination rooms must be care-fully considered. To ensure staff commitment to the practice waste management policies, ideally practice managers, and staff should work together to think about which specific waste bins are required in specific areas.

Along with a clinical waste bin, a landfill waste bin should be conveniently posi-tioned in the decontamination area, thus simplifying the correct management of waste at source. Handwashing sinks in clinical areas should have both a landfill and a clinical waste bin. Best practice in patient waiting areas would be to have a clearly labelled general waste bin and a recycling bin. In areas accessible to the public, clinical waste bins should be kept to a minimum as the public are unlikely to be familiar with the implications of using the bins inappropriately.

The size of the waste bin provided should be appropriate for the expected volume of waste. Office staff might benefit from having a larger recycling bin for their office waste and a smaller bin for their landfill waste. To help save waste storage space, larger dental practices might consider the purchase of a waste compactor for their cardboard waste.

In short, the dental team must consider the size and location of their recycling and landfill waste bins. These bins must be clearly labelled, and staff must receive regular training to ensure that waste is disposed of correctly.

10.6 Performing a Waste Audit

Waste audits, even when they are not a legal requirement, are considered to be one aspect of good working practice for healthcare providers [61]. Along with the mandatory audit (in the United Kingdom), dental practices can undertake an in-house comprehensive waste audit or a less onerous bin placement survey. Both processes will help identify how appropriately waste is being categorised in the practice.

To conduct a comprehensive waste audit practices will need appropriate PPE/clothing, weighing scales, filled waste bins, paperwork to record the survey findings, a table, and a camera.

Step 1: Each filled sample waste bin should be weighed and the weight recorded.
Step 2: Carefully empty each individual sample waste bin. Allocate the contents into their correct waste stream container, for example, clinical, non-clinical, food, or recycling waste.
Step 3: Repeat weighing of each waste bin [21].
From this process, the practice will be able to gauge how effectively their waste management systems are being adhered to and consider whether any staff familiarisation ortraining is required.

To conduct a basic bin placement survey:

Step 1: Identify the activities that take place in the area being surveyed.
Step 2: Consider which waste bins that specific area needs, for example, clinical, landfill, and recycling.
Step 3: Decide on the most appropriate size of each bin required.
Step 4: Devise clear, concise labelling for each bin [63].

10.7 The Impact on Human Health of a Single Dental Appointment

Tables 10.3 and 10.4 showed the environmental and human health impacts of processing 1000 kg of various dental waste streams, but how does this translate to the waste that is produced by a dental practice each day? Kahatab (2020) [63] conducted a waste audit (with thanks to A/Prof Alison Dougal) of dental clinics in an Irish dental setting. Waste was collected from central sterilisation, two dental

Table 10.5 Human health impact of dental waste management per patient appointment in DALYs (audit from National Coagulation Centre dental units) [63]

	Food waste stream	Contaminated waste stream	Municipal//landfill waste stream	Cardboard waste stream	DALYs totals
Total DALYs per patient appointment (in hours 2sf) (Cycle 1)	0.000051	0.00019	0.000075	–	0.00031
Total DALYs per patient appointment (in hours 2sf) (Cycle 2)	0.00000059	0.00017	0.000012	0.000021	0.00021

surgeries and a consultation room over a period of 3 days. The audit focused on contaminated waste (healthcare risk waste or HCRW) and landfill waste (healthcare non-risk waste or HCNRW), but other potential waste streams were identified during the audit, such as recyclable waste and food waste. Kahatab et al. found that in the first cycle of the audit an average of 342.75 g of landfill waste and an average of 201.75 g of contaminated waste was produced per patient. This audit allows us to calculate the DALYs lost per patient appointment for each waste stream. Table 10.5 shows that the processing of the contaminated waste stream contributed to a loss of 0.00019 healthy hours per patient (about 7/10ths of a second) whereas landfill waste only contributed to loss 0.000075 healthy hours per patient (less than 3/10th of a second).

Kahatab et al.'s audit highlights the importance of correctly segregating clinical waste. Cycle 2 of the audit occurred following staff training and changes being made to signage in the clinical areas. A recycling bin was also added to clinical areas. Cycle 2 showed improved waste segregation and a reduction of 0.0001 healthy hours (approximately 4/10th of a second) per dental patient seen (Table 10.5).

Richardson et al. (2016) [61] conducted a similar audit in a mixed NHS/private dental practice in North Devon. Waste was collected over four (session 1) and five (session 2) days. The waste collected in session 1 was multiplied by 25% to estimate waste collection over 2 full weeks. The purpose of the audit was to investigate how much non-clinical waste was being disposed of in the contaminated waste stream. Richardson et al. did not specify how many patients were seen during their week of data collection; it has therefore been estimated that 15 patients were seen per day [64]. Table 10.6 shows that the waste from both sessions contributed 0.000042 h of DALYs (approximately 2/10th of a second) if it is all disposed of in the contaminated waste stream. However, by correctly separating the waste (in this case, disposing of sterile paper and plastic instrument packaging separately), 1/100th of a second of DALYs is saved per patient appointment.

These small numbers of DALYs rapidly become significant when you consider the millions of dental appointments that occur each year.

Table 10.6 Human health impact of dental waste management per patient appointment in DALYs (calculated using 'What's in a bin' waste audit) [61]

	Contaminated waste stream	Plastic waste stream	Cardboard waste stream	DALYs totals
Total DALYs per patient appointment in hours (2sf) (using only contaminated waste bin)	0.000042	–	–	0.000042
Total DALYs per patient appointment in hours (2sf) (when waste is correctly segregated)	0.000038	0.00000085	0.00000042	0.000040

10.8 Changing Waste Disposal Behaviours in the Dental Setting

10.8.1 Barriers to pro-environmental behaviour

Barriers to staff adopting sustainable waste management procedures can be grouped into three separate categories: lack of personal understanding, too much trouble and lack of commitment/accountability [65].

10.8.1.1 Lack of Understanding

When appropriate waste disposal facilities and processes are in place, if staff do not understand the importance of waste management or the processes involved, they may dispose of waste incorrectly or disengage from the process entirely. Abstract knowledge of environmental issues may motivate improved recycling and waste segregation behaviours, but concrete knowledge, such as which items belong in which bins, and which items can be recycled, has been shown to be a much better predictor of behaviour [65]. Dental teams should be aware of the financial and planetary costs associated with waste streams, and the actions they can take to reduce these. Staff training resources relating to waste management should be made available to the practice's lead person on waste management. University students (undergraduate and postgraduate) would also benefit from waste management instruction being part of their curriculum and work with curriculum change is underway [66–68].

10.8.1.2 Too Much Trouble

Even staff with the knowledge and motivation to dispose of waste correctly are less likely to do so if it is perceived to be too much trouble [69]. If recycling facilities are not readily available in surgery, the additional effort of remembering, saving, and transporting recyclable material to a different location in the practice may be prohibitive for a busy associate or dental nurse. Where there is limited space to store waste, mixed dry recycling (where various dry recyclable materials are allocated to the same waste stream.) could be considered. Stackable recycling bins would also reduce the amount of floor space required for waste containers. Vermiculture (worm farms) for the disposal of food waste can be very space efficient.

10.8.1.3 Lack of Commitment/Accountability

Individual values are as important as external infrastructure to promote recycling behaviours. In additional to intrinsic motivation, staff must feel that any behaviour change is a collective action with the involvement of the whole team. Grose suggests that changes in waste management policy should not be seen as just a top-down approach and that staff should feel motivated to report practice waste management concerns/issues [70]. They should also be able to be proactive/innovative in line with current guidance.

To assist in this process, one identified staff member should:

- Act as the main point of contact for practice waste management improvement suggestions.
- Implement relevant changes to current procedures.
- Ensure practice waste management processes are communicated effectively to all members of staff [21, 22].

In line with relevant legislation, practices should formulate a policy on the management of waste detailing all practice procedures. The policy should encompass, for example, staff guidance/training on each waste category, waste bin placement within the practice, instruction on how waste should be separated, along with a reduce, reuse, and recycle element explaining the practice's approach to waste reduction.

10.8.2 Enablers of pro-environmental behaviour

External drivers for improving waste management have been categorised by Pietzsch [71].

10.8.2.1 Discussions with Industry

There is a need for discussions between the dental profession, the waste management industry, and product manufacturers to identify possible routes to encouraging consumer waste behaviour change. Numerous environmental benefits could be achieved if manufacturers redesigned their products to increase use of renewable materials, minimise the level of toxic components, reduce unnecessary packaging, and enhance the products' useful life. See Chap. 9.

10.8.2.2 Incentives and Disincentives

Waste management financial incentives (e.g. subsidies) and disincentives (e.g. penalties/taxes) have proven to be effective in some areas [71].

10.8.2.3 Legislation

Internationally, most countries have legislation to ensure waste is managed appropriately. In England, for example, it is an offence to dispose of waste without an environmental permit. Hazardous waste must be appropriately segregated, packaged, and labelled [72]. Currently, European directives exist relating to the treatment of various waste materials; packaging, electronic/electrical items, and spent batteries [73]. Dental practices in Scotland have a legal requirement to recycle as much of their waste as possible and dispose of their waste safely. Local authorities and waste contractors must also adhere to high recycling standards—paper, card, metal, plastic, and glass waste must be separated appropriately for waste collection. If weekly food waste levels exceed 5 kg, this must also be separately presented for collection [74].

Box 10.1 provides some useful considerations regarding waste disposal practices.

Box 10.1 Encouraging Positive Waste Disposal Behaviours in the Dental Practice
There are many opportunities to encourage pro-environmental behaviour which can be applied to the dental practice, and they have been shown to have high levels of effectiveness ranging from 66% to over 80% [75].

Education and Awareness involves providing information materials for staff and patients in the form of leaflets, posters, and other reading materials. This is a popular approach since it is easy and does not require significant resource [75]. In practice, this could mean placing a poster above the recycling bins depicting which items can be disposed of in each receptacle. *Education and Awareness* is more effective in people who are already motivated to behave in sustainable ways but lack the required knowledge.

Social Influence relies on the influence that people have on their peers. It can be effectively implemented in practice through the identification of motivated volunteers or 'Champions' who can demonstrate correct waste disposal behaviour and promote sustainability in the practice. *Social influence* has been shown to positively impact household garden waste disposal behaviours that were sustained for up to a year! [76].

Nudges gently suggest a particular choice by making it easier, or the default option. Nudges are often very successful as they require little conscious thought or intrinsic motivation [75]. Plastic cup recycling by university students increased when the recycling bins were made larger and more visible compared to general waste bins [77]. This could work particularly well in an office or administrative environment in the dental practice.

Incentives—evidence on the success of this approach is contradictory. *Incentives* can be monetary or non-monetary and are used to reward people for carrying out a desired behaviour. However, since *Incentives* don't improve the intrinsic motivation to carry out sustainable behaviours, the behaviours may cease when the incentives do. Further research is needed to identify which incentives are most likely to encourage pro-environmental behaviour and how long those incentives should be provided for [78].

Take Home Points for the Dental Team

- Practices produce significant amounts of recycling, landfill, offensive hygiene, clinical, hazardous, and food waste.
- Disposal of dental waste can have significant impact on population health as well as the environment—correct segregation of waste can reduce these impacts.
- The dental profession needs to: (a) reduce the amount of waste generated, (b) categorise and segregate waste appropriately, and (c) make staff/individuals aware of the financial and sustainability benefits of appropriate waste management.
- The dental team can encourage positive waste disposal behaviour through education, waste champions, subtle environmental changes, and incentives.

References

1. Dictionary. www.dictionary.com. Accessed July 2021.
2. Towards the circular economy. World Economic Forum. http://reports.weforum.org/toward-the-circular-economy-accelerating-the-scale-up-across-global-supply-chains/1-the-benefits-of-a-circular-economy/. Accessed July 2021.
3. Circular economy in conjunction with treatment methodologies in the biomedical and dental waste sectors. https://link.springer.com/article/10.1007/s43615-020-00001-0. Accessed July 2021.
4. Zero waste international alliance. www.zwia.org. Accessed July 2021.
5. Duane B, Ramasubbu D, Harford S, Steinbach I, Swan J, Croasdale K, et al. Environmental sustainability, and waste within the dental practice. Br Dent J. 2019;226(8):611–8.
6. Department of Health. Environment and Sustainability. Health Technical Memorandum 07–01: Safe management of healthcare waste. 2013.
7. Government of the United Kingdom. Hazardous Waste. https://www.gov.uk/dispose-hazardous-waste. Accessed July 2021.
8. Government of the United Kingdom Legislation. Environmental Protection Act (1990). http://www.legislation.gov.uk/ukpga/1990/43/section/34. Accessed July 2021.
9. Government of the United Kingdom Legislation. The Controlled Waste (England and Wales) Regulations. 2012. http://www.legislation.gov.uk/uksi/2012/811/contents/made. Accessed July 2021.
10. Government of the United Kingdom. The carriage of dangerous goods and use of transportable pressure equipment (amendment) regulations. 2011. http://www.legislation.gov.uk/uksi/2011/1885/contents/made. Accessed July 2021.
11. Allen R. Disposing of clinical and dental waste. BDJ Team. 2015;1:14038. https://doi.org/10.1038/bdjteam.2014.38.
12. Williams S. Waste management. BDJ Pract. 2021;34(3):39.
13. Lets recycle com. 2021. Composting. https://www.letsrecycle.com/prices/composting/windrow-ivc-and-ad-prices-2021.
14. Lets recycle com. 2021. Glass prices. https://www.letsrecycle.com/prices/glass/glass-prices-2021/.
15. Lets recycle com. 2021 Plastic bottles. https://www.letsrecycle.com/prices/plastics/plastic-bottles/plastic-bottles-2021/.
16. Lets recycle com. 2021 Merchant prices. https://www.letsrecycle.com/prices/waste-paper/merchant-prices/2021-merchant-prices/.
17. GPT The Waste Solution. Food Waste Gate Fees Are Dropping As Ad Capacity In The Uk Increases. https://gptwaste.com/food-waste-gate-fees-are-dropping-as-ad-capacity-in-the-uk-increases/. Accessed July 2021.

18. Lets recycle com. EfW, landfill, RDF 2021 gate fees. https://www.letsrecycle.com/prices/efw-landfill-rdf-2/efw-landfill-rdf-2021-gate-fees/ accessed July 2021.
19. Royal College of Nursing. Freedom of Information. Follow up Report on Management of Waste in the NHS. https://www.rcn.org.uk/professional-development/publications/pdf-006683.
20. Currency Converter. https://www.xe.com/currencyconverter/convert/?Amount=1&From=GBP&To=EUR. Accessed July 2021.
21. Environmental Protection Agency: Greenhealthcare. Reducing Waste in Irish Healthcare Facilities. 2014. https://www.epa.ie/pubs/advice/green%20business/Reducing-waste-in-Irish-Healthcare-Facilities-waste-guidance-booklet-reduced-size.pdf. Accessed July 2021.
22. Royal College of Physicians. Less waste, more health: a health professional's guide to reducing waste. 2018. https://www.rcplondon.ac.uk/projects/outputs/less-waste-more-health-health-professionals-guide-reducing-waste. Accessed July 2021.
23. Richardson J, Grose J, Manzi S, Mills I, Moles D, Mukonoweshuro R, Nasser M, Nichols A. What's in a bin: a case study of dental clinical waste composition and potential greenhouse gas emission savings. Br Dent J. 2016;220(2):61–6.
24. Ecoinvent. https://ecoinvent.org/the-ecoinvent-database/data-releases/ecoinvent-3-7-1/.
25. World Health Organisation. The Global Health Directory. Disability-adjusted life years (DALYs). https://www.who.int/data/gho/indicator-metadata-registry/imr-details/158. Accessed July 2021.
26. DEFRA. Guidance on applying the Waste Hierarchy. https://assets.publishing.service.gov.uk/government/uploads/system/uploads/attachment_data/file/69403/pb13530-waste-hierarchy-guidance.pdf.
27. Healthy Hospitals Healthy Planet Healthy People. World Health Organisation; https://www.who.int/publications/i/item/healthy-hospitals-healthy-planet-healthy-people. Accessed Aug 2021.
28. West Kent Primary Care Trust. Paper Policy. http://map.sustainablehealthcare.org.uk/west-kent-primary-care-trust/paper-policy. Accessed July 2021.
29. NHS Supply Chain. NHS saves thousands of trees and enough water to fill 161 Olympic size swimming pools. 2020. https://www.supplychain.nhs.uk/news-article/nhs-saves-20000-trees-and-enough-water-to-fill-161-olympic-size-swimming-pools/. Accessed July 2021.
30. Information Commissioner's Office. https://ico.org.uk/for-organisations/guide-to-the-general-data-protection-regulation-gdpr/. Accessed July 2021.
31. Environmental Paper Network. Paper Calculator. http://c.environmentalpaper.org/home. Accessed July 2021.
32. UK Government. Research and analysis. Dental prescribing dashboard 2020. https://www.gov.uk/government/publications/dental-prescribing-dashboard-2018. Accessed July 2021.
33. FGDP. Antimicrobial Prescribing in Dentistry. https://www.fgdp.org.uk/sites/fgdp.org.uk/files/docs/in-practice/amps-online/FGDP%20AMP%20Ed3%202020%20online%20v1.pdf. Accessed July 2021.
34. Martuzzi A, Mitis F, Forastiere F. Inequalities, inequities, environmental justice in waste management and health. Eur J Pub Health. 2010;20(1):21–6. https://doi.org/10.1093/eurpub/ckp216.
35. World Health Organisation. Antibiotic Resistance. https://www.who.int/news-room/fact-sheets/detail/antibiotic-resistance. Accessed July 2021.
36. Wieczorkiewicz SM, Kassamali Z, Danziger LH. Behind closed doors: medication storage and disposal in the home. Ann Pharmacother. 2013;47(4):482–9. https://doi.org/10.1345/aph.1R706. Epub 2013 Mar 27.
37. Agnihotry A, Thompson W, Fedorowicz Z, van Zuuren EJ, Sprakel J. Antibiotic use for irreversible pulpitis. Cochrane Database Syst Rev. 2019;5(5):CD004969. https://doi.org/10.1002/14651858.CD004969.pub5.
38. Thompson W, Tonkin-Crine S, Pavitt S, McEachan R, Douglas G, Aggarwal V, Sandoe J. Factors associated with antibiotic prescribing for adults with acute conditions: an umbrella review across primary care and a systematic review focusing on primary dental care. J Antimicrob Chemother. 2019;74(8):2139–52. https://doi.org/10.1093/jac/dkz152.

39. Mullot JU, Karolak S, Fontova A, Levi Y. Modeling of hospital wastewater pollution by pharmaceuticals: first results of Mediflux study carried out in three French hospitals. Water Sci Technol. 2010;62:2912–9.
40. Herwadkar A, Singh N, Anderson C, Korey A, Fowler W, Banga AK. Development of disposal systems for deactivation of unused/residual/expired medications. Pharm Res. 2016;33(1):110–24.
41. Byrne D, Saget S, Davidson A. et al, Comparing the environmental impact of reusable and disposable dental examination kits: a life cycle assessment approach. Br Dent J 2022;233: 317–25. https://doi.org/10.1038/s41415-022-4912-4.
42. Siu J, Hill A, MacCormick A. Systematic review of reusable versus disposable laparoscopic instruments: costs and safety. Aust N Z J Surg. 2017;87(1–2):28–33.
43. United States Environmental Protection Agency. Reducing and Reusing Basics. https://www.epa.gov/recycle/reducing-and-reusing-basics. Accessed July 2021.
44. NHS Case Study. https://www.warp-it.co.uk/nhs.aspx. Accessed July 2021.
45. The Freecycle Network. https://www.freecycle.org/. Accessed July 2021.
46. Gumtree Website. https://www.gumtree.com/freebies. Accessed July 2021.
47. Warp it. https://www.warp-it.co.uk/.
48. Government of United Kingdom. Environmental management. Waste. https://www.gov.uk/dispose-hazardous-waste. Accessed July 2021.
49. Sustainable Healthcare. Introducing recycling operating theatres. https://map.sustainablehealthcare.org.uk/oxford-radcliffe-hospitals-nhs-trust/introducing-recycling-operating-theatres.
50. Green Healthcare. Reducing food waste in Irish hospitals results, guidance and tips from a 3-year programme. Dublin: Green Healthcare Programme, Environmental Protection Agency; 2013. 24p. http://hdl.handle.net/10147/324073. Accessed Nov 2021.
51. EPA (United States) Overview of greenhouse gases overview of greenhouse gases. https://www.epa.gov/ghgemissions/overview-greenhouse-gases. Accessed July 2021.
52. Moulta J, Allanc S, Hewitta C, Berners-Lee M. Greenhouse gas emissions of food waste. https://eprints.lancs.ac.uk/id/eprint/124861/1/Moult_et_al_2018.pdf. Accessed July 2021.
53. Duane B, Ramasubbu D, Harford S, Steinbach I, Swan J, Croasdale K, Stancliffe R. Environmental sustainability and waste within the dental practice. Br Dent J. 2019;226(8):611–8. https://doi.org/10.1038/s41415-019-0194-x.
54. Jagtap S, Garcia-Garcia G, Duong L, Swainson M, Martindale W. Codesign of food system and circular economy approaches for the development of livestock feeds from insect larvae. Foods. 2021;10(8):1701. https://doi.org/10.3390/foods10081701.
55. https://www.euro.who.int/__data/assets/pdf_file/0012/268779/Safe-management-of-wastes-from-health-care-activities-Eng.pdf.
56. Gautam V, Thapar R, Sharma M. Biomedical waste management: incineration versus environmental safety. Indian J Med Microbiol. 2010;28(3):191–2. https://doi.org/10.4103/0255-0857.66465.
57. Nzihou A, Themelis NJ, Kemiha M, Benhamou Y. Dioxin emissions from landfill solid waste incinerators (MSWIs) in France. Waste Manag. 2012;32(12):2273–7.
58. Viel J, Floret N, Deconinck E, Focant J, De Pauw E, Cahn J. Increased risk of non-Hodgkin lymphoma and serum organochlorine concentrations among neighbors of a landfill solid waste incinerator. Environ Int. 2011;37(2):449–53.
59. Fiordelisi A, Piscitelli P, Trimarco B, Coscioni E, Laccarino G, Sorriento D. The mechanisms of air pollution and particulate matter in cardiovascular diseases. Heart Fail Rev. 2017;22(3):337–47. https://doi.org/10.1007/s10741-017-9606-7.
60. Tait PW, Brew J, Che A, Costanzo A, Danyluk A, Davis M, Khalaf A, McMahon K, Watson A, Rowcliff K, Bowles D. The health impacts of waste incineration: a systematic review. Aust N Z J Public Health. 2020;44(1):40–8. https://doi.org/10.1111/1753-6405.12939. Epub 2019 Sep 18.
61. Richardson J, Grose J, Manzi S, Mills I, Moles DR, Mukonoweshuro R, Nasser M, Nichols A. What's in a bin: a case study of dental clinical waste composition and potential greenhouse gas emission savings. Br Dent J. 2016;220(2):61–6. https://doi.org/10.1038/sj.bdj.2016.55.

62. Environmental Protection Agency Greenhealthcare. How-to-guide. Undertaking a Bin Placement Survey. http://www.greenhealthcare.ie/wp-content/uploads/2014/05/How-To-Undertake-a-Bin-Placement-Survey-revised.pdf. Accessed July 2021.
63. Taking special care to manage our waste sustainably—an audit of the waste management practices in Ireland's National Coagulation Centre. https://www.researchgate.net/publication/350963709_International_Association_for_Disability_Oral_Health_Research_Symposium_2020_RESEARCH_SYMPOSIUM_2020_Proceedings_Abstracts_2_International_Association_for_Disability_Oral_Health_Research_Symposium.
64. Brunton PA, Sharif MO, Creanor S, Burke FJ, Wilson NH. Contemporary dental practice in the UK in 2008: indirect restorations and fixed prosthodontics. Br Dent J. 2012;212(3):115–9. https://doi.org/10.1038/sj.bdj.2012.92.
65. Barnosky, E and Delmas, M and Huysentruyt, Marieke. The circular economy: motivating recycling behavior for a more effective system. 2019. SSRN: https://ssrn.com/abstract=3466359 or https://doi.org/10.2139/ssrn.3466359
66. Duane B, Dixon J, Ambibola G, Aldana C, Couglan J, Henao D, Daniela T, Veiga N, Martin N, Darragh JH, Ramasubbu D, Perez F, Schwendicke F, Correia M, Quinteros M, Van Harten M, Paganelli C, Vos P, Moreno Lopez R, Field J. Embedding environmental sustainability within the modern dental curriculum. Exploring current practice and developing a shared understanding. Eur J Dent Educ. 2021;25(3):541–9. https://doi.org/10.1111/eje.12631.
67. E learning for Healthcare. https://www.e-lfh.org.uk/e-den/. Accessed July 2021.
68. Academy of Medical Royal Colleges. Protecting Resources, Promoting Value: a doctor's guide to cutting waste in clinical care. In: Maughan D, Ansell J, editors. Academy of Medical Royal Colleges; 2014. https://www.aomrc.org.uk/reports-guidance/protecting-resources-promoting-value-1114/. Accessed July 2021.
69. Derksen L, Gartrell J. The Social Context of Recycling. Am Sociol Rev. 1993;58(3):434–42.
70. Grose J, Burns L, Mukonoweshuro R, Richardson J, Mills I, Nasser M, Moles D. Developing sustainability in a dental practice through an action research approach. Br Dent J. 2018;225(5):409–13.
71. Pietzsch N, Ribeiro J, de Medeiros J. Benefits, challenges and critical factors of success for Zero Waste: a systematic literature review. Waste Manag. 2017;67:324–53.
72. United Kingdom Legislation. The Environmental Permitting (England and Wales) Regulations. 2007. https://www.legislation.gov.uk/uksi/2007/3538/contents/made. Accessed Nov 2018.
73. European Council. Waste and Recycling. https://ec.europa.eu/environment/topics/waste-and-recycling/waste-framework-directive_en.
74. United Kingdom Legislation. The Waste (Scotland) Regulations. 2012. https://www.legislation.gov.uk/sdsi/2012/9780111016657/contents. Accessed Nov 2018.
75. Grilli G, Curtis J. Encouraging pro-environmental behaviours: a review of methods and approaches. Renew Sust Energ Rev. 2021;135:110039.
76. Cobern MK, Porter BE, Leeming FC, Dwyer WO. The effect of commitment on adoption and diffusion of grass cycling. Environ Behav. 1995;27(2):213–32. https://doi.org/10.1177/0013916595272006.
77. Cosic A, Cosic H, Ille S. Can nudges affect students' green behaviour? A field experiment. J Behav Econ Policy. 2018;2(1):107–11.
78. Maki A, Burns R, Ha L, Rothman A. Corrigendum to "Paying people to protect the environment: a meta-analysis of financial incentive interventions to promote proenvironmental behaviors". J Environ Psychol. 2016;47:242–55.

11 The Future of Dentistry Products: How Can We Redesign the Products We Create

Willmar Ricardo Rugeles Joya, Eleni Pasdeki-Clewer, Brett Duane, and Laura Alejandra Peñuela

11.1 Innovating to Improve Sustainability

Dental product manufacturing and disposal contributes significantly to environmental damage. Current practices in 'sustainable' dental products and waste management fall short of meeting the sector's responsibility for sustainability. Innovation will play a major role in enabling meaningful sustainable solutions to enter the dental marketplace.

Sustainability needs to become the main driver for evolving manufacturing processes. It needs to *drive change* and not be the unintended co-beneficiary of efficiency-driven changes. Sustainability needs to become the new north star of manufacturing. These changes will not only impact on manufacturers but also on consumers and their established patterns of consumption, often based on convenience and habit. Consumers need to accept their share of responsibility in supporting sustainable change and their role in co-producing sustainable solutions.

This chapter provides examples of how companies (but also consumers) can embrace the concepts of innovation to drive sustainable outcomes. It also provides examples of innovation, how the process of innovation came about and,

W. R. R. Joya (✉)
Department of Architecture and Design, Pontificia Universidad Javeriana, Bogotá, Colombia
e-mail: rugeles-w@javeriana.edu.co

E. Pasdeki-Clewer
Independent consultant, Amersham, UK

B. Duane
Trinity College Dublin, Dublin, Ireland
e-mail: brettdu@tcd.ie

L. A. Peñuela
Javeriana University, Bogota, Colombia
e-mail: uela@javeriana.edu.co

    197
B. Duane (ed.), *Sustainable Dentistry*, BDJ Clinician's Guides,
https://doi.org/10.1007/978-3-031-07999-3_11

consequently, the products that were developed. The processes used to drive innovation are shared with the intention to inspire and ignite imagination and creativity amongst our readers.

In this chapter, we challenge all industry to move away from a risk-averse mentality *[resistance to change]* to an opportunity-driven mentality *[constructive challenge]*. Through this change of behaviour and practice, manufacturers can work with consumers to realise/bring about both tangible and intangible benefits to their companies.

The innovations described are not listed in any order of priority and can be scaled up or down as appropriate. They range from small changes (e.g. using a new material) to radical changes that fundamentally alter the way in which consumers view, select, use, or dispose of a product.

11.1.1 Starting with Something Simple

Innovation does not always need to radically change the components that go into the manufacture of a product. Sometimes, small steps can create big impacts. **Incremental innovation** [1] looks at a process step by step and analyses the life cycle of the product from cradle to grave. Ideally, each constituent/stage of a product's manufacture would be measured using a life cycle assessment process (see Chap. 1) which will help identify objectively where environmental contributions originate. Such detailed analysis is not always necessary; for example, if we swap coal-based energy for solar or wind power we can assume that environmental gains will be made (see Chap. 4).

Small changes may involve substituting a material with a more easily recyclable alternative. For example, replacing the primary packaging of hand gel from PVC (a complex polymeric material) to PE (a mono-polymeric material) makes the product packaging much easier to recycle. Alternatively, and even better, substitute the complex polymeric packaging with compostable polymers. Such material substitutions may benefit with the addition of education, i.e. manufacturers proactively informing users how to dispose of the products/packaging. Small changes could even include gradual reductions in energy use or switching to a greener form of energy.

To summarise companies can start by introducing small changes and improvements that are focused on specific parts of the production process. Cost-driven quick wins can act as a stepping-stone towards a larger scale, more sustainable change.

11.1.2 Simplifying Forms, Materials, and Processes

Although this seems like the first step of incremental innovation, the principle is really about finding the simplest way to solve a problem. The process of simplification is the opposite of the well-trodden, set ways that people generally use to solve a problem [2]. Simplification of processes can be at (1) a **political level** {e.g. to enforce public policies or promote change in the entire sector}, (2) a **social level** {to influence change in consumer behaviour}, (3) **a productive level** {e.g. to reduce process inputs or change the energy used in production}, or (4) **a technical level** {e.g. to change the aesthetics of the products or the type of energy used}—see Fig. 11.1.

Generally, in industrial processes, the path of least resistance is to seek substitutes or find shortcuts/quick solutions to satisfy customer demand and other external factors. As a matter of course, pre-consumer waste, by-products, and other unwanted resources are seen as useless material only fit for landfill. By comparison, in nature, all components have value and purpose and are used as a resource (e.g. food or energy). This brings us to the third principle:

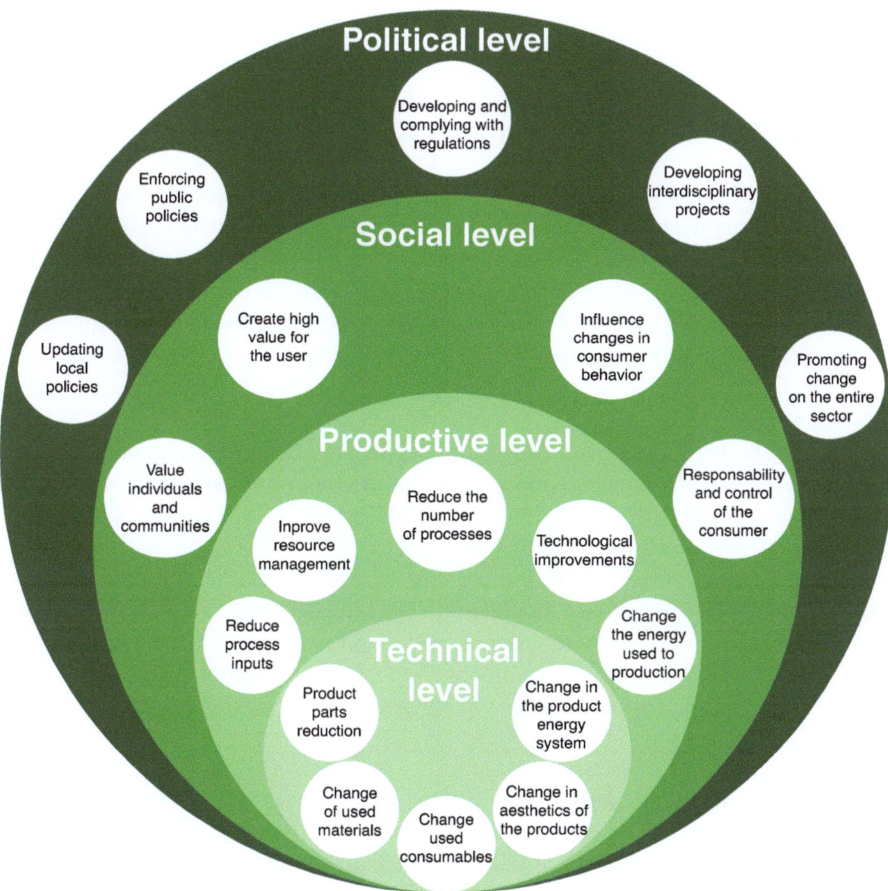

Fig. 11.1 Impact levels in changes introduced in the company

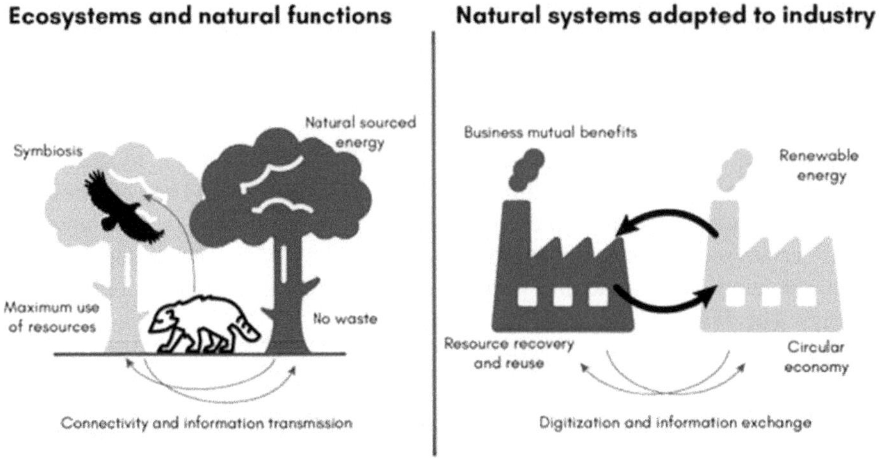

Fig. 11.2 Application of biomimicry in the company

11.1.3 Copying Nature: Biomimicry [3]

For millions of years, evolution has allowed planet earth as an entity to value, verify, and find the best ways in which resources are produced, used, and reused.

In nature, there is no waste (see Fig. 11.2). Each element of the biosystem provides resources for another element of the same system—a perfect closed-loop system. This third mechanism is about applying the principles of biomimicry in industrial settings and processes to identify different ways to generate value, for example, by diversifying the product base or managing it to better integrate resource efficiency.

This principle relates to considering and analysing the more complex opportunities in the production process. There is no longer talk of small changes, or reductions, or even testing what has already worked before. The company moves away from incremental innovation and instead focuses on introducing disruptive and radical changes, using processes from other areas or industries, making unique adjustments or changing routes—or fundamentally challenging conventional processes. This will require some moderate resource without necessarily being an extraordinary drain in terms of money or numbers of people. The only thing that is needed is an open mind to test and validate new processes without saying an outright 'no'.

11.1.4 Industrial Ecology

Up to now, we have explored individual, not necessarily interconnected changes. The fourth opportunity/mechanism/principle is to consider the company as part of an open system (systemic design) [4], as if the company were a living being (industrial ecology). In this scenario, the product is part of a complete ecosystem

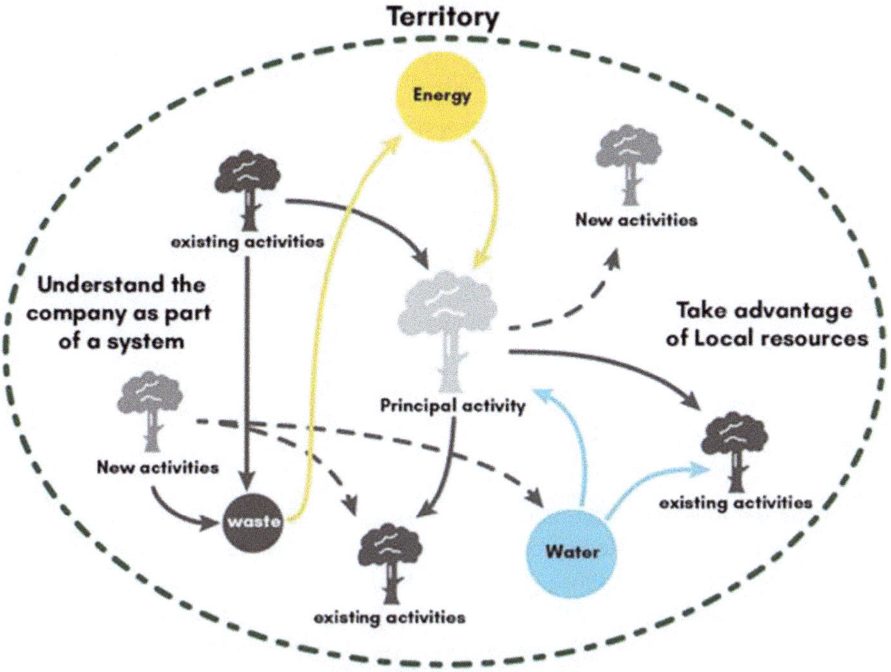

Fig. 11.3 The company as part of a system within the territory

surrounded by every element impacting on and influencing the others. Instead of the 'tree', we are looking at the forest (see Fig. 11.3).

When thinking of a product-specific incremental change (such as the ones described in step one), these they are likely to have only limited impact on resource consumption and waste generation. However, when thinking of a product as part of an industrial ecosystem, we can consider drastic changes to influence the way the product interacts with the industrial ecosystem as a whole.

Process changes can be applicable to a whole sector, inviting new companies to be part of the model, and generating a rapid transition to more system-wide sustainable ways of working.

11.1.5 Develop Sustainable Product-Service Systems (SPSS)

The last mechanism/principle seeks to move away from processes focused on the sale of products to offer solutions that are not necessarily material based. A sustainable product-service system (SPSS) [5], is one where dematerialisation (the elimination of the need for products) is a clear option, moving to *servitisation* [6] or service design processes. Consider tooth cleaning products (e.g. toothbrushes, floss) whose main purpose is to eliminate the accumulation of plaque—any other way in

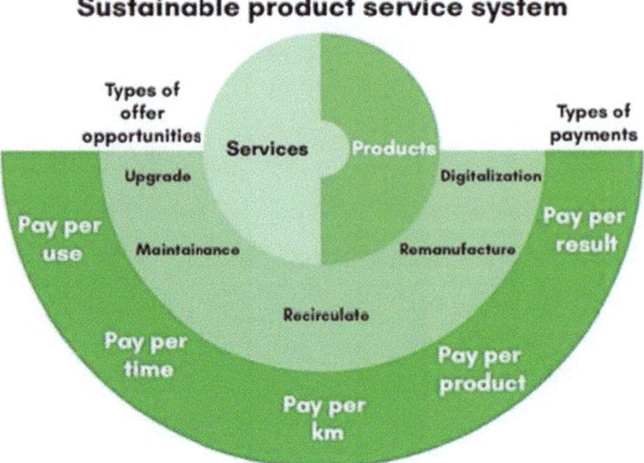

Fig. 11.4 Payment methods and service opportunities in SPSS

which we might achieve an oral cavity free from bacterial build up/accumulation of bacteria is a dematerialised solution, e.g. a specialist (yet to be invented) chewing gum could serve this purpose. Such a solution would then remove the need for toothbrushes ~~(materiality of the brush)~~ to be manufactured, packaged, transported, sold, and disposed of. Unfortunately—one step at a time—the chewing gum itself will still need to be manufactured, packaged, etc.!

As can be seen in Fig. 11.4, there are ~~also~~ other *payment models for outcomes received* possibilities. In this case, payment is no longer equivalent to physical exchange (pay per things), but it corresponds to the value of the alternative service received or result obtained. We could pay a company to provide us with a gown service (instead of paying gown by gown); this would then encourage (with appropriate sustainability incentives) manufacturers to provide the most durable gowns, washed, or recycled in the most environmentally sustainable way. The contract of care could include sustainable upgrades (as part of a robust circular economy), maintenance, remanufacturing, etc.

This moves us away from ownership of products to receipt of services of equivalent or superior planetary health outcomes. Consider, for example, replacing a family's set of toothbrushes to a model where a family pays for instruction/software for a 3 D printer. The family could then use the 3-D printer ad infinitum to print their own toothbrushes at home using existing, appropriate, household waste products—therefore cutting out the need for factory production costs, packaging, and shipping. Effective procurement of solutions together with contract management of the corresponding services are critical in ensuring effective delivery and maintenance of standards of care.

The SPSS model is a supply model that provides an integrated mix of products and services. These can meet a particular consumer need in order to deliver a 'satisfaction unit', measured by the interactions between the various elements of the supply system. In this scenario, the economic and competitive interest of suppliers is to continuously seek beneficial solutions.

11.2 Case Studies in Innovative Sustainability

Applying innovation to product development processes can be done in different ways, all of which open opportunities to influence and improve the company and create lasting changes in the environment that surrounds it. The goal is to have a positive impact on the environment, ideally without additional life-time costs.

The following case studies demonstrate how sustainable innovation can be applied in different projects.

11.2.1 Case Study 1: A Company Makes Small or Rapid Changes

In the first case study, a company has a typical situation that is faced by many. The company carries out a materiality assessment into sustainability, market analysis on others' successful approaches, and decides on small and/or rapid changes to improve its impact.

This approach can bring about several challenges. Firstly, from a sustainability perspective, it is necessary to carry out comprehensive research into the feasibility of changing manufacturing processes within the industry.

This could be as simple as analysing the environmental emissions of resource use (e.g. the energy source of electricity coal/natural gas/renewable, etc.) but may require more complicated holistic analysis—e.g. conducting LCA (life cycle assessment)—see Chap. 1. The company then needs to ensure that it communicates the change and its impacts effectively and factually with its stakeholders. Companies must avoid making sustainability claims that they cannot substantiate see Box 11.1 and Fig. 11.5:

Box 11.1 Greenwashing
Greenwashing is the term used to describe a communication and or marketing process where ecological arguments are used to project an environmentally responsible image—though a detailed analysis would provide a different image [7].

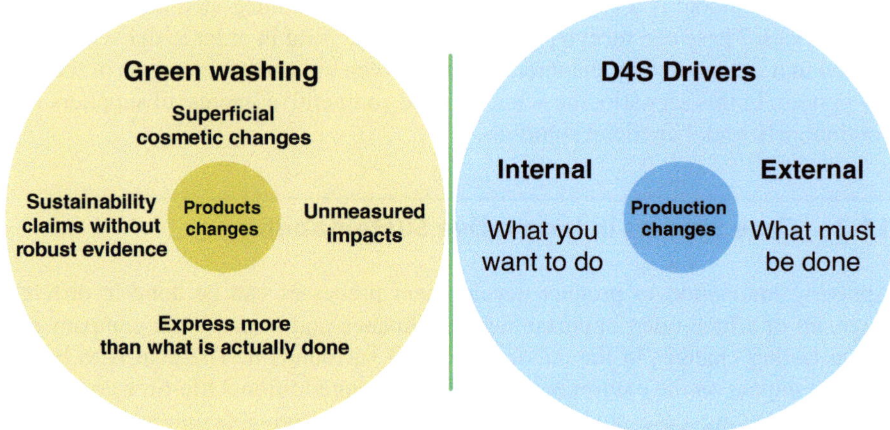

Fig. 11.5 Superficial vs. real engagement

Greenwashing claims may include superficial engagement, i.e. where companies make changes with little environmental impact, e.g. they change the colour of their packaging, or replace current materials with similar ones that generate little environmental improvement, or simply add environmental labels with limited information or unmeasured impacts. In extreme cases, companies knowingly claim environmental benefits which cannot be backed up with evidence. Companies need to ensure that they express appropriate ASARA (as sustainable as reasonably acceptable) commitment with measurable SMART (specific, measurable, achievable, realistic, and timely) indicators that allow for monitoring the improvements implemented; this should be reflected in a transparent communication strategy. Over time, this drive to become more sustainable may need companies to strike a balance between internal and external drivers [8], identifying what elements should be considered in the preparation of strategies to manage sustainability. Examples of these that can be seen in Box 11.2.

Box 11.2 Internal and External Drivers

Internal drivers	External drivers
Reach new consumers	Public opinion
Reduce costs	Pressure from community groups
Increase brand reputation	Pressure from other organisations
Opportunities to create value	Requirements of local legislation
A true and strong environmental concern	Ecological credit, for example, ecolabel
Generate improved opportunities at a social level for staff, for population health, etc.	Subsidy schemes
	Competition in the market
	Pressure from external suppliers
	Pressure from customers
	Pressure from wholesalers

Once the drivers that promote actions for change have been identified, adjustments in the process can take on a greater weight at a strategic level. In this way (based on consumers' perception of increased company value), the drivers can become a key incentive for the company's continued improvement.

Companies such as Curaprox use recyclable materials for a particular brush. In Slovakia, they have put a recovery process for these toothbrushes to the test, with collection bins strategically located in stores to encourage appropriate recycling. Toothbrush bristles are removed (these are usually complicated for recycling) and the heads are separated from their handles which are subsequently recycled into small litter bins that are sent to selected schools across the country for environmental education purposes [9]. These recovery processes are accompanied in some cases by incentives that promote repurchase, with discounts for new brushes also accompanied by a podcast on the importance of dental care and the planet. This is a clear example of a well-managed process that creates value for the company in the long term.

11.2.2 Simplification, Reduction, and Maximising the Lifespan of the Toothbrush

In a world increasingly focused on the aesthetics of products, style has become a key differentiator for companies. Style should not be just about aesthetics; simplicity, purposefulness and resource efficiency are key considerations in optimising product design. This is about redefining aesthetics, with environmental impact minimisation being seen as part of a product's appeal. An ideal product has fewer components which are easily disassembled and recycled and fewer parts that can fail (see Fig. 11.6).

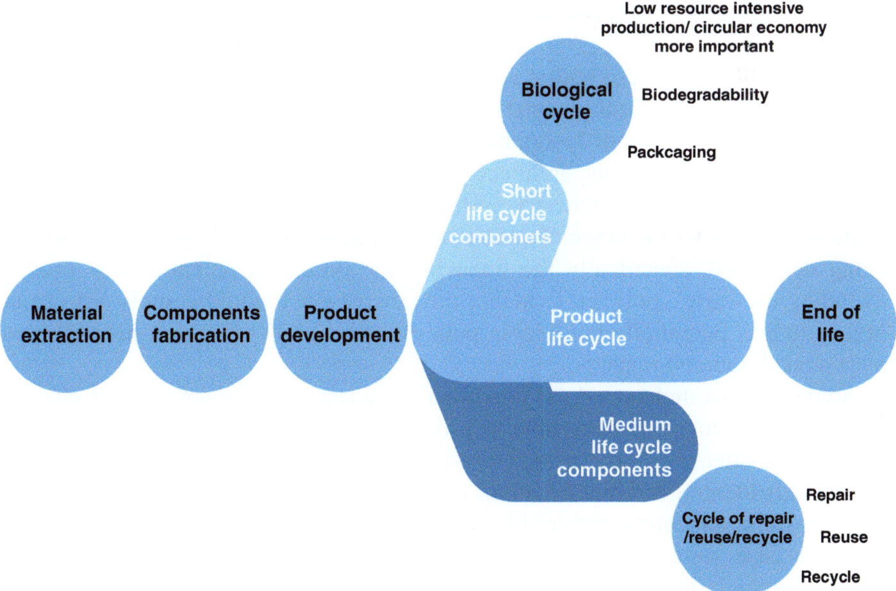

Fig. 11.6 Life cycle possibilities of materials and components

Components of products that of necessity need to be short-lived (e.g. for hygiene or effectiveness of care purposes) should be designed using minimal resources to manufacture and dispose of (e.g. be biodegradable). Parts that are intended for extended use should be designed with robustness and reliability in mind thus reducing the need for premature replacement. Toothbrush-bristle recycling is currently not considered to be a viable option because of the extensive cleaning requirement prior to being recycled. Toothbrush bristles, for example, should then be biodegradable/compostable. Any production of short-term products—such as bristles—needs to have a low overall environmental impact.

Medium lifespan components need to be part of a repair/reuse/recycle pattern, thus maximising the products useful lifespan. For example, an aluminium toothbrush handle would be expected to last much longer than a normal plastic brush handle, be reused countless times, thus reducing the number of products that end up in waste.

Manufacturers must also consider product packaging which is, by definition, short-lived. Packaging design should be purpose-driven, minimise unnecessary marketing or promotional aspects, and avoid bonded or complex materials. There are clear opportunities for companies to promote the reduced environmental impact of their products through minimalist packaging design, educating users in the process [e.g. 'sustainable' toothbrush packaging which avoids excessive packaging, bleached products, and bright colours]. Resource-intensive packaging should be the producer's responsibility to manage (e.g. through take-back schemes).

11.2.3 Case Study 2: Producing an Alternative to Non-recyclable Gloves

For the third case, we use nature as the main element, understanding the ways in which we can use a natural planetary resource to guide us.

Within the University of Javeriana (Bogotá, Columbia) design centre, the dental team works with industrial architects and designers to develop a system more aligned to one seen in a planetary system. This biomimicry initiative encourages students to consider the range of anticipated impacts generated by any new product being developed, specifically the financial (the cost of a potential new product including its waste), political (whether the new product would comply with existing, or future, potentially modifiable policy), and social (whether it fits with people's considerations) impacts.

Students must understand the functional requirements of a potential product. In this example, gloves must be able to provide an effective barrier for the user, be elastic, cost-effective, and prevent cross-infection between patients and staff.

Students identify how nature solves similar problems (e.g. how water is purified, how a toxic or dangerous material is degraded) and take this into account.

In this case, students identified the high use of PPE within dental healthcare settings (as recently published by Almutairi) [10].

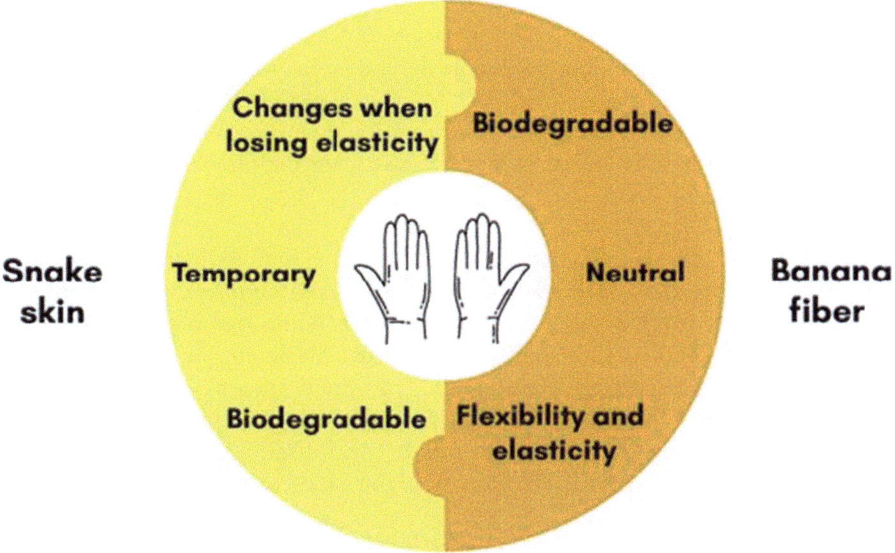

Fig. 11.7 Natural characteristics used in the product

Latex or nitrile gloves are de facto single-use products with low environmental impact recovery rates. In order to understand potential replacements, the team of students studied two natural compounds whose properties included elasticity and could be used as hand protection, i.e. snake skin and banana fibre (see Fig. 11.7).

Both products are natural and biodegradable. However, snakeskin when shed loses elasticity, discounting its use, but banana fibres remain flexible and resistant. Analysing both these products demonstrated that elastic compounds could be developed that could be applied in liquid form, drying fast, and allowing the dentist's hands to be coated and that, after drying, could be removed from the hand as if it were a glove. Once used however this substance would need to be collected in a separate waste stream, treated for pathogens (shredded, autoclaved), and then disposed of at a point where it is biodegraded, just as in nature these elements end up in an environment that helps facilitate its decomposition.

11.2.4 Case Study 3

The last scenario refers to the development of a sustainable product and services systems (SPSS) that develops sustainable products and associated services using a system approach.

In this case study, we propose a teledentistry model and personalised treatment is hard to access geographically remote regions. Teledentistry tools are used to carry out a pre-examination/treatment analysis of a patient. This approach helps reduce the number of visits needed to the dental practice by offering the level of care required remotely, including behavioural counselling, conditioning, etc.

This model seeks to:

- Provide better access to care for people in rural isolated regions far from specialised care centres.
- Reduce the resources required for the provision of surgical dentistry services.
- Reduce the processes and resources necessary for the provision of sustainable preventive care.

Many rural Colombian communities (some with a high indigenous population who in turn generally have high caries rates) have significant difficulties in accessing health services with cost and distance being the main barriers. The country has a model of rural practice supported by health students in the last semester of their university qualification, in which students must relocate to these remote areas. However, students find resources lacking (equipment and consumables) and, therefore, cannot provide specialised care. The people being targeted in these remote areas are often at high risk of caries and require considerable preventive care.

The model is unsustainable because, due to lack of on-site resources and specialist knowledge, treatments that could be carried out rurally are, of necessity, being carried out in big urban centres, creating financial and environmental repercussions.

This rural location model can also generate additional expenses for the communities themselves because sometimes it is necessary to move equipment from location to location, staff are needed elsewhere, and patients need to travel far to seek care. This travel can take several days depending on location of clinics, resources, etc. In Colombia, these additional costs significantly reduce the funds available for preventive care and treatment. If care is limited to several infrequently performed types of care, this increases the chances that low value disposable instruments are used, with the related large amounts of packaging and other materials associated with non-reusable equipment. Purchasing such products then transfers the waste problem to rural areas with less controls and processes to dispose of complex materials.

To solve this problem, the proposed SPSS model would focus on improving the production of local renewable supplies from local producers, taking advantage of the region's resources, and couple this with adequate digital tools that can connect patients with health professionals, or health professionals with colleagues. An electronic follow-up system will allow appropriate follow-up care. Teledentistry would allow more complicated care/advice to be provided to some patients to reduce travel.

In this example of SPSS (Fig. 11.8), small companies would provide local care and support health students in their final year of training and include:

- Local sustainable equipment
- Equipment needed could be produced simply and made out of local resources (e.g. a portable collapsible wooden/recyclable plastic dental chair). Where appropriate, at the end of life, products could be shredded, autoclaved, recycled, and reconstituted locally.
- High sugar foods would be disincentivised

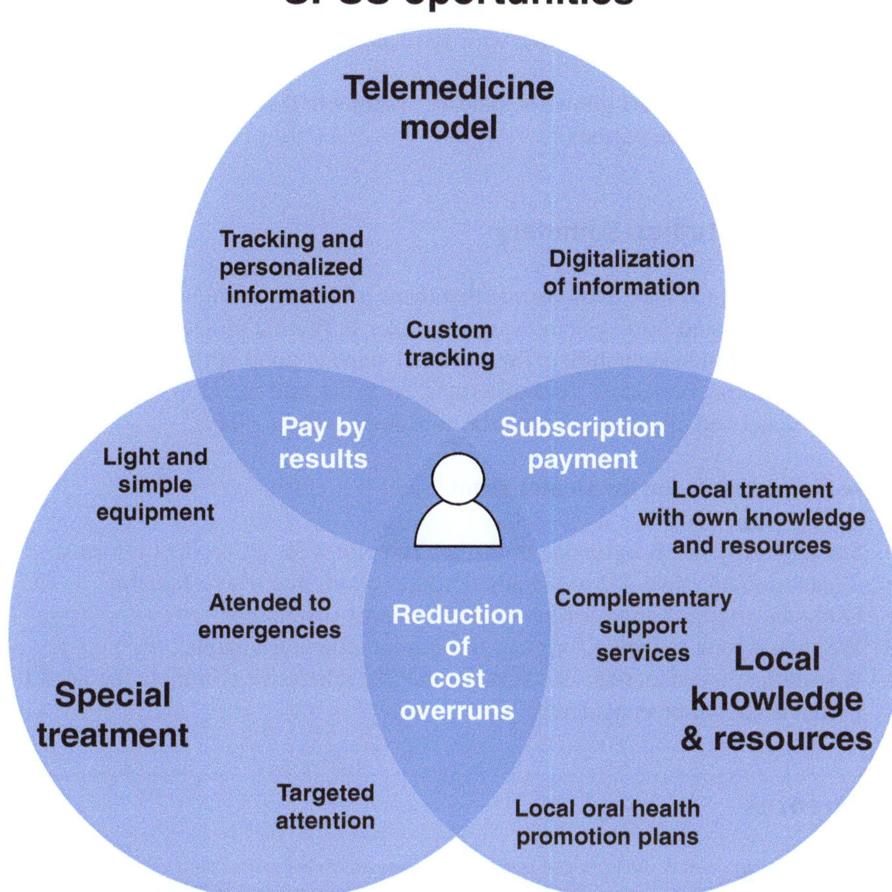

Fig. 11.8 SPSS opportunities

- Accompanying this model would be policies designed to reduce the consumption of high sugar foods (e.g. via sugar taxes) and, in turn, supporting the consumption of local, low-sugar and unprocessed foods.
- These sugar taxes can be used to subsidise the entire model, taking care of health and allowing good oral health as was recently suggested in England [11].
- Environmental waste would be penalised
- Within this system producers of dental products could be financially penalised depending on the environmental impact of their waste. For products which are actively recycled into reusable products, no charges would be incurred. Additional environmental taxes would be included in transport costs (at the cost of 258 USD ton of carbon dioxide emissions) [12].
- This model, using a system of financial incentives or penalties, can improve sustainability in a local area; those who generate waste pay the penalties, local producers (with less travel needs) are prioritised, and low sugar healthy production is promoted, thus supporting the diversity of the local economy.

The locally made payment model not only covers this aspect of oral health but could cover the creation of subsidised preventive products (subsidies based on their preventive element—see Chap. 5), with local production incentivised by realistic carbon charges.

Essentially, this model allows healthcare systems in the main cities to offer specialised services in the regions.

11.2.5 Case Studies: Summary

The cases presented here demonstrate that there is no single way that sustainability can be incorporated into system design. Neither is there a single way to face the problems faced in sustainability. Taking small steps is good at the beginning—but we must commit ourselves, as businesses, to grow and develop strategies with greater impact and engagement with the consumer and the planet.

Take Home Points for the Dental Team

- Sustainability needs to be one of the key principles for all product reforms.
- Greenwashing exists—critique any products claim that it's sustainable.
- Often the simplest approach/process is the most sustainable.
- We should look to nature for ideas to become more sustainable.
- A sustainable product-service systems (SPSS) where we eliminate the need for products should be considered.

References

1. Donald A, Verganti R. Incremental and radical innovation: design research vs. technology and meaning change. Des Issues. 2014;30(1):78–96. https://doi.org/10.1162/DESI_a_00250.
2. Maeda J. The laws of simplicity. Brilliance audio. 2006. http://lawsofsimplicity.com/.
3. Benyus J. Biomimicry: innovation inspired by nature. Harper Perennial; 2002.
4. Bistagnino L. Systemic design, Design the production and environmental sustainability. Slow Food. 2011.
5. Vezzoli C, Kohtala C, Srinivasan A, Diehl J, Fusakul S, Xin L, Sateesh D. Product-Service System Design for Sustainability. Greenleaf. 2014. ISBN: 978-1-906093-67-9.
6. Ecocanvas. https://ecologing.es/ecocanvas/. Accessed 16 Sept 2021.
7. You matter. Greenwashing definition—what is greenwashing? https://youmatter.world/en/definition/definitions-greenwashing-definition-what-is-greenwashing/. Accessed 16 Sept 2021.
8. Crul M, DIEHL J. Design for sustainability, a practical approach for developing economies. Delf University of Technology; 2009.
9. European Union. European Circular Economy Stakeholder Platform. https://circulareconomy.europa.eu/platform/en/good-practices/curaprox-collecting-used-toothbrushes-slovakia. Accessed 16 Sept 2021.

10. Almutairi W. The Planetary Health Effects of Covid 19 Dental Care (Life Cycle Assessment Approach). 2021. Submitted to BDJ-Confirm with BDJ.
11. O'Dowd A. Call for slice of sugar tax revenue to help oral health. Br Dent J. 2019;226:638. https://doi.org/10.1038/s41415-019-0334-3.
12. Bressler RD. The mortality cost of carbon. Nat Commun. 2021;12:4467. https://doi.org/10.1038/s41467-021-24487-w.

Sustainability: The Need to Transform Oral Health Systems

Brett Duane, James Coughlan, Carlos Quintonez, Bridget Johnston, Julian Fisher, Eleni Pasdeki-Clewer, and Paul Ashley

12.1   Introduction

This chapter provides information on how a sustainable (profession-wide) oral healthcare system might be created for populations. It also includes a consideration of social accountability and dentistry's social contract in the context of sustainability.

The original version of the chapter has been revised. The last name of James Coughlan was unfortunately published with an error. The initially published version has now been corrected. A correction to this chapter can be found at https://doi.org/10.1007/978-3-031-07999-3_14

B. Duane (✉) · B. Johnston
Trinity College Dublin, Dublin, Ireland
e-mail: brettdu@tcd.ie; bjohnst@tcd.ie

J. Coughlan
European Dental Students' Association, Amsterdam, The Netherlands
e-mail: James.coughlan1@nhs.net

C. Quintonez
University of Toronto, Toronto, ON, Canada
e-mail: Carlos.Quinonez@dentistry.utoronto.ca

J. Fisher
Charité Zahnklinik, Berlin, Germany
e-mail: julian-marcus.fisher@charite.de

E. Pasdeki-Clewer
Amersham, England, UK

P. Ashley
University College London, London, UK
e-mail: p.ashley@ucl.ac.uk

B. Duane (ed.), *Sustainable Dentistry*, BDJ Clinician's Guides,
https://doi.org/10.1007/978-3-031-07999-3_12

The chapter will be relevant to dental organisations and policy makers who are considering how they might provide dental and oral health care in a more sustainable and equitable way—now and into the future. It positions sustainability in its broadest sense, meaning environmental, economic, and social sustainability that goes beyond not only maintaining or conserving an ecological balance (such as through the appropriate and wise use of resources), but as something that can be upheld, defended, and/or justified.

Dentistry like much of health care is at an inflection point in its history. Firstly, it is finally being recognised as an important component of good general health. The United Nations has recognised oral diseases—among other important non-communicable diseases—as pivotal to the universal health coverage agenda. Similar recognition to the importance of good oral health has been given by the World Health Organization's Executive Board and World Health Assembly [2, 3]. The Lancet has published a series of articles on oral health care as an often historically neglected part of health and healthcare policy internationally. There is evidence that oral diseases reduce quality of life, and affect employment and social mobility, thus highlighting the need for the creation of universal health care to reduce inequality. Oral diseases are a risk factor for non-communicable diseases (such as cardiovascular diseases and diabetes see Peres [4]) and excluding dentistry from universal health systems reduces long-term population health outcomes.

Unfortunately, current models to deliver dentistry are inherently flawed. In a number of countries, the business of dentistry is predicated on an uncomfortable tension between dentistry as health care and dentistry as a small business enterprise. Dentistry can meet both individual and population health threats but is also needed for wellness desires and/or aesthetics.

Despite evidence behind the effectiveness of both community and clinical preventive care, the focus for many oral healthcare systems (e.g. the NHS dental system in England) is on providing treatment only with little incentive to reduce caries. As we said, we believe the model of dentistry is flawed, with no evidence behind 6-monthly check-ups [5] and with items that help prevent disease (such as fluoride) often not being funded.

The current COVID-19 pandemic has also created new infection prevention and control requirements for the safe delivery of oral health care which arguably makes it even less sustainable from an environmental perspective. To some extent, and within this area, dentistry was already unsustainable given the considerable quantities of waste we produce. With Covid measures in place, the large volumes of unit dose packaging and sterilisation bags have been further burdened by additional volumes of personal protective equipment. Given this, leaders in dentistry are now slowly turning to how we can practice dentistry more environmentally sustainably.

At no other time have calls for reform been so active, both within and outside of dentistry globally. Even organisations like the FDI World Dental Federation, the Australian Dental Association, and Canadian Dental Association—traditionally conservative bastions of dentistry—have become more progressive in their suite of policy statements and activities, suggesting/explicitly noting concern over the social and commercial determinants of health, the need to rethink dentistry as a profession and system of care, and consider how to incorporate environmental sustainability [6–8].

This chapter presents this broad vision of sustainability in dentistry by coupling sustainability with dentistry's social contract, or the mutual commitments and reciprocal obligations that dentistry shares with society by virtue of being a regulated health profession. A number of system characteristics need to be considered from an environmental, fiscal, and social perspective.

Healthcare systems need to be more focussed on efficient, appropriate treatment (based on evidence) to not only become more efficient but also to reduce their overall environmental impact [1].

12.2 Six Health Systems Framework Building Blocks

The WHO developed the six main building blocks (see Fig. 12.1) that describe health systems. Sustainability of oral health services and care—the ability to be maintained at a certain rate or level—can be viewed through the lens of these six building blocks for health systems strengthening [9].

1. Service delivery
2. Health workforce
3. Health information systems
4. Access to essential medicines
5. Financing
6. Leadership/governance

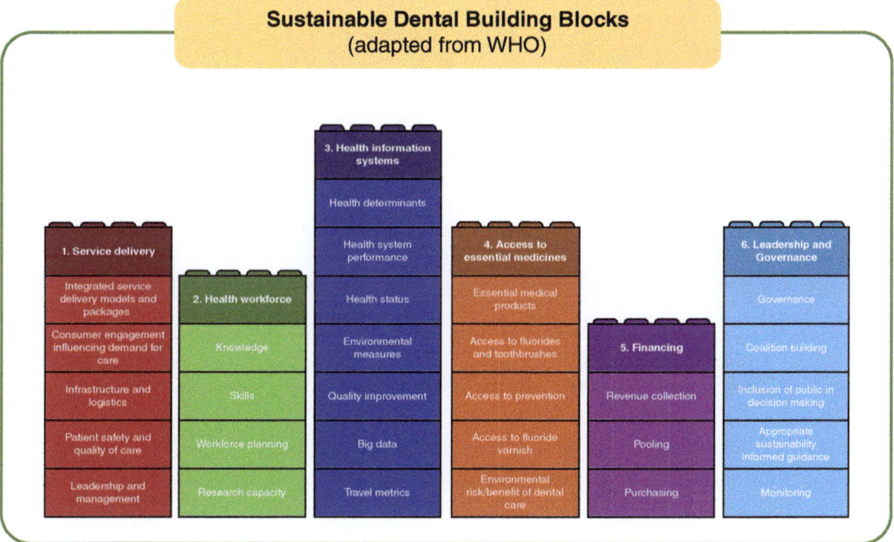

Fig. 12.1 Sustainable dental building blocks

12.3   Building Block: Service Delivery

A universal health system is one which is broadly defined as all individuals having access to high quality health services without financial hardship [10].

A universal healthcare system means no healthcare unit can specifically target or cater to the wealthy, meaning that the scarce healthcare resources (including, in many cases, healthcare staff who have been trained with at least some public money) can be fully utilised to provide an equitable service to all. Exactly what constitutes a universal healthcare service is widely debated. The evidence suggests that when people have a universal healthcare service it increases their life expectancy and reduces societal inequality [11].

We know from the work of Stockton that a successful service delivery model includes the following headings [12]:

12.3.1 Integrated Service Delivery Models and Packages

In dentistry, this would ensure we have integration between sustainable preventive programmes offered in the community and less sustainable preventive/operative programmes offered within the clinic.

12.3.2 Consumer Engagement Influencing Demand for Care

Stockton's review highlights the need for any new system to have extensive consultation and engagement (including engagement with vulnerable groups, who are in most need of a universal healthcare system).

12.3.3 Infrastructure and Logistics

We need smart IT systems that encourage sustainable, efficient referral pathways achieved with minimal travel requirements (an IT system which normalises teleconsultation for patients who live far from the care centre).

12.3.4 Patient Safety and Quality of Care

We need to highlight that patient safety is not just about adding layers of questionable low evidence-based decontamination and PPE, but also about the impact that this care has on planetary health and, indirectly, on patient health.

12.3.5 Leadership and Management

We need strong leadership and management. See also leadership/governance.

Within the heading of service delivery, we also need to ensure that dental practices have systems, rehearsed in order that they can cope with planetary event. For example, we need to be able to cope with rising temperatures, more frequent heat waves, potential flooding, and supply changes, i.e. where we source our dental products from.

Resource usage matters, therefore we also need to consider the environmental impact of services. The United States produces far more sulphur dioxide, more particulate matter, more greenhouse gases, and more nitrogen than the UK. The UK only surpasses the USA in its use of water. This is despite spending twice as much per capita compared with Canada and the UK [13], while having similar life expectancies and worse access, quality, and amenable rates of mortality [14, 15].

According to Bressler [16], the amount of carbon equivalent emissions released by the international health system corresponds to 141,000 excess deaths per year.

The climate change impact of the international healthcare system is 1.3 billion DALYS or, in simple terms, the healthcare system takes 2 months off all our lives.[1] As such, the environmental impact of services must be weighed equally to the financial and conventional health impacts.

Recent studies have highlighted low value care which is routinely carried out, such as routine 6-month examinations (as opposed to risk-adjusted intervals) [17] and scale and polish for healthy patients [18]. Notably, while these interventions can be considered low value in their contribution to oral health outcomes, patients valued the interventions and were willing to pay for them [19]. Some countries have taken steps to ensure only evidence based high value care is funded. Denmark, for instance, introduced a new dental contract which required risk assessed recall intervals [20]. Wales has acted similarly [21].

In a publicly funded system with scarce resources, there is a compelling argument that care which does not improve health should not be prioritised ahead of more cost-effective interventions which do have health benefits; especially when they provide societal benefits and have a reduced carbon footprint. Prioritising cost-effective interventions can increase value (and potentially decrease costs, for example, by reducing referrals to secondary or tertiary care centres), thus helping to create sustainable health systems for the future [22].

12.4 Building Block: Health Workforce

The core elements of this block are knowledge, skills, workforce planning, and research capacity.

---

[1] 1,420,220,285 kilotonnes of carbon. Multiplying this by 3.07136E-06 using the RECIPE formula.

12.4.1 Knowledge

A well-performing *health workforce* is one that works in responsive ways, that is fair and efficient to achieve the best health outcomes possible given available resources and circumstances. In order to advance sustainability within the oral healthcare system, there is a core knowledge required from the wider oral health workforce. Duane (2021) proposed a dental curriculum that encompassed eight key areas [23]. While this curriculum was intended for dentists, many of the competencies are applicable to the wider team:

1. Energy use
2. Pedagogy
3. Waste
4. Prevention
5. Biodiversity
6. Procurement
7. Decontamination
8. Travel.

Some of these key areas, such as prevention and decontamination, are crosscutting issues that are generally incorporated into the education of oral health professionals, while others are more sustainability specific. Teaching in these areas should be incorporated into undergraduate and postgraduate curricula, and also in continuing professional development learning outcomes.

Figure 12.2 shows how universities and educational providers can begin to implement such education on sustainability into the curriculum of oral health professionals.

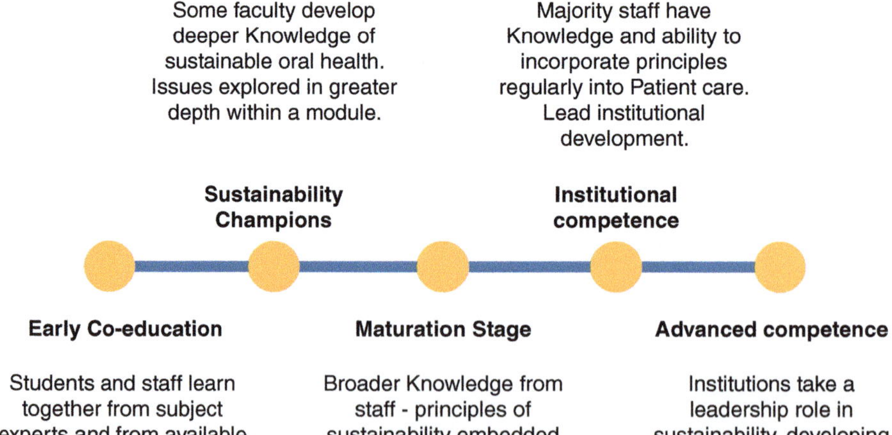

Fig. 12.2 Implementation process of a sustainable oral health curriculum. With thanks to Coughlan, Hegenauer, and Volkmann (2021)

12.4.2 Skills

To provide suitable health care, we need a diverse dental team. Staff need to be appropriately trained, motivated, and willing to deliver the best possible care for their patients, and this includes having training in sustainability [24]. While there is a core knowledge requirement, the workforce must be able to apply this knowledge in practical situations to reduce their footprint. Examples from previous chapters are abundant, but include the inclusion of key skills, such as audit or quality improvement exercises, application of sustainability principles to treatment planning and effective waste disposal practices.

12.4.2.1 Scope of Practice

In the UK, the General Dental Council's 'scope of practice' describes the areas in which dental professionals have the knowledge, skills, and experience to practice dentistry. This includes the provision of fluoride varnish by suitably trained dental professionals. As fluoride varnish application is regulated by the GDC, there is no scope for other practitioners, such as suitably qualified health visitors, to apply this product. A clinic which could provide a number of evidence-based products/examinations for vulnerable people, could be established. However, to facilitate such common risk approach clinics, other competent healthcare providers—with appropriate training—need to be able to apply fluoride varnish.

A sustainable healthcare system would ensure that holistic prevention could be carried out by a diverse community health work force, for example, by multi-skilled health visitors, or community health workers in LMICs.

In addition, a sustainable healthcare system needs to encompass oral health skills to be better integrated into areas where traditionally oral health is not taught, nor preventive programmes integrated into systemic health care.

12.4.2.2 Oral Health Care Integrated into Allied Health Training

From a western perspective, and from our anecdotal experience oral health is rarely integrated into the training programmes of community health workers, medical school students, or allied health providers. Currently, GPs (general practitioners) receive no oral health training; therefore, patients are often moved from one healthcare provider to another before receiving the care they need. This is not sustainable! Knowledge and understanding of oral health for non-dental healthcare workers would help facilitate efficient signposting to appropriate services and alert health staff to the symptoms of dental emergencies, avoiding duplication of care.

12.4.3 Workforce Planning

The WHO strategy in oral health argues that in most countries insufficient attention is given to planning the oral health workforce to address population oral health needs. Previous models of workforce planning (which have focussed on a ratio of dentists to population) are unsustainable in low- and middle-income countries experiencing rapid population growth. They are also inefficient in high-income countries because existing inequities in access based on the availability of services, ability to pay, and geography are not being addressed (i.e. the epidemiological transition has resulted in a large group of younger, healthier patients and a smaller group of older, high-needs patients) [25]. Instead, sustainable workforce planning must be adaptable to changes in demography, developments in the epidemiology of oral diseases, as well as to the reality of labour markets in each country which vary considerably.

Birch et al. proposed four key considerations for workforce planning [25].

1. The population that is covered—who is eligible for cover.
2. The epidemiology—the burden of oral diseases.
3. Service provision—what evidenced-based services are covered.
4. Productivity—how the services are provided.

This provides a framework around which policy makers can assess the needs of the current and future workforce.

12.4.4 Research Capacity

There are various actions which could be taken by appropriate agencies to build research capacity (see Table 12.1).

Table 12.1 Organisations which could build research capacity

Agency	Role
Infection control agency/ Department of Health Universities	Financial support (public and private sector) for priority areas of research, including seed funding to support innovation
	Development of centres of excellence for sustainable health care to bring public health, health practitioners, and sustainability/data analysis/industrial ecology experts together. Ideally, such centres would have close ties to teaching and research establishments.
Developers of guidance, for example, SDCEP (Scottish Dental Clinical Effectiveness Programme)	Ensuring that dental-based research or evidence-based guidelines include an environmental analysis with appropriate expertise
Research agencies	Financial support (public and private sector) for priority areas of research, including seed funding to support innovation
Professional Associations	Financial support (public and private sector) for priority areas of research, including seed funding to support innovation
Researchers	Investigating the complex internal drivers and external forces that influence sustainability. Undertaking broad and specific LCA or equivalent assessments for dental products and procedures to identify and address 'hot spots'. This analysis should include the provision of evidence for deciding between single- and multiple-use instruments

12.5   Building Block: Health Information Systems

12.5.1 Health Determinants, Health System Performance, and Health Status

A well-functioning *health information* system is one that ensures the production, analysis, dissemination, and use of reliable and timely information on health determinants, health system performance, and health status. These can be collected at a local level to enable practices to assess their energy use, as well as at the system level to enable policy learning and guide oral health system improvements.

Within dentistry and the broader public health system, we are accustomed to measuring oral health status (e.g. caries, periodontal health, oral cancer), as well as conducting a parallel process of measuring some health determinants such as sugar consumption, deprivation, child poverty, and tobacco consumption. With the current environmental crisis, we also need to measure the sustainability process (processes which cause reduced sustainability). A dental team familiar with quality improvement processes will be aware that an integral part of quality improvement is the use of measurement (you cannot manage what you do not measure) [26].

12.5.2 Environmental Measures

Generally, the most straightforward things to measure are energy levels and type. Dental practices should be encouraged to collect information on electricity and gas use (kWh), a sample of patient and staff travel details, and procurement.

The carbon footprint can be calculated by converting these data into emissions using the DEFRA (Department for Environment, Food and Rural Affairs) or SDU figs [27, 28]. This methodology is used within the Scottish and English carbon footprint studies and discussed in various publications [29–31].

From a patient perspective, measurable and simple to understand elements of sustainability could be presented on patient information boards within the dental practice. Such displays simultaneously educate staff and patients [32]. Waiting room posters have proved to be effective in helping people remember health promotion messages, they might also be used to teach sustainability.

12.5.3 Quality Improvement

Embedding sustainability into a healthcare setting is an aspect of quality improvement [33, 34]. There are various indicators that can be recorded in order to measure sustainability within the dental practice. Like any other quality improvement indicator, these should be SMART:

> SMART objectives courtesy of the BDJ
>
> - Specific: the measure should quantify an important result (e.g. kWh of electricity used).
> - Measurable: the indicator can be measured (using an actual unit, such as kWh).
> - Achievable: this should be a realistic target, otherwise people may get disincentivised by failure (e.g., aim for a 10% reduction in energy use, as this is achievable in most cases).
> - Relevant: that is, related to sustainability (energy use is related to sustainability).
> - Time specific: for example, over 1 year (the target of a 10% reduction will take place over a 1-year period).

The Greener NHS has developed a series of integrated metrics for use in both primary and secondary care which are applicable within the dental setting [35]. SMART indicators that dental practices could consider are:

> - Energy use per unit activity (e.g. unit of dental activity [UDA] or patient appointment).
> - Travel per unit activity.
> - Procurement (purchases) per unit activity.
> - Organisation water use per unit activity or patient appointment.
> - Organisation waste in kg or bags to landfill per unit activity or patient appointment.

12.5.4 Big Data

At the system level, there is a vast amount of data produced by oral healthcare systems, from electronic health records, insurance claims, mobile devices [36], and even social media. Known as 'big data', these offer insight that can be used to guide need-based workforce planning, the location of new services (or the relocation of current services), and economic analysis of oral health services among many others. This is crucial from a sustainability point of view. Making use of routinely collected data effectively at a system level can help ensure that the services provided (and the financial, physical, and human resources used to do so) are being deployed efficiently to maximise oral health at minimal cost to purchaser and the environment.

12.5.5 Travel Metrics

Given that travel is a key consideration in the sustainability of oral health services, the geospatial quality of provider level data can help those setting up or commissioning services to locate them in areas which require least travel for the maximum number of people, or ideally in locations close to public transport links.

12.6 Building Block: Access to Essential Medicines and Technologies

12.6.1 Essential Medical Products

A well-functioning health system ensures equitable access to essential *medical products, vaccines, and technologies* of assured quality, safety, efficacy, and cost-effectiveness, based on the evidence. Dentistry in common with medicine will need access to analgesics and antibiotics.

12.6.2 Access to Fluorides and Toothbrush

We also believe, however, that in a society where the consumption of high sugary foods is a norm, there should be guaranteed access to fluoride (either water, varnish or as a dentifrice) and a toothbrush as they are fundamental to prevention and management of dental caries and gum disease. At a global level, this has been advanced by the World Health Organization, where fluoride toothpaste, sodium diamine fluoride, and glass ionomer cement have been added in a new dental section to the list of essential medicines [37, 38], which is used as a guide for medicines which should be available to all in the population.

12.6.3 Access to Prevention

We know how expensive caries oral diseases can be, both individually and across the wider healthcare system [4]. We know from public health care that prevention is cost-effective, provides value for money, and produces financial/health gains in the longer term. In broader health care, community-type prevention programmes can be managed at five times less cost than individual interventions.

In Chap. 5, we highlighted the comparatively low environmental footprint of one of the most successful cariostatic preventive programmes in dentistry, i.e. water fluoridation (WF). We also discussed other preventive programmes such as fluoride varnish (FV), both in the community and practice setting, and programmes which facilitated increased access to fluoride toothpaste and toothbrushes. Scotland has operated a successful oral health improvement programme like this for 15 years [39].

12.6.4 Access to Fluoride Varnish

We would advocate a system where the provision of professional fluoride such as fluoride varnish was available in community centres, thus allowing FV to be applied within a community setting (and reducing travel). We would take this principle a step further and advocate that health workers should receive training to be able to apply FV in vulnerable populations.

12.6.5 Considering the Environmental Risk/Benefit of Dental Care

Currently, the true cost of producing one ton of carbon is $258. When considering the environmental footprint of preventive programmes against the much higher footprints of an examination or a crown preparation, you can understand the confusion/controversy/conundrum when you consider that the relatively low environmental footprint procedures are the ones which seem to be less prioritised by most funding bodies (water fluoridation = 443 g, community fluoride varnish = 3331 g, examination = 5500 g, a restoration = 14,750). Please note that an exact comparison of these carbon dioxide emissions is difficult to gauge as the more recent figs. (WF, CFV) use LCA modelling, whereas the exam, fissure sealant, and restorative procedures use a less accurate financial input-output approach.

In order to underpin this process, we argue that **without any additional total cost**, dentistry could be funded quite differently if it was based on a sustainable model which also took into account the true environmental costs. The establishment of a new system of preventive-focussed dentistry demands an emphasis on how a low transport, preventive programme would work. Dental team leaders would require participants to bring together their explicit local knowledge to ensure a system is created which is appropriate [40].

12.7 Building Block: Financing

Globally, the financing of dental care varies significantly, but it is a fundamental consideration in the advancement of oral health as a universal right. When considering the funding of oral healthcare, significant emphasis has been placed on total expenditure, yet relatively less has focussed on other functions or goals integral to efficient and equitable financing, and sustainable outputs and outcomes of the system. The historic split between medicine and dentistry is strongly apparent, with most dental care being both privately funded and delivered by private providers.

Financing functions in health care can be split into three main areas, (1) revenue collection, the process of raising funds for health, (2) pooling, the process of equitably sharing financial risk across the population, and (3) purchasing, the procurement of health services [41]. The functioning of these is heavily influenced by the political economy of the health system.

12.7.1 Revenue Collection

The source of funding for dental care varies significantly, but is widely characterised by high private expenditure, either through private health insurance (PHI) or out of pocket (OOP), and low public spending from general taxation and social health insurance (SHI). This is in sharp contrast to the prevailing consensus among health economists that funding for health should predominately come from public sources, specifically general taxation [42]. General taxation consists of a variety of tax instruments, each with different equity and efficiency considerations.

Even in traditional welfare states, such as the UK, private expenditure (either in the form of co-payments or full private payments) comprised 51% of total dental expenditure. Germany had the lowest private expenditure, with 17% of contributions coming from PHI and 24% OOP [43].

Some authors have highlighted the potential for revenue from 'health taxes' (or 'sin taxes') to fund preventative dental services, such as those targeting tobacco and sugar, noting that funding from SSB (sugar sweetened beverage) taxes across the world have already been earmarked for physical education, water, and healthy eating programmes [44]. The intrinsic appeal of this is clear. While earmarked taxes for health can provide an injection of funds for dental services, especially in the short term, experience of other areas of health suggest that this can sometimes result in reductions from other sources of revenue [45]. This an acute risk given the low political priority that oral health is given globally [46]. Furthermore, if consumers and producers alter their behaviour away from sugary drinks (which is the primary goal of the policy), then there will also be reductions in revenues. As such, while health taxes are strongly encouraged as a public health intervention, care must be taken to protect existing sources of funding for dental care.

12.7.2 Pooling

The risks of poor oral health are not equal across society; there is greater need among the old, as well as disadvantaged and vulnerable groups [47]. Pooling of funds involves taking the revenue from different sources and combining it so that the financial risk is distributed away from those with high health needs and low ability to pay. As such, the ideal pool is large (ideally 1) and combines high- and low-risk members with high- and low-income contributors, namely a single payer system. Consequently, systems relying on PHI and OOP are the most inefficient and inequitable, with small, fragmented pools and poor protection from impoverishing or catastrophic health spending [48].

Impoverishing health spending is where families spend a significant amount of their disposable income on health care to the extent that they are foregoing spending on other necessities. Impoverishing spending is when households are pushed below, or further below, the poverty threshold [49]. A recent report from the WHO European Region found dental care is a main driver of Catastrophic Health Expenditure (CHE) [50], while an analysis of out-of-pocket dental expenditure in Low-to-Middle-Income Country (LMIC)s found that costs of dental care from OOP prevented expenditure on necessities and forced families below the poverty line although not as much as medications, hospitalisations, and outpatient care [51]. The financial burden associated with dental care across the WHO European Region is driven to a large extent by low levels of public funding for such services.

12.7.3 Purchasing

Purchasing is the process by which healthcare services, including dental services, are paid for. This includes the payment mechanisms by which healthcare workers and institutions are remunerated. In the context of sustainability, strategic purchasing provides a tangible opportunity to align the goals of the system (e.g. improved oral health, need-based procurement, and sustainable practice), with the incentives of those delivering the service.

There is a clear mismatch between the oral healthcare purchased (based around a restorative, high travel and high carbon paradigm, and funded by wealthier patients paying privately) and that which is required—namely a preventative, community-based approach funded by public sources. Such preventative programmes are effectively carbon neutral, while having good evidence of return on investment.

For example, Public Health England found water fluoridation to have a return on investment of £21.98 for every £1 spent, targeted toothbrushing programmes had £3.66 return and fluoride varnish £2.74. In Scotland, the Childsmile programme, which incorporated brushing in schools and targeted prevention of high needs children, led to national savings of around £4,000,000 per year after introduction, with the figure rising each year [52]. These are all low travel, low carbon options, which maximise investment by governments.

There are also opportunities for remuneration targeting quality (known as Pay For Performance), where high value, low carbon interventions are monitored through health information systems, and where practices that carry these out regularly are paid part of their contract value on the basis these are carried out. As noted in the workforce section, this could feasibly be routinely carried out by trained dental nurses in practice, as well as community health workers or health visitors in community settings, or where numbers of dentists are low.

Recent focus on purchasing has emphasised value-based care as a model [53], which at its crux is 'patient-based outcomes per dollar spent' [54], with global interest in health technology assessments which explicitly consider cost-effectiveness and patient value. This principle has also been advanced in relation to dental care [55], but while patient value and cost have driven has the recent discourse and analysis, there is a compelling argument that environmental costs should also be included [20].

There are difficulties in assessing notions of value in oral health, with the most commonly used outcome measure that explicitly incorporates patient values (QALYs), being difficult to relate to oral health conditions [56]. Early efforts at economic evaluations of dental interventions have generally been of low quality [57]. Recent evaluations, however, have been of a higher standard and do provide information about the cost and/or benefits of dental interventions [58].

When developing health reforms and deciding on entitlements, a package of care which explicitly considers value should be a part of the process. In order to do so, more high-quality economic evaluations using a cost-utility analysis or cost-benefit analysis are required, as these are generally required by health technology assessment organisations [59].

12.8 Leadership/Governance

Leadership and governance involves ensuring the existence of policy frameworks combined with effective oversight, coalition building, regulation, attention to system design, and accountability.

12.8.1 Governance

We argue that a dental system needs to be appropriately funded to enhance sustainability, with appropriate sustainability-informed guidelines and a quality management system to ensure patients receive optimal health care at the least cost to planetary health.

12.8.2 Coalition Building

Appropriate oral health care requires appropriate coalition. Coalitions should be multi-sectoral, include actors working at different health system levels and their actions could include surveillance, the coordination of a wide range of diverse but supporting health improvement activities, and monitoring health and wellness [60].

In the Childsmile programme, for example, there is both formal and informal coalition between health visitors (delivering oral health improvement advice), education providers (providing advice but also a setting for oral health interventions), with NHS Scotland Trusts monitoring oral health, and with ISD Scotland collecting and reporting on data. Within NHS England, managed clinical networks bring together a coalition of workers to ensure representation from a wide range of clinicians supports appropriate care. Integrated care systems have been set up in England to focus on collaboration with emphasis on places and local populations as the driving forces for improvement [61].

12.8.3 Inclusion of Public in Decision-Making

We referred to the need for a new system to have extensive consultation and engagement with vulnerable groups, see Sect. 12.3.2.

12.8.4 Appropriate Sustainability Informed Guidelines

In health care, an evidence-based approach is considered to be the most desirable option to select when choosing between different therapies. Moving from evidence to implementation is a complex multi-step process which is governed by a range of different frameworks and organisations around the world. As well as efficacy, other measures such as patient preference, economic impact, and resource impact are considered and factored in when recommending a healthcare intervention. Sustainability is not yet routinely considered.

With growing evidence of the potential harm of healthcare systems and processes, this is a time to debate the need for an environmental impact assessment to accompany evidence-based guidelines. In industry, the responsibility to give equal consideration to profit, environment and social impact is often referred to as the 'triple bottom line'. We advocate that healthcare policy should consider their own 'triple bottom line' to ensure they produce evidence-based guidelines that are not only clinically effective, but also make economic and environmental sense.

12.8.5 Monitoring

Monitoring the effectiveness of interventions on health outcomes is important to ensure a system is both equitable and efficient (in terms of quality, cost, and sustainability). This, however, makes it difficult to compare the effectiveness of one intervention against another. Within the oral health system there can still be considerable improvement made on how we understand the effectiveness of both public health and health system interventions [62].

12.9 How Do We Influence Dentistry?

Influencing dentistry, like any system, comes under the heading of service delivery, we need to ensure that dental practices have plans, rehearsed in order that they can cope with planetary event. For example, we need to be able to cope with rising temperatures, more frequent heat waves, potential flooding, and supply changes, for example, where we source our dental products from.

In order to influence health systems effectively, advocates must consider specifically what they want to achieve, who has the power to implement such a change, and plan strategies to achieve this. Theoretical models of policy change can provide a framework for enacting change. Kingdon's 3 streams model stipulates that for effective policy change there should be an alignment of the problem, policy (solution), and political will to implement change [63]. Meanwhile Sabatier's Advocacy Coalition Framework pits opposing coalitions against each other based on long-term beliefs rather than short-term interests, with an emphasis on the importance of policy coalitions [64]. Beliefs are shaped by policy learning, which are said to change over a timespan of 10 years or longer. The importance of framing, the means by which an issue is presented, was proposed by Shiffman, who specified the importance of the internal frame—the level to which different actors agree on the problem definition and the solution, as well as the external frame—the way in which the issue is presented to those who control resources [65].

These theories and frameworks emphasise that simply generating evidence of effective intervention is not enough, and that attention must be paid to how issues and ideas climb the policy agenda, how they are framed by different political actors, the power dynamics between these political actors, the temporal sequences of events, and the relevant resources used by these groups.

Previous chapters have outlined the content of policy changes that need to be made, from sustainable financing of oral health care to the reduction of waste and the shift towards walking and public transport. We will therefore focus on policy context and process, as well as the actors involved.

Actors are people and groups involved in policy processes. Different actors have varying intrinsic motivations, resources, decision-making power or influence, and strategies. The table below sets out many of the actors and actions they can take, but these can also be used by advocates to identify policy actors with which they can engage to advocate for such change.

Once advocates have identified the actors involved in policy change, they should investigate how and where policy change occurs. It is important that when the so-called policy windows, or periods when the issue gains the attention of decision-makers, occur, that advocates are prepared to engage with these decision-makers, and have credible and politically astute arguments, as there is limited time with which to engage to try to enact policy change before another issue comes to the political fore [65]. This might be identifying open consultations by the ministry of health, professional associations, or other devolved governmental organisations.

As mentioned, simply presenting evidence of a problem is unlikely to lead to policy change, so researchers should proactively engage with policy makers. Evidence finds that structured engagement between policy and academia helps to facilitate the increased and better use of research findings [66]. This is an area where effective policy and entrepreneurs and advocacy coalitions can facilitate forums within which policy makers and researchers can align.

Framing is also important; practising sustainable dentistry in the context of the climate crisis is a professional obligation and should be discussed as such. Framings should convey the sense of urgency, as well as the fact that unsustainable practices can and should be changed.

We all need to influence education providers, healthcare system administrators, legislators, commissioners, dental team members, professions, specialists, industry, and waste management systems. Increasingly, it is the younger dentists who are demonstrating the need for widespread change. Some authors have been involved with and are watching with interest the development of the Youth for Sustainable Oral Health manifesto which asks people to pledge these actions (see Fig. 12.3).

Considering this picture gives an understanding of how complex a system of change in dentistry might be; but what if we broke it down; what if we all took actions which made change more simple.

Within the following tables, we suggest options for different organisations to become leaders within sustainability. Although there is considerable overlap between people delivering dentistry, and those involved in education, and research there is a role for all of us (Table 12.2).

The point being is that what we need in sustainability is leaders.

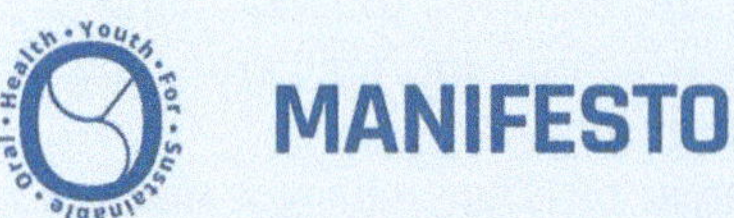

Who are YSOH?

The Youth for Sustainable Oral Health (YSOH) is a movement of young oral health professionals around the world who want to make oral health more sustainable, in line with the United Nations Sustainable Development Goals (SDGs). Youth are clear that action on climate change and sustainability is needed now, and we aim to ensure that the oral health community is at the forefront of this action.

What is the problem?

We see that the current situation is not good enough. Oral health services consume resources at a massive rate; water, metal, plastic and electricity. As a community, we unnecessarily produce millions of tonnes of plastic waste, and millions more of CO_2 emissions. As students, both in undergraduate and beyond, we learn nothing about the impact of our profession on the environment, or about planetary health and climate change, the greatest collective threat humanity has ever faced.

The burden of oral diseases has remained constant for decades with little improvement. 3.5 billion people live with untreated dental disease. Millions live their lives with the intense pain of oral diseases every day, not able to eat, to smile at their children, to talk to their friends. These people can be found in every country in the world, often the poorest and most vulnerable of our communities. They do not have the option of expensive treatment. Does our current education properly prepare us to help solve these challenges, or future ones on the near horizon?

Business as usual is not working. Change is needed, and it is needed now. We, as young oral health professionals, have a unique opportunity through the 2021 WHO Oral Health Resolution to shape the future we want, centred on sustainable, equitable and person centred oral health for all. Now is the time to act, to reform our institutions and our profession at the local, national and global level.

How Can I Help?

Change is required at every level. We therefore call for:

- **Students and professionals** to act together, advocating and working within their schools and communities to promote oral health equity and climate justice.
- **Universities and Educational Institutions** to provide comprehensive education on how to reduce waste and energy consumption in students' future daily practice. In line with the WHO Oral Health Resolution, students should learn to treat patients holistically, considering prevention, the social determinants of health and planetary health. Working with students, they should also make their clinics less wasteful and support quality improvement exercises around sustainability.
- **Dental Councils and Regulators** to set ambitious standards for oral health professionals' knowledge and skills, and require continuing professional development on planetary health and (the provision of sustainable oral health services) sustainable clinical practice.
- **Chief Dental Officers** to drive policy change within government to ensure that climate neutral oral health provision is incentivised and encouraged.
- **Professional and Specialist Societies** to adopt policies, set guidelines and release recommendations on how their fields can become more sustainable and take account of planetary health.
- **Research Funders** to increase funding opportunities for oral health research relating to sustainability, and to incentivise widespread knowledge transfer between academia, clinical practice and policy.
- **Industry**, as a key actor in sustainability, to invest in designing effective, accessible and affordable oral health products that reduce single use packaging and shipping emissions, recognising that waste is a human health and planetary health issue.

If you agree that immediate change is needed, we urge you to **sign** this manifesto and take action!

www.ysoh.info

Fig. 12.3 Youth for Sustainable Oral Health manifesto

Table 12.2 People involved in dentistry

Organisation	Leadership action
Academic Journals	Support high quality new research in this area. The British Dental Journal has been publishing in this area for a number of years (Nature 2019)
Commissioner of Dentistry	Drive change within dentistry by requiring sustainable metrics within contractual agreements and quality domains
Dental Associations	The dental associations across the world pledge to be sustainable, influencing their industry-based journals and publications, their members, etc.
Dental Councils/ Education Authorities	Support the development of peer-to-peer networks that work with other health areas in this field
Dental Councils/ Education Authorities	Mandate the inclusion of sustainability within the undergraduate and postgraduate curriculum. For example, the UK General Medical Council has introduced a sustainability component into its curriculum (Sustainable Healthcare Education 2019)
Dental Schools	Dental students write letters to their head of school demanding for sustainable change; asking the school to educate them, and asking the hospital that trains them to make a pledge to be the most sustainable
Dental Team Member	The dental team member pledges to be educated, to be informed, and that by 2022 (s) he will only work for a dental practice that does everything in their power to be sustainable
Dentist	Pledge to do all he/she can make his/her practice the most sustainable dental practice ASARP
Developers of guidance, for example, SDCEP (Scottish Dental Clinical Effectiveness Programme)	Ensure that dental-based research or evidence-based guidelines includes an environmental analysis with appropriate expertise
Education Agency	Fund sustainability scholars. For example, Health Education England has supported the funding of sustainability scholars (Centre for Sustainable Healthcare 2019)
	Ensure sustainability is embedded in learning outcomes at all levels of dental education
Everyone	Ensure sustainability is included in governance of the dental team
Everyone	Have an internal sustainability policy
Government	Involve dental professionals in developing sustainable dentistry policy to increase its relevance
Government	Offer regulatory or policy incentives for manufacturers to develop sustainable healthcare goods or require manufacturers to provide information on energy use
	Provide subsidies and energy buy-back schemes for solar-generated electricity
Government Bodies/ Education Sectors	Develop joint cross-cutting professional guidance for dental teams. For example, https://sustainablehealthcare.org.uk/dental-guide
Head of the Dental School/Hospital	Pledge to make the school the most environmentally friendly across both education and hospital services
Infection Control Agency/Department of Health	Financial support (public and private sector) for priority areas of research, including seed funding to support innovation

(continued)

Table 12.2 (continued)

Organisation	Leadership action
Infection Control Agency/Department of Health	Revise all infection control policies ensuring sustainability, environmental emissions, and indirect patient harm (e.g. DALYs) are published with recommendations
Manufacturers	Dental manufacturers agree to be the most sustainable ever and form cooperatives to understand the life cycle analysis of their products, and swiftly form working groups, to amend, innovate, consider their waste products and to truly evolve into an industrial ecological system that rapidly removes inefficiencies in their systems and works with their consumers to revolutionise their product base Embed into policy developing the evidence base for sustainable products Encourage transparency or standardisation of measurement or reporting of the environmental credentials of a product
Professional Associations	Financially support (public and private sector) for priority areas of research, including seed funding to support innovation Support and incentivise practitioners to become more sustainable, for example, the FDI is developing consensus statements to help lead within this area Increase the knowledge of dental teams in sustainability (British Dental Association 2019) through the association journal (Nature 2019) [67]
Research Agency	Financially support (public and private sector) for priority areas of research, including seed funding to support innovation Prioritise sustainability/planetary health
Researchers	Investigate the complex internal drivers and external forces that influence sustainability. Undertaking broad and specific LCA or equivalent assessments for dental products and procedures to identify and address 'hot spots'. This analysis should include the provision of evidence for deciding between single- and multiple-use instruments
Specialists	Pledge to analyse their own areas of dentistry. For example, within endodontics the authors have already started this work, analysing ways of making endodontics less environmentally harmful by measuring the environmental footprint of the processes but also by looking at the ways of avoiding carrying out traditional RCT [68]
University	Develop centres of excellence for sustainable health care to bring public health, health practitioners, and sustainability/data analysis/industrial ecology experts together. Ideally, such centres would have close ties to teaching and research establishments Create an internal sustainable policy. For example, https://www.tcd.ie/about/policies/assets/pdf/sustainability-policy-15112017.pdf Declare a climate emergency. For example, https://www.irishtimes.com/news/environment/irish-academics-among-11-000-scientists-declaring-climate-emergency-1.4073664 Divest in fossil fuels Drive sustainable changes across all internal schools

Take Home Points for the Dental Team

- In order to make a sustainable healthcare system, we need a transformation.
- We need an appropriate service delivery model, workforce, health information system, preventive care, financing, and leadership.

References

1. Hensher M, Tisdell J, Canny B, Zimitat C. Health care and the future of economic growth: exploring alternative perspectives. Health Econ Policy Law. 2020;15(4):419–39. https://doi. org/10.1017/S1744133119000276.
2. World Health Organisation. Oral Health 148th Meeting. https://www.dentalhealth.ie/assets/ files/pdf/oral_heatlh_who_148th_meeting_jan_2021_-_report_by_director_general.pdf.
3. World Health Organisation. https://www.who.int/news/item/27-05-2021-world-health-assembly-resolution-paves-the-way-for-better-oral-health-care.
4. Peres MA, Macpherson LMD, Weyant RJ, Daly B, Venturelli R, Mathur MR, Listl S, Celeste RK, Guarnizo-Herreño CC, Kearns C, Benzian H, Allison P, Watt RG. Oral diseases: a global public health challenge. Lancet. 2019;394(10194):249–260. https://doi.org/10.1016/ S0140-6736(19)31146-8. Erratum in: Lancet. 2019;394(10203):1010.
5. Sheiham A. Is there a scientific basis for six-monthly dental examinations? Lancet. 1977;2(8035):442–4. https://doi.org/10.1016/s0140-6736(77)90620-1.
6. FDI Sustainability in Dentistry. https://www.fdiworlddental.org/sustainability-dentistry.
7. Australian Dental Association. Dentistry and sustainability. https://www.ada.org.au/ Professional-Information/Policies/Dental-Practice/6-21-Dentistry-and-Sustainability.
8. Canadian Dental Association. https://cda-adc.ca/en/about/media_room/news_ releases/2009/11_16_09.asp.
9. World Health Organization. Monitoring the building blocks of health systems. https://www. who.int/WHO_MBHSS_2010_full_web.
10. Primary health care on the road to universal health coverage: 2019 monitoring report. Geneva: World Health Organization; 2019. https://www.who.int/healthinfo/universal_health_coverage/ report/uhc_report_2019.pdf?ua=1.
11. Masterclass. What is universal health care? https://www.masterclass.com/articles/ what-is-universal-health-care#what-are-the-advantages-of-universal-health-care.
12. Stockton DA, Fowler C, Debono D, Travaglia J. World Health Organization building blocks in rural community health services: an integrative review. Health Sci Rep. 2021;4(2):e254. https://doi.org/10.1002/hsr2.254.
13. Peterson-KFF Health System Tracker. Health spending. https://www.healthsystemtracker.org/ chart-collection/health-spending-u-s-compare-countries/.
14. Peterson-KFF Health System Tracker. Life expectancy. https://www.healthsystemtracker.org/ chart-collection/u-s-life-expectancy-compare-countries/#item-le_life-expectancy-at-birth-in-years-2017_dec-2019-update.
15. Peterson-KFF Health System Tracker. Quality US healthcare. https://www.healthsys-temtracker.org/chart-collection/quality-u-s-healthcare-system-compare-countries/#item-healthcare-quality-and-access-haq-index-rating-2016.
16. Bressler RD. The mortality cost of carbon. Nat Commun. 2021;12(1):4467. https://doi. org/10.1038/s41467-021-24487-w.

17. Fee PA, Riley P, Worthington HV, Clarkson JE, Boyers D, Beirne PV. Recall intervals for oral health in primary care patients. Cochrane Database Syst Rev. 2020;2020(10)

18. Ramsay CR, Clarkson JE, Duncan A, Lamont TJ, Heasman PA, Boyers D, et al. Improving the quality of dentistry (IQuaD): a cluster factorial randomised controlled trial comparing the effectiveness and cost-benefit of oral hygiene advice and/or periodontal instrumentation with routine care for the prevention and management of perio. Health Technol Assess (Rockv). 2018;22(38):vii–143.

19. Clarkson JE, Pitts NB, Goulao B, Boyers D, Ramsay CR, Floate R, et al. Risk-based, 6-monthly and 24-monthly dental check-ups for adults: the interval three-arm rct. Health Technol Assess (Rockv). 2020;24(60):1–138.

20. MacNeill AJ, McGain F, Sherman JD. Planetary health care: a framework for sustainable health systems. Lancet Planet Heal. 2021;5(2):e66–8.

21. Public Health Wales. ACORN Assessment of Clinical Oral Risks & Needs For Routine Patients. 2020. http://www.primarycareone.wales.nhs.uk/sitesplus/documents/1191/Routine patient ACORN.pdf.

22. World Health Organization regional office for Europe. The case for investing in public health: the strengthening public health services and capacity—a key pillar of the European regional health policy framework health 2020. 2014.

23. Duane B, Dixon J, Giwa A, Aldana C, Couglan J, Henao D, et al. Embedding environmental sustainability within the modern dental curriculum—exploring current practice and developing a shared understanding. Eur J Dent Educ. 2021;25(3):541–9.

24. Patel K, Jenkyn I. An introduction to clinical governance in dentistry. Br Dent J. 2021;230:539–43. https://doi.org/10.1038/s41415-021-2839-9.

25. Birch S, Ahern S, Brocklehurst P, Chikte U, Gallagher J, Listl S, et al. Planning the oral health workforce: time for innovation. Community Dent Oral Epidemiol. 2020;49:17–22.

26. Lighter DE. How (and why) do quality improvement professionals measure performance? Int J Pediatr Adolesc Med. 2015;2:7–11.

27. Sustainable Development Unit. Reporting on sustainability. Available on request from Greener NHS. https://www.england.nhs.uk/greenernhs/. Accessed May 2019.

28. Department for Business, Energy & Industrial Strategy. Greenhouse gas reporting: conversion factors 2017. https://www.gov.uk/government/publications/greenhouse-gas-reporting-conversion-factors-2017. Accessed May 2019.

29. Duane B, Hyland J, Rowan JS, Archibald B. Taking a bite out of Scotland's dental carbon emissions in the transition to a low carbon future. Public Health. 2012;126:770–7.

30. Duane B, Berners Lee M, White S, Stancliffe R, Steinbach I. An estimated carbon footprint of NHS primary dental care within England. How can dentistry be more environmentally sustainable? Br Dent J. 2017;223:589–93.

31. Grant P, Bailey SL. Calculate the carbon footprint of your hospital. BMJ. 2010;341:c2366.

32. Wicke DM, Lorge RE, Coppin RJ, Jones KP. The effectiveness of waiting room notice-boards as a vehicle for health education. Fam Pract. 1994;11:292–5.

33. Mortimer F, Isherwood J, Wilkinson A, Vaux E. Sustainability in quality improvement: redefining value. Future Healthcare J. 2018;5:88–93.

34. Mortimer F, Isherwood J, Pearce M, Kenward C, Vaux E. Sustainability in quality improvement: measuring impact. Future Healthcare J. 2018;5(9):4–97.

35. Sustainable Development Unit. An integrated metrics approach module. https://www.england.nhs.uk/greenernhs/. Accessed May 2021.

36. Listl S, Chiavegatto Filho ADP. Big data and machine learning BT. In: Peres MA, Antunes JLF, Watt RG, editors. Oral epidemiology: a textbook on oral health conditions, research topics and methods. Cham: Springer International Publishing; 2021. p. 357–65. https://doi.org/10.1007/978-3-030-50123-5_23.

37. World Health Organization. World Health Organization Model List of Essential Medicines—22nd List. Geneva; 2021.

38. World Health Organization. World Health Organization Model List of Essential Medicines for Children—8th List. 2021.

39. The shame in a failure to introduce a comprehensive child dental health programme throughout all of the United Kingdom Perspect Public Health. 2019;139(1):15–16. https://doi.org/10.1177/1757913918815428.
40. Langley J, Wolstenholme D, Cooke J. Collective making as knowledge mobilisation: the contribution of participatory design in the co-creation of knowledge in healthcare. BMC Health Serv Res. 2018;18:585. https://doi.org/10.1186/s12913-018-3397-y.
41. Kutzin J. Health financing for universal coverage and health system performance: concepts and implications for policy. Bull World Health Organ. 2013;91(8):602–11. http://www.who.int/entity/bulletin/volumes/91/8/12-113985.pdf.
42. Yazbeck AS, Savedoff WD, Hsiao WC, Kutzin J, Soucat A, Tandon A, et al. The case against labor-tax-financed social health insurance for low- and low-middle-income countries. Health Aff (Millwood). 2020;39(5):892–7.
43. Allin S, Farmer J, Quiñonez C, Peckham A, Marchildon G, Panteli D, et al. Do health systems cover the mouth? Comparing dental care coverage for older adults in eight jurisdictions. Health Policy (New York). 2020;124(9):998–1007.
44. Bedi R. The sugar tax: a leadership issue for the dental profession and an opportunity to demonstrate that oral health is part of general health. Contemp Clin Dent. 2018;9:149–50.
45. Cashin C, Sparkes S, Bloom D. Earmarking for health: from theory to practice. Geneva: World Health Organization; 2017. https://apps.who.int/iris/rest/bitstreams/1082540/retrieve.
46. Benzian H, Hobdell M, Holmgren C, Yee R, Monse B, Barnard JT, et al. Political priority of global oral health: an analysis of reasons for international neglect. Int Dent J. 2011;61(3):124–30.
47. Peres MA, Macpherson LMD, Weyant RJ, Daly B, Venturelli R, Mathur MR, et al. Oral diseases: a global public health challenge. Lancet. 2019;394(10194):249–60. https://doi.org/10.1016/S0140-6736(19)31146-8.
48. Ottersen T, Elovainio R, Evans DB, McCoy D, McIntyre D, Meheus F, et al. Towards a coherent global framework for health financing: recommendations and recent developments. Heal Econ Policy Law. 2017;12(2):285–96.
49. Wagstaff A. Measuring financial protection in health. Policy Research Working Paper Series 4554. 2008. https://openknowledge.worldbank.org/handle/10986/6570.
50. Spending on health in Europe: entering a new era. Copenhagen: WHO Regional Office for Europe; 2021. License: CC BY-NC-SA 3.0 IGO. https://www.euro.who.int/en/publications/abstracts/spending-on-health-in-europe-entering-a-new-era-2021.
51. Bernabé E, Masood M, Vujicic M. The impact of out-of-pocket payments for dental care on household finances in low and middle income countries. BMC Public Health. 2017;17(1):1–8. https://doi.org/10.1186/s12889-017-4042-0.
52. Anopa Y, McMahon AD, Conway DI, Ball GE, McIntosh E, Macpherson LMD. Improving child oral health: cost analysis of a national nursery toothbrushing programme. PLoS One. 2015;10(8):1–18.
53. World Health Organization. From value for money to value-based health services: a twenty-first century shift. 2020. https://www.who.int/choice/publications/vbhs.pdf?ua=1.
54. Porter ME. What is value in health care? N Engl J Med. 2010;363(26):2477–81. https://doi.org/10.1056/NEJMp1011024.
55. Listl S. Value-based oral health care: moving forward with dental patient-reported outcomes. J Evid Based Dent Pract. 2019;19(3):255–9. https://doi.org/10.1016/j.jebdp.2019.101344.
56. Kastenbom L, Falsen A, Larsson P, Sunnegårdh-Grönberg K, Davidson T. Costs and health-related quality of life in relation to caries. BMC Oral Health. 2019;19(1):1–8.
57. Public Health England. York Health Economics Consortium. A rapid review of evidence on the cost-effectiveness of interventions to improve the oral health of children aged 0–5 years About Public Health England. 2016. https://assets.publishing.service.gov.uk/government/uploads/system/uploads/attachment_data/file/560972/Rapid_review_ROI_oral_health_5_year_old.pdf.
58. Eow J, Duane B, Solaiman A, Hussain U, Lemasney N, Ang R, et al. What evidence do economic evaluations in dental care provide? A scoping review. Community Dent Health. 2019;36(2):118–25.

59. Sharma D, Aggarwal AK, Downey LE, Prinja S. National healthcare economic evaluation guidelines: a cross-country comparison. Pharmacoecon Open. 2021;5(3):349–64. https://doi.org/10.1007/s41669-020-00250-7.
60. Janosky JE, Armoutliev EM, Benipal A, et al. Coalitions for impacting the health of a community: the Summit County, Ohio, experience. Popul Health Manag. 2013;16(4):246–54. https://doi.org/10.1089/pop.2012.0083.
61. Kings Fund. Integrated Care Systems explained. https://www.kingsfund.org.uk/publications/integrated-care-systems-explained#what-are-ICSs.
62. European Commission. Tools and methodologies to assess the efficiency of health care services in Europe. https://ec.europa.eu/health/sites/default/files/systems_performance_assessment/docs/2019_efficiency_en.pdf.
63. Kingdon J. The reality of public policy making. In: Danis M, Clancy CM, Churchill LR, editors. Ethical dimensions of health policy. Oxford: Oxford University Press; 2002. p. 97–116.
64. Sabatier PA. An advocacy coalition framework of policy change and the role of policy-oriented learning therein. Policy Sci. 1988;21(2/3):129–68. http://www.jstor.org/stable/4532139.
65. Shiffman J, Smith S. Generation of political priority for global health initiatives: a framework and case study of maternal mortality. Lancet. 2007;370:1370–9. www.thelancet.com.
66. Parkhurst J. The politics of evidence: from evidence-based policy to the good governance of evidence. Routledge; 2017. p. 1–182.
67. BDJ. Nature. Sustainable dentistry. https://www.nature.com/collections/djidaaddgi/.
68. Duane B, Borglin L, Pekarski S, Saget S, Duncan HF. Environmental sustainability in endodontics. A life cycle assessment (LCA) of a root canal treatment procedure. BMC Oral Health. 2020;20(1):348. https://doi.org/10.1186/s12903-020-01337-7.

Conclusion

13

Brett Duane

This textbook, has taken you through a diverse number of topics. The subject matter is rapidly changing, and I would expect a plethora of new material to continue to be published in this area. This is a good thing as it means we will rapidly be able to do much more than we suggest here.

The greatest change I've seen in the last 12 years since my journey in sustainable dentistry began is the normalisation. We all broadly recognise the need to become more sustainable in everything we do, and all around us the damaged planet is letting us know how we are failing it. And it's acceptable to speak on sustainability and fine to research on it.

To summarise this book, I will use principles first outlined by Mortimer in 2010 [1].

We need to radically redesign the system of care of dentistry to be better at preventing illness. We envisage therefore a system focussed on prevention, with vulnerable groups supported by delivery within the community (e.g. a Childsmile approach) and finally embedded in everything we do clinically. We should give greater responsibility to patients in managing their health; aligning ourselves with public health principles of patient empowerment (making access to dental care easy, making home-based prevention easy and affordable), patient involvement (service co-design) community engagement (encouraging active participation in our communities to improve oral care systems). Everything we do has to be based on lean principles of maximising customer value while reducing, eliminating waste. Lean means creating high quality care for our population with as little resource as possible [1]. Finally, we need to use technology with the lowest environmental resources.

B. Duane (✉)
Trinity College Dublin, Dublin, Ireland
e-mail: brett.duane@dental.tcd.ie

This wording of this has been changed from Mortimer's original paper, as we should not just be (unfortunately) focussed on just zero carbon; to be truly sustainable, we need to focus on the overall environmental impact.

Reference

1. United Nations. Sustainable development goals. https://www.un.org/sustainabledevelopment/development-agenda/.

Correction to: Sustainability: The Need to Transform Oral Health Systems

Brett Duane, James Coughlan, Carlos Quintonez, Bridget Johnston, Julian Fisher, Eleni Pasdeki-Clewer, and Paul Ashley

Correction to: Chapter 12 in: B. Duane (ed.),
Sustainable Dentistry, **BDJ Clinician's Guides,**
https://doi.org/10.1007/978-3-031-07999-3_12

The last name of James Coughlan was unfortunately published with an error. The initially published version has now been corrected.

The updated version of this chapter can be found at https://doi.org/10.1007/978-3-031-07999-3_12